*Care and Treatment of the Mentally Ill
in North Wales, 1800–2000*

Care and Treatment of the Mentally Ill in North Wales, 1800–2000

PAMELA MICHAEL

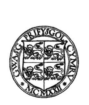

UNIVERSITY OF WALES PRESS
CARDIFF
2003

British Library Cataloguing-in-Publication Data.
A catalogue record for this book is available from the British Library.

ISBN 0–7083–1740–5

Typeset by Bryan Turnbull
Printed in Great Britain by MPG Books Ltd, Bodmin, Cornwall

Contents

List of Illustrations

Preface

This book is the fruit of research carried out initially (1993–6) in the School of History and Welsh History in the University of Wales Bangor, with financial support from the Wellcome Trust (Grant no. 038862). I wish to acknowledge the Trust's financial investment in this project, along with the opportunity given to me to discuss substantive issues in the research of madness with other scholars in the field. I acknowledge the support and co-operation of Clwyd Health Authority and the Clwydian Health Trust for allowing me access to records and for their support of the project.

My sincere thanks to my colleagues in University of Wales, Bangor, to Professor R. Merfyn Jones, Dr William Griffith and Dr David Hirst. They devised the project and then gave me the freedom to pursue the research. I have gained immensely from their support and collaboration. They are, however, in no way responsible for the views expressed in this book, nor answerable for any of the deficiencies. My own personal approach will be obvious.

I do not believe that any researcher can be wholly objective, but that the closest we can get is to acknowledge our own involvement and subjectivity. As Liz Stanley and Sue Wise have pointed out 'the presence of the researcher's self' is central in all research.[1] Therefore a brief statement of my own engagement with this history is called for, in order that readers understand from the beginning my own involvement and place in this history.

I paid my first research visit to the 'Denbigh Hospital' on 12 November 1993. It was a cold, crisp morning, but bright. When I drove down Castle Hill and turned the corner, and caught my first solitary glimpse of the asylum, the picture before me almost caught my breath. The asylum faces east and, as the wintry sun rose over the hill, it was bathed in a deep golden light. The stonework of this Jacobean-style structure is naturally of a mellow amber, but the rays of sun amplified the contours, and made the vast solid walls of the structure, set in parkland tinged that morning with frost, somehow ethereal. At this moment was born an enduring fascination with the architecture of asylumdom.

I had visited the asylum once before, for the official ceremonial 'launch' of the project, but on that occasion the day was flat and colourless, and the building looked grim, and somehow more institutional. On this second occasion, my first visit as a lone researcher, I met the two duty charge nurses (as they then were), Clwyd Wynne and Gwynfor Jones. I could not have received a warmer or more courteous introduction to the hospital. I was taken in and given tea in the reception room, where patients were taken on arrival to go through the formal admission process. It was equipped with an examination couch, screens, a sink and a table well stocked with tea, coffee and biscuits. This undoubtedly coloured my first impressions of the hospital. I both identified with the newly arrived patient and felt reassured and set at ease by the softly spoken staff and the relaxed atmosphere. Clearly they were experts in judging the mood and psychological profile of each new patient, and I sensed that they were taking stock of me in the same way.

I soon discovered that they had a passionate interest in the story of the asylum. They had acquired a fund of expert knowledge, ran a history society within the hospital, and often gave talks and slide shows in the locality. They told me that they had been 'collecting a few things'.

This was a day of introductions, and Clwyd took me across to Gwynfryn, a pleasant Victorian house on the opposite side of the road, which was then being used as the Academic Unit, and introduced me to the secretary, Anne Hayes. The office was cosy, the window open and whilst we were there a squirrel came onto the window sill to eat the nuts that she placed on a little saucer. Anne too was fascinated by the history of the hospital, and had been typing up notes from the early case records of patients admitted to the asylum, some of which are used in this history.

Thus, on my first visit, I only saw a small part of the hospital. Clwyd Wynne explained that it would really require a few hours to give me a complete tour. This, along with the surprise that was to be in store for me regarding the 'little collection', was to be for another time. On future visits I was to appreciate the vast amount of work that had gone into what turned out to be a vast collection of photographs and documents concerning the history of the hospital. I was also to have the privilege of learning much more about the hospital from retired staff members, especially John D. Williams and Dai Bryn Jones. I also learned a great deal of local history from Bobi Owen. Their input into this book has been enormous and their enthusiasm a constant source of inspiration.

Meanwhile I visited the county archives, and gradually became familiar with the collection of material deposited there, which had already been listed and ordered. The service offered by Clwyd Archive Service (later Denbighshire Record Office) has been second to none. This has probably been the largest and longest-running project they have ever encountered. It has at many times caused them trouble and inconvenience. For the efficient and professional service offered, and for the congenial company and warm and friendly atmosphere, I am deeply grateful. I offer special thanks to Kevin Mathias, who throughout has been in charge of the archive office, and to Jane, Mavis, Karen, Catrin, David and Rowland. My warmest thanks to Alice Langford Jones for her dedication to preparing a large historical database, which forms a lasting legacy of this project. Thanks, too, to Dr David Healy for a shared enthusiasm for the value of this database of case histories and for many fruitful discussions.

Throughout I have received moral support from my family and especially from my husband Dai, without whose encouragement and assistance this book would not have been completed.

The author and publisher gratefully acknowledge the permission of Denbighshire Record Office to reproduce photographs and document extracts from their collection.

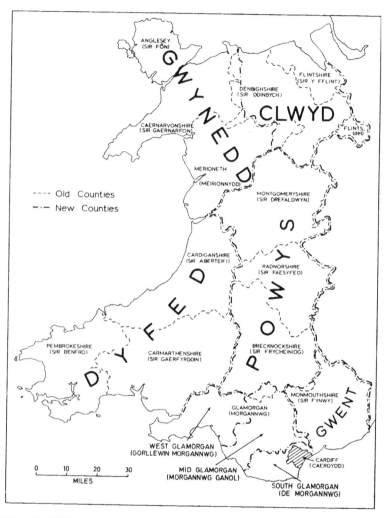

Map of the Welsh counties before and after local government reorganization in 1974. Further reorganization in 1996 led to the restoration of the county name of Denbighshire, though with altered boundaries.

Archival Sources

The main depository for the records of the North Wales Hospital, Denbigh, is the Denbighshire Record Office at Ruthin.[1] The key reference number for the collection is HD/1. The first deposit was made in February 1974, the second in December 1980, two in 1986, others in 1989 and 1993, and a final miscellaneous collection was transferred to the archive in 1996 when the hospital closed. The earlier deposits were each catalogued at different dates following transfer to the archives, but the latest deposit has yet to be catalogued.[2] The ordering of the schedule reflects this time sequence so that, for instance, the annual reports are variously filed as HD/1/1–14, HD/1/88–9 and HD/1/131–3. There is an almost full run of annual reports, and issues missing from the sets of bound volumes in the hospital collection have been found elsewhere (for example, in other collections at the DRO, and in the library of the University of Wales, Bangor). The bound volumes cease in 1939, although some subsequent reports are available in the hospital collection up until 1955. For the years 1950–60 use was made of the Board of Control Reports held at the Public Record Office, MH95/1.

The minute book of the founders (DRO HD/1/81) provides a detailed account of the activities of the subscribers and founders in setting up and building the hospital. The minute books of the various committees provide a detailed picture of the day-to-day running of the asylum and of the complex decision-making processes at work in the institution (HD/1/15–56, 83–7, 151–63). They also minute various issues that were discussed at sub-committee level, but did not surface in the annual reports (for example, the discussions over sterilization of female patients).

The Rule Books outline the formal structure of the asylum and are located at HD/1/69–80. Staff ledgers provide details of salaries, wages, staff applications, working conditions, superannuation, length of service, payments to widows and orphans, etc. (HD/1/116–30). A collection of account books, cash books and ledgers offer a detailed picture of the financial management of the institution (HD/1/90–115, 246–66). Separate accounts were kept for the farm, as well as milk registers and stock books (HD/1/136–50).

Probably the most valuable and certainly the most voluminous sections of the collection are the records relating to patients – the patient registers, certification papers and case notes. The admission registers provide details of every patient admitted, whether private or pauper, male or female, giving age, address, occupation, cause of insanity, diagnosis, where first confined and whether or not a first admission. When patients were admitted more than once, they were assigned a new admission number each time, but dates of previous admissions were usually entered. There were separate registers of discharges and deaths, although generally the date of death or discharge was pencilled into the admission register. Together these ledgers provide basic data for a comprehensive profile of patient admissions. The admissions details for all patients entering the asylum in each decennial census year were entered into a database for analysis as part of this research project. Admissions registers are located at HD/1/294–328; discharge registers at HD/1/387–90, 394–409 and HD/1/275; registers of deaths at HD/1/415–26 and 430.

Until 1930 patients could not enter the hospital on a voluntary basis and for legal 'certification' documentation providing written evidence of behaviour considered symptomatic of insanity witnessed prior to committal had to be completed.[3] The reception orders are bundled in sequence and retained in large archive boxes (HD/1/455–505). Each certificate has to be carefully unfolded and some certificates enclose further information or letters. The clerical staff at the Denbigh Asylum copied most of the salient details from the certification papers into the patient case books. Only a small sample of certificates was analysed for this study, in order to verify that for the most part details were faithfully transcribed into the case books.

Patient case notes form the basis of the detailed descriptions of patients in this book. On admission the medical officer would examine a patient and write a summary in the case book. The certification details were transcribed and certain basic information was also entered, for example, whether the patient was suicidal on admission, whether epileptic, state of nutrition, catamenia, etc. Case notes were compiled to meet the needs of government and institutional bureaucracy and kept as records of clinical judgements.[4] Case histories do not offer us a full or rounded portrait of the patient but rather a series of snapshots seen through the eyes of a medical observer. Nonetheless they do offer an opportunity for historical researchers to develop a social epidemiology of asylum patients, which is crucial to a fuller understanding of the institution. For without knowing 'more about (those) who were admitted, when, and what became of them, it is impossible to generalize about the social function of the asylum'.[5] A 10 per cent sample of all patients admitted to the asylum between 1875 and 1937 was entered into a database for quantitative and qualitative analysis. The entire case notes were entered into a free text database and although extensive use has been made of individual patient histories in this book these only constitute a small fraction of the total. Patient case notes are located at HD/1/331–86 and HD/1/506–19. For all the case notes mentioned in chapter 6, see the typed transcript of case notes, arranged in alphabetical order, in DRO Denbigh Hospital uncatalogued deposit.

When the hospital was closing vast quantities of paperwork had to be cleared from the building. The logistics of this operation were awesome. In the basement the case files of every patient admitted to the hospital since 1937 were stored. The files of all patients who had died in the hospital since that date were stored in the attic and were known simply as the 'dead files'. There was also an enormous collection of outpatient records. Owing to statutory requirements governing the retention of medical records the hospital was obliged to retain all case files relating to any patient who had received treatment within the previous twenty-five years, and to retain patient records for twelve years after death. Consequently it was necessary to identify only those records not falling into these categories before destroying any patient case files. The timescale for clearing the hospital site did not allow for selection of files eligible for destruction according to these criteria. Consequently all of the case records were temporarily retained and removed in lorry loads from the Denbigh hospital and deposited with the new health trusts and hospitals. Some of the records transferred to the Hergest Unit at Ysbyty Gwynedd have since been destroyed, but a 10 per cent sample was retained and deposited at Gwynedd Archives. At the time of going to press records stored at the Princess Alexandra Hospital in Rhyl also face destruction.

Central government records relating to the Denbigh hospital are located at the Public Record Office at Kew and located mainly amongst the records of the Lunacy Commissioners and the Board of Control. Newspapers provide another valuable source and *The Times*, the *Carnarvon and Denbigh Herald* and the *North Wales Chronicle* were chiefly consulted for this study. A collection of newspaper cuttings kept by the hospital (HD/1/284) proved especially useful.

Some photographs were deposited by the hospital at the Denbighshire Record Office (HD/1/442–51), but the hospital history group gathered many more photographs and these provide a superb visual record of the history of the hospital. So many people over the years have contributed to securing the safe custody of all the hospital records used in this study. Their efforts deserve recognition.

List of Abbreviations

AR	Annual Report
ECT	Electroconvulsive Therapy
DRO	Denbighshire Record Office
GRO	Gloucestershire Record Office
MOR	Medical Officer's Report
NHS	National Health Service
NLW	National Library of Wales
OT	Occupational Therapy
PP	Parliamentary Papers
PRO	Public Record Office
RCV	Report of the Committee of Visitors
RMS	Report of the Medical Superintendent
RVC	Report of the Visiting Commissioners
UCNW	University College of North Wales (now known as UWB or University of Wales, Bangor)

Throughout the text the hospital is referred to in a variety of ways. The official name underwent a number of changes. Opened in 1848 as the North Wales Lunatic Asylum, in 1858 it became the North Wales Counties Lunatic Asylum. Following the 1913 Mental Deficiency Act it dropped the term 'lunatic' and became the North Wales Counties Asylum. Following the 1930 Mental Treatment Act it became the North Wales Counties Mental Hospital. With the creation of the National Health Service in 1948 responsibility passed from the counties to central government and so the hospital then became the North Wales Mental Hospital. Following the 1959 Mental Health Act the name was changed to the North Wales Hospital. Sometimes it is referred to by its colloquial name of the Denbigh asylum or the Denbigh hospital to avoid tedious repetition. The official titles have occasionally been abbreviated to:

NWLA	North Wales Lunatic Asylum
NWCLA	North Wales Counties Lunatic Asylum
NWCMH	North Wales Counties Mental Hospital
NWMH	North Wales Mental Hospital

Introduction

The history of insanity has attracted many scholars over recent decades, stimulated by the exhilarating intellectual debates that cluster around so many aspects of this subject. Researchers from a variety of disciplinary backgrounds have entered the field, ranging from psychiatrists to social historians, social scientists and philosophers. The growth of a hegemonic system of institutional care for the mentally ill was a modern phenomenon of international significance. Its ascendancy has been interpreted by some as an essential feature of the modernization of capitalist society. Primarily, researchers fall into two opposing camps. One sees the growth of institutional care in 'Whiggish' terms as the development of a more humanitarian approach to the insane, the result of pioneering and progressive endeavour based to a large degree on altruism.[1] The opponents see asylums as a repressive feature of modern society, serving the needs of the developing capitalist system and promoting the interests of a small professional group of experts.[2] The first interprets the development of hospital care as a great benefit to mankind; the other sees it as a 'disaster for the insane'. The latter view interprets the demise of the large mental institutions as a feature of late capitalism,[3] determined by the structural imperative of the economic system, whilst the former interprets it as part of an evolving progression towards a more benign, humane approach delivered through the vehicle of 'community care'. The post-structuralist philosophical writings of Michel Foucault introduced a radical perspective on the history of insanity, promoting the notion of madness as a social construct, and viewing changing methods of treating the insane as the embodiment of shifting discourses of knowledge and power.[4] Foucault's imaginative motifs of the medieval 'ship of fools' and the 'great confinement' of the insane of the eighteenth century have both been criticized by historians.[5] For Britain, in particular, it has been shown that his dramatic scenario does not 'fit' the objective reality of historical periodization. Some critics have complained at his demotion of the material reality of much illness. Yet his 'ways of seeing' and of conceptualizing the social experience of madness have become enormously influential. Certainly, his focus on the power dimension of medical discourse to produce categories of persons and on the expansion of state surveillance in this process have provided valuable insights which have informed the present study. As the result of these new approaches, it has become increasingly unfashionable to look at the history of an individual asylum and to take at face value the avowed intentions of its founders. It is even more out of step with current historiographical trends to look sympathetically at the evolution of institutional provision and view the establishment of hospital care for the mentally ill as a great 'humanist project'. If this book appears to support such an unfashionable approach, it is not a position adopted lightly, but after considerable reflection over several years of study. Although this book's account of the history of the North Wales Asylum may be critical of some aspects of institutional care, there is nonetheless an implicit assumption that, on the whole, the primary goal of the institution was to relieve the sufferings of its patients. That stated, the readers may make of this history whatever they want. As far as possible I have attempted to document and describe changes and events in terms of the way they were represented or understood at the time and to allow the reader some space for interpretation.

The book provides a regional case study in the social history of madness and at the same time a history of a single institution within that region. It aims to address current debates concerning the diversity of experience in the pattern of institutional provision for the insane as this developed in Britain in the nineteenth century. What might once have been seen as a monolithic system is now perceived to have had marked regional variations.[6] Until recently, England was taken to be the norm but new research on Ireland and Scotland has revealed that, within the wider historiography of insanity, England offers but one example.[7] Scotland has a different history both in terms of policy and legislation and of 'welfare mix', with a greater emphasis on domestic care of the insane and a more influential voluntary sector.[8] In Ireland the rapid proliferation of asylums in the wake of the Famine years is inevitably seen in more political terms, for the expansion of state provision resulted in Ireland's having the highest rates of incarceration of any country in western Europe.[9]

Whilst Wales was subject to the same legislative and administrative directives as England, this did not preclude some measure of difference. Hitherto a small but significant body of work has begun to explore both the contribution of Wales towards the changes in legislation and the particular histories of different asylums.[10] The growth of institutional provision in Wales followed a rather different chronology from that of England. Whereas in England the 'trade in lunacy' had flourished, prompting the establishment of many private madhouses during the eighteenth and early nineteenth centuries, in Wales there were few. The first madhouse in Wales seems to have been May Hill's House in Swansea, a small venture catering for the 'melancholy effects of Mental Disease', opened in 1815.[11] A few licensed premises were established in the mid-nineteenth century, namely Vernon House in Briton Ferry, opened in 1843, and Amroth Castle in Pembrokeshire, opened in 1853, but there is no evidence of other private ventures in Wales.[12] The first county asylum in Wales was the small Pembrokeshire Asylum, opened in 1824 in the old gaol in Haverfordwest,[13] described by the Metropolitan Lunacy Commissioners in 1844 as 'totally unfit for its purpose'.[14] Subsequently Pembrokeshire entered into a joint agreement with Cardiganshire and Carmarthenshire for the establishment of a Joint Counties Asylum at Carmarthen, finally opened in 1865. The Monmouthshire County Asylum at Pen-y-Fal near Abergavenny began to operate in 1851, and the Glamorgan County Asylum at Bridgend in 1864.[15] The asylum for Brecon and Radnor, situated at Talgarth, was opened in 1903. Therefore the construction of public asylums in Wales occurred considerably later than in England, and was slow to follow even the 1845 legislation requiring counties to make provision for the insane. The North Wales Lunatic Asylum, opened in 1848 and a subject of this book, was the first Welsh asylum to be established following the Asylums Act of 1845. As will be shown, however, its origins predated this Act and were intimately associated with the progress of the reformist activity culminating in that legislation.

A second feature that marks Wales off from England is the fact that only the industrial counties of Glamorgan and Monmouthshire supported their own individual county asylums. Other Welsh counties made a variety of arrangements to secure provision for their insane poor and, besides entering into alliance with other counties in Wales, they made agreements with English border counties such as Shropshire and Herefordshire. The rural Welsh counties were neither sufficiently populous, nor wealthy enough to be able to support asylums of their own. In north Wales one asylum was established to provide for the insane poor of five counties, namely Anglesey, Caernarfonshire, Merioneth, Flintshire and Denbighshire. A sixth county, Montgomery, took part in early discussions, but did not join the alliance, opting instead to enter into agreement with Shropshire.[16]

A further important characteristic that distinguished much of Wales from England was the language of communication of the patients, for a proportion of all those admitted from Wales were Welsh-speaking.[17] In the nineteenth century Welsh-speaking patients were in the overwhelming majority in the North Wales Lunatic Asylum, reflecting the linguistic profile of the communities from which they came. The whole of north Wales formed a language zone where Welsh predominated, except for a narrow band running adjacent to the English border and encompassing the towns of Holywell and Wrexham.[18] In 1851, whereas on average two out of three of the inhabitants of Wales spoke Welsh, in the counties of north-west Wales the proportion was considerably higher.[19] The first language census of 1891 showed that 93 per cent of the populations of Anglesey, Caernarfonshire and Merioneth spoke Welsh. In Merioneth and Caernarfonshire over 70 per cent of the people remained monoglot Welsh-speakers. By 1901 the proportion of monoglot Welsh-speakers in Anglesey had fallen to 48 per cent, but that of Welsh-speakers still stood at 92 per cent. All three western counties (Anglesey, Caernarfonshire and Merioneth) remained predominantly Welsh-speaking and as late as 1931 one in five of the population in these counties was recorded as monoglot Welsh.[20] In the eastern counties of north Wales the proportion of Welsh-speakers overall was never as high, with 65 per cent of the population of Denbighshire recorded as Welsh-speakers in 1891 and 33 per cent unable to speak English. In Flintshire 68 per cent of the population was Welsh-speaking in 1891 and 26 per cent were monoglot Welsh-speakers. The pattern varied considerably from one locality to another. Within the counties of Denbigh and Flint there were towns and communities where the Welsh language remained dominant, others where English was in the ascendant.[21] The issue of the language was fundamental to the establishment of the North Wales Lunatic Asylum.[22]

North Wales formed a distinctive economic, social and cultural region.[23] Over the 200 years covered by this study many transformations have occurred in the relative fortunes of different towns and districts. There is sufficient diversity within the region for it to be usefully analysed in terms of a series of subregions, the dynamics of which have changed over time.[24] There were essentially two industrial regions, each centred on an extractive industry, slate in the north-west and coal in the north-east. Merioneth's woollen industry and Anglesey's copper mines fell into rapid decline in the early nineteenth century, leaving Anglesey predominantly rural and Merioneth with one large industrial settlement based around the slate mines of Ffestiniog. Linguistic and religious differences have often intersected with economic and social divisions. Kinship links remained particularly strong, especially in rural Welsh-speaking areas, where they extended to relatives of both the second degree and third degree (such as siblings of grandparents, second cousins and the children of nephews and nieces). In many areas families (and local doctors and parish overseers) would have an intimate knowledge of a locality and everyone in it. An illness in the family would bring many callers, a tradition still alive in the 1940s and later when if 'someone is so ill as to require constant attention the neighbours are always ready with their offers to come to watch ("gwylio") at night'.[25] Traditional methods of farming and customs of reciprocity underpinned the emphasis on family allegiance and filial responsibility. In a rapidly secularizing society religion could still remain central to the system of social care, whether emanating from the paternalistic Anglican church or from the more democratic, if patriarchal, chapel denominations. Religion might also be interpreted as supporting the same pattern of responsibility and obligation towards relatives and members of the community. Of course, there was another side to Welsh religiosity of the nineteenth and early twentieth centuries. Many of the personal case histories of patients admitted to the Denbigh asylum seem to support K. O. Morgan's contention that 'at its worst, Welsh Nonconformity helped generate tensions, frustrations and fantasies, feelings of sub-conscious guilt and sexual deprivation'. Tangible hints of the corrosive effect of 'a peculiarly sombre Sabbatarianism' on individual psyches may be derived from some of the illustrative case histories cited in this book.[26] Nevertheless, for all the underlying tensions, the nexus of cultural, social, religious, familial and linguistic links was fundamental to the support systems of social care in north Wales.

Whilst it would be wrong to speak of a distinctively 'Welsh system' of provision for the insane, there were recognizable differences to the pattern in England. Even after public asylums were opened, a significantly higher proportion of 'pauper lunatics' in Wales continued to receive care at home or with relatives than were sent to either the asylum or the workhouse. In Wales institutional provision did not become the norm until around the turn of the twentieth century. The strength of family commitment was crucial to this system of community care, which continued to exist alongside that provided by the asylums for most of the second half of the nineteenth century.

The first two chapters of this book are devoted to an examination of pre-institutional patterns of care. The others are more concerned, though not exclusively, with the history of one institution, the North Wales Lunatic Asylum at Denbigh (later known simply as the North Wales Hospital), within its regional context and over its entire working life. Such a long time period inevitably encompasses many changes, not only in terms of administration and personnel, therapies and treatments, but also with regard to the philosophy of care, and social and cultural contexts within which the institution functioned. Legislative changes had an impact on both the management and funding of the asylum. Evolving official policy and philosophies of treatment influenced the criteria upon which patients were confined or admitted to the asylum. Vital shifts in the economic and social structure of the region directly impacted on the men and women who were admitted for treatment. Patients brought with them their individual histories and tragedies, their language, religion and beliefs, and their personal, family and kinship ties. George Eliot reminds us in her novel *Felix Holt* that 'there is no private life which has not been determined by a wider public life'.[27] So, in this sense, every part of this book remains a regional study, reflecting the social conditions and public events that have shaped the lives of the individuals who became subjects of this institution. Patients far outnumbered staff, and while they may have been subordinate in terms of power, they influenced the character of this hospital just as much as the doctors and attendants who

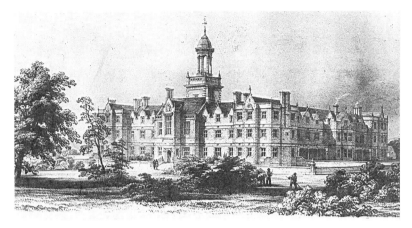

1. Lithograph reproduction of the architect's impression of the 'Hospital for the Insane, Denbigh' – Thomas Fulljames, 1845. Denbighshire Record Office

staffed the institution. Historians are increasingly beginning to recognize the role of patients' families in the shaping of the workhouse and the asylum.[28] Despite this, the contribution of patients themselves has received little attention. If there is a difference in the character of the institutions in different regions and nations within the United Kingdom, then this is likely to be the result of differences not only in local management, but also in the social profile of the people for whom the hospitals provided.

The book throughout seeks to address the 'top–down, bottom–up' forces which gave this institution its own unique character, balancing the influence of locale and region against the imperative of central inspection and legislative change. The conduct of 'everyday life' within the asylum is treated as a 'negotiated order', the product of the interactions between patients and staff. The asylum operated according to formal rules and structures, but within this imposed regime staff and patients pragmatically built their daily lives. In the early years staff as well as patients resided in the asylum and were subject to the routines and regulations ascribed by the rules. There is a need to examine the balance or tension 'between the formal and the informal' within such institutions.[29] Some patients stayed in the Denbigh asylum for a short time, some for years, and some remained for the majority of their lives, even as long as forty to fifty years. Equally some staff served the institution for much of their adult lives. Were they merely passive subjects of this highly ordered and disciplinary structure? Or were they active agents, able to influence or mediate the authoritarian structures through everyday interactions? How repressive was the institution? To what extent were patients 'stripped of their identity'? The type of observational analysis of a total institution made by Erving Goffman cannot be replicated in a historical study. Official records, which provide the main source for asylum studies, are not the ideal starting point for conducting a sociological enquiry into the everyday life of any organization, for that life is invariably 'taken for granted' when records are compiled. Nonetheless, an attempt has been made to tease out information that can throw light on the daily round and the 'underlife' of the Denbigh asylum.

This study does not claim to be written 'from the patient's perspective'. It is a rounded history of an institution. However, it does attempt to place patients at the centre of the study and thereby contribute to a newer genre of institutional studies. For despite the burgeoning of studies of the asylum system one area remained until recently strangely neglected, for of 'what it meant to be an asylum patient – or to be mad – less is known'.[30] The patient case notes provide the opportunity to explore the career of patients within the institution. Some 2,000 case histories have been analysed for this study and, although only a small fraction of the individual case histories are cited in this book, the intimate personal details have provided a basis for much of the interpretation.

Finally, from inside the institution it is possible to look outward to the society beyond the perimeter walls. Ideas about what constituted mental illness and what caused it have changed over time, as have the ways in which illness manifested itself or was experienced by the sufferer. Anne Digby has argued that for historians there is a great deal to be learnt by looking at the changing notions of what caused and above all what defined mental illness. The value of this, she argues, 'resides not so much in supplying accurate information on causation as in throwing light on broad changes in mentalité and attempting to gain an insight into the general evolution of con- temporaries' views on mental illness'.[31] The boundaries between acceptable and 'deviant' behaviour can tell us a great deal about the norms and cultural expectations of any society. Exploring the way illness was viewed and experienced within a Welsh context may help to reveal some of the broader societal changes which have taken place in Wales over the past two centuries.

In writing this book I have tried to avoid an overly academic style of presentation or plummeting into the more arcane areas of psychiatric practice and controversy. My aim has been to construct a narrative that will be of interest to various audiences, including health workers, any student of the history of Wales, and historians of medicine. Above all the book is intended to be accessible to the people of north Wales, knowing that this last category must include many former patients and ex-staff of the North Wales Hospital, Denbigh, and their families. In trying to fulfil this ambition of addressing diverse audiences I have, however, come to realize, with some humility, that there is actually only a single audience for any study of mental illness, since 'everyone who is born holds dual citizenship, in the Kingdom of the well, and in the Kingdom of the sick'.[32]

✻

CHAPTER ONE

The Insane Poor

Despite a substantial literature on madness and society in eighteenth-century England and Scotland,[1] there has been little historical coverage of the topic for Wales in that period. Without some sense of the customary methods of caring for the insane in earlier decades, it is difficult to evaluate the changes that came about later. This chapter will outline the pre-asylum care of the insane in north Wales. First, it will provide a brief account of the welfare system provided by the Old Poor Law and then it will move on to consider the New Poor Law of 1834.

Before the nineteenth century, making provision for the care of those suffering from mental disability or insanity in Wales was primarily a private and family affair. However, the plight of the individual lunatic or idiot presented an issue for the community and the local parish whenever a family became impoverished, or when relatives were unable, or unavailable, to cope. Under the system of the Old Poor Law local ratepayers, through representatives on the parish vestry, could give consideration to the needs of a stricken individual or family and were empowered to make arrangements where necessary. The Elizabethan Poor Law Act of 1601 left much to initiative at local level, and in Wales there was a great deal of variation in the operation of this Act, not only from county to county, but also from parish to parish.[2] However, some parishes in north Wales which did not formally operate the terms of the Old Poor Law simply left the poor and infirm to rely on older, communal forms of assistance and charity. In parts of Anglesey there was no official organization for the relief of the poor until the mid-eighteenth century.[3] This absence of official disbursement of relief reflects the durability and persistence of customary methods of assistance, based on kinship and reciprocity (*cymorth*).[4] When a couple married they would be given help to set up a home through the custom of 'biddings', whereby relatives and neighbours contributed essential items for the new household. On the birth of an illegitimate baby, informal arrangements were made for the father to provide support, and communal sanctions applied in cases of default. Whilst care must be taken not to romanticize such a system, given the scale of need and suffering, the durability of these older customs of reciprocity and obligation does set Wales apart. Collections for the needy, and for specific causes, would often be made in church. In 1759 William Bulkeley of Brynddu, Anglesey, recorded in his diary contributing 5*s.* towards the upkeep of 'John Rowland the Idiot whom the parish maintains by paying his sister 3 pounds a year for boarding and lodging of him', at the same time complaining about the 'stingy and ungenerous nature of the people of this parish' who had given only a total of 2*s.*, rendering it necessary to consider raising a poor rate for the first time.[5] A system based entirely on goodwill could prove haphazard, parsimonious and uncertain.

The usual strategy in Wales was for the parish vestry to offer a small allowance to the family of an insane person for help with care and upkeep. In the absence of anyone in the family available to cope, a neighbour, a distant relative, or another poor person in the parish would be paid for the task of caring.[6] Farmers and households requiring extra labour would take in an insane or idiot pauper, in return for a small fee. Sometimes the individual so placed could make a useful contribution to unskilled but laborious tasks. The parish made a higher payment in the case of elderly or infirm paupers or those of unsound mind who were incapable of work. In order to keep the level of payment to a minimum some parishes sought competitive bids for contracting out the care and upkeep. The Royal Commission of Inquiry, conducted as a prelude to the reform of the Poor Law in 1834, found that: 'In one or two parishes, such as Dolgelley and Llanykil [*sic*], in Merioneth-shire, the impotent are put up to auction in the vestry, and farmed out to those who will maintain them on the cheapest terms.' [7]

An inability to work or to settle down was a characteristic commonly associated with insanity, and amongst wandering beggars there were always individuals with mental health problems. They slept in outbuildings, or under hedges, and depended upon the charity of local inhabitants. In calculating the level of weekly parish relief, it was common in Wales for the amount that an insane pauper could obtain through begging to be taken into account.[8] In cases where vagrants were 'furiously mad' or so far disordered in their senses 'that they may be dangerous to be permitted to go abroad', the justices of the peace were empowered under the Vagrancy Act of 1744 to order that they be apprehended, and 'kept safely locked up in some secure place' and, if necessary, 'to be there chained'.[9] The number of vagrants grew during the food shortages and economic crises following the Napoleonic Wars.[10] Government determination to reduce reliance on begging as a means of support meant that it was necessary to differentiate between the able-bodied and those who were roaming or sleeping outdoors as a result of insanity. As reforms were introduced prohibiting the detention of the insane in gaols and workhouses, the establishment of county lunatic asylums offered the only means of legally apprehending the wandering insane.

If a pauper lunatic cared for at home or in lodgings became violent or otherwise unmanageable, then it was sometimes necessary to consider sending them away to a lunatic asylum. Parishes were loath to enter into this sort of arrangement because of its high cost. The expense could become a burden upon the ratepayers so was resisted except in the most dire of circumstances. If a decision was taken to send a lunatic away to an asylum, this entailed arranging for transportation to one in England. Considerations of distance and language militated against this, particularly in those western regions furthest from the English border. As late as 1847 all insane paupers of the Dolgellau Poor Law Union were boarded out or living with relatives and in the growing slate quarrying area of Ffestiniog 94 per cent of the insane were similarly placed.[11]

A refractory insane pauper could present an intractable problem for parish overseers. Freeholders and other inhabitants of the parish of Llangollen were called together in September 1809 to consider the case of Rice Evans, a pauper 'being in an Incene state'. Following consultation it was agreed that 'two Medical Men' examine him and each was paid 2 guineas. Subsequent entries in the Vestry Book record a payment of £9. 4s. 6d. to Thomas Jones, 'Lunacy Surgeon at Trawscoed' (which may relate to surgical treatment administered to the patient); another of 10s. 0d. to Edward Edwards, overseer, for a journey to Mrs Benion concerning Rice Evans; 6s. 0d. for a journey to William Jones of Llanarmon concerning Rice Evans; 5s. 0d. for a journey to Nanteos looking for a place for Rice Evans; and a further journey to Mrs Jones of Llanarmon costing 6s. 0d. Rice Evans died soon after this flurry of activity to find him a placement, and the parish records indicate numerous legal transactions following his death, and involving his widow.[12] The responsibilities placed upon the parish overseers under the old Poor Law system were onerous and, although they could claim expenses, they were not salaried officials. In the absence of any madhouse or county asylum, overseers relied for expertise in these matters on a small number of specialist doctors, and possibly on a few experienced carers, as the foregoing example suggests. Attending to Rice Evans certainly proved to be both troublesome and expensive.

If the insane person was considered manageable and a workhouse was available in the area then that invariably was the option chosen. At a vestry meeting held in Llangollen in May 1798, an agreement for the coming year was made between the parishioners and John Jones of Llangollen, inn-keeper, for a contract price for the maintenance of all paupers currently in the workhouse and any others who might be delivered there. They took the precaution of nominating a committee of parishioners who, during the year, would be allowed to come to an agreement with John Jones, regarding 'such extra expense of the maintenance of Insane persons which may probably be delivered into the workhouse'.[13] The cost of food and clothing and other items such as medical attention could prove expensive in the case of insane paupers. The overseer's accounts also record earlier payments of £4. 5*s*. 1*d*. for 'Elizabeth Parry of Llangollen, Singlewoman when she was Insane', and of £9. 0*s*. 11*d*. for 'Robert Edwards, Bachelor and on his account being Insane'.[14]

Glimpses such as this shed some light on local attempts to make arrangements for the insane. Throughout north Wales the emphasis under the Old Poor Law system was on 'outdoor relief' rather than workhouse care. This meant supporting paupers in their own homes or 'in the community'. Parishes gave assistance towards the payment of cottagers' rents and granted abatements on the rates. Paupers would be helped with the purchase of clothing, and in times of dire need given a sack of oats or seed potatoes to plant. This system of domestic relief for the poor went hand in hand with the domestic care of the insane.

Major structural changes were taking place in the economy of the United Kingdom, with both north and south Wales becoming integral parts of a burgeoning capitalist system. Radical changes in agricultural practice and primary production reflected an orientation towards changing markets. The average size of farms was increasing, and many cottagers and smallholders were finding it difficult to survive without entering the labour market. The industrial revolution led to a growth in commerce and saw entrepreneurs open up coal mines, slate quarries and mineral workings. The iron industry took off in north-east Wales, stimulating further demand for coal. When slumps occurred in trade and workers were laid off, or firms went bankrupt, wage labourers had few means of survival. The pressure to provide poor relief increased, especially in the economic downturn following the boom stimulated by the Napoleonic Wars. Expenditure on poor relief in the five counties of north Wales doubled between 1803 and 1832.[15]

As costs escalated throughout England and Wales, political pressure grew for a thorough reform of the system of poor relief. It was feared that the provision of outdoor relief was encouraging dependency, for some to have large families which they could ill afford, and for women to have children out of wedlock. A new system was proposed, the cornerstone of which was to be the workhouse. Instead of being provided with outdoor relief, the poor were to be sent into a forbidding institution, where they were to be subjected to a strict disciplinary regime intended to act as a deterrent. The payment of labourer's rents was no longer to be lawful under this new legislation. The Poor Law Amendment Act of 1834 introduced a new model of administration. Parishes were amalgamated into Poor Law unions, large enough to support the building of a workhouse. The system was to be staffed by paid officials called 'relieving officers', who superseded the parish overseers. The legislation of 1834 did not directly alter the legal framework for the management of pauper lunacy. Nonetheless, as the foregoing description of outdoor relief in north Wales makes clear, the welfare system provided under the Poor Law remained central to the upkeep of the insane poor. The New Poor Law introduced a scheme of medical relief, and Poor Law medical officers became responsible for monitoring the condition of pauper lunatics. Even before that the Madhouses Act of 1828 initiated a system whereby parishes were required to submit an annual list of 'Lunatics and dangerous idiots'. In 1842 the responsibility for this, and for providing a description of the condition and arrangements made for the care of each individual lunatic or idiot, passed to the clerk to the Poor Law union.[16] One of the key aspects of the New Poor Law system was that it introduced a much more centralized state bureaucracy, with powers to gather information, to inspect and to enforce changes. It undermined local autonomy and diversity that had permitted the type of ad hoc provisions so characteristic of rural Wales.

The commissioners administering the new system in Wales faced considerable opposition, and had a hard time in enforcing the radical changes required. William Day, appointed assistant Poor Law commissioner for north Wales counties in 1836, was struck particularly by the extent of poverty he witnessed. He faced extraordinary political and practical difficulties in communicating with a Welsh-speaking populace and in trying to enforce a regime for which there was little sympathy. In north Wales both ratepayers and labourers vociferously denounced the system as inappropriate to local needs, alien to the economy and to the social and cultural mores of Welsh society. Its most strident critics warned that it would lead to starvation and infanticide.[17] During a later period of office in south-west Wales, William Day encountered disturbances and insurrection, and objectors attempted to burn down the new workhouse at Narberth.[18] The Rebecca rioters, who destroyed the tollgates, and the protesters who ransacked the workhouse in Carmarthen were angered by the increasing burden of costs associated with the upkeep of roads and the maintenance of the poor. Resistance to the New Poor Law in north Wales was less forthright but still bitter. In 1840 the main topic of conversation was said to be the effect of the Poor Law Amendment Act, 'with the ratepayers complaining about the burden of the rates and the poor complaining about the terrible hardships they had to endure'.[19] Compliance with the new system was achieved slowly and with difficulty. Over 250 parishes were formed into seventeen Poor Law Unions, each to have its own workhouse. However, by 1844 the only unions in north Wales that had built workhouses were Pwllheli, Ruthin, Holywell, St Asaph and Corwen.[20]

The salaried relieving officers arranged for medical consultations and placements for the pauper insane, and processed payments. Many harmless idiots and lunatics were placed in workhouses, or received financial assistance under the New Poor Law, either to stay with relatives or be placed in lodgings. Once the North Wales Lunatic Asylum was opened, a Poor Law relieving officer usually accompanied the patient on the journey to the asylum, having first obtained a medical opinion and the signatures of two magistrates on the certification documents. Hence the Poor Law system was directly involved in lunacy provision and administration. The new asylum and the local poor law administration interlocked, for the asylum system 'was built on the poor law administrative structure'.[21]

One of the principles of the new workhouse system was that the poor should be 'classified' according to their need and status. The elderly, the sick and children were to be separated. All of those capable were to be put to work, carrying out minor chores or performing laborious tasks such as stone-breaking and picking oakum. The institution was to be strict and repressive, orderly and regulated. Into this inappropriate environment an increasing number of imbeciles, idiots and pauper lunatics were placed. The 1834 Act, however, reaffirmed earlier legislation that 'dangerous' lunatics and idiots were not to be kept in the workhouse, but were to be removed and sent to either a public or a private lunatic asylum.[22]

The foregoing account has emphasized the extent to which, under the Old Poor Law, the system in Wales differed from that of England. The degree of diversity that existed throughout England in the operation of the Poor Law has been the focus of recent research, and it has been suggested that there was no entirely consistent or national Poor Law.[23] There were essentially two macro-regions, first, the south-east of England, which offered a wider entitlement and more generous relief and, second, the north and west of England where lower standards of relief operated and the system was more ramshackle and parsimonious. The Poor Law regime in north Wales approximates most closely to that of the north-west region of England. A comparative approach could usefully be employed in Wales, and the suggestion that we think about 'poor law systems' and 'regional states of welfare' is a valuable one.[24] Wales as a region can 'hardly be said to constitute a unified and uniform Poor Law system', but appears to exhibit a number of marked subregional variations.[25] This brief chapter has tended towards generalization, and a more detailed examination would undoubtedly indicate differences within and between north-east and north-west Wales. Broadly, the evidence supports the view that there was considerable variation at local level.

For Wales, the New Poor Law represented a significant break with the past. It completely restructured the units of administration, and forced Wales to conform more closely to a standardized system, equivalent in scope to England's, both in terms of operation, staffing and levels and types of relief. These changes were to be fundamental in facilitating the transfer of patients to a public asylum, and in bringing about a gradual reduction of what had previously been almost sole reliance on outdoor care of the insane. Peter Bartlett has argued that the reform of the Poor Law was a prerequisite for the adoption of a universal system of pauper asylums.[26] Jonathan Andrews identifies the reform of the Poor Law as being crucial to the growth of a system of public asylums in Scotland. He has shown how legislative enactment to reform the poor laws in Scotland was introduced later, and only after that did a shift occur towards publicly funded institutional care for the insane.[27] As the nineteenth century progressed, different welfare systems were gradually harmonized as the central state enforced ever more uniformity, and a new philosophy of care was inculcated and finally adopted across all regions of England and Wales.

Yet, even as the centralization of powers proceeded, the traditional characteristics of the system continued to differentiate Wales from England until late in the nineteenth century. Workhouses in Wales never played the same role as those in England with regard to long-term detention of the insane poor, whilst lunatic wards were a rarity. By 1862 only three Poor Law unions in Wales, namely Cardiff, Corwen and Pwllheli, provided special lunatic wards, as compared with 113 in England.[28] Relatives, neighbours and paid carers in the community continued to provide a large proportion of the care for the lunatic and idiot poor in Wales. At the close of the nineteenth century an English Poor Law inspector was ruefully to admit that in Wales 'out-door relief has always been the rule and not the exception'.[29] This applied not simply to the care of the lunatic poor, but to welfare provision generally. Anne Digby has pointed out that, whereas in England and Wales as a whole slightly more than one half of all relief expenditure was disbursed as outdoor relief, in Wales alone the proportion was more than four-fifths.[30]

The introduction of a system of institutional care for the insane has to be set against this background of continuing community-based care in north Wales. However, the nationwide coordination of the Poor Law system and the inauguration of a centralized system of lunacy inspection were pre-requisites to the establishment of a comprehensive network of public asylums. As the following chapter will show, progress toward parliamentary legislation was influenced by a consideration of the condition of the insane poor in Wales.

✻

Chapter Two

Investigating North Wales

Estimating the Extent of Pauper Lunacy

Reformers acknowledged that the difficulty of ascertaining the number of insane poor hindered informed discussion. In an attempt at quantification the Parliamentary Select Committee of 1806–7 arrived at an estimate of 2,248 pauper lunatics and idiots in the whole of England and Wales. This figure was challenged by Sir Andrew Halliday, a Scotsman devoted to gathering information about the condition of the insane in Great Britain and Europe.[1] Following his intervention a clause was inserted in the 1828 Asylums Act requiring justices of the peace in each county to obtain returns on the number of insane persons receiving parish support.[2] When the first set of returns appeared Halliday seized on this opportunity to analyse and publicize the findings.[3] His report of 1829 analysed the incidence of pauper insanity, alongside a description of the topography, agriculture and industries of each shire. Halliday showed that in the six counties of north Wales (including Montgomeryshire) there was a total of 373 insane paupers, comprising 314 idiots and just 59 lunatics.[4] This represented a proportion of one insane person to every 850 persons in the total population of these counties. In south Wales the proportion of the insane was even higher, being one to every 750 persons in the population, based on the return of 523 insane persons; and there were eight and half idiots recorded for every person termed a lunatic. This high proportion of idiots intrigued Halliday, who formed the opinion that in Wales, as in Scotland, this was due to the way of living in the agricultural districts, since:

> where the people labour hard and fare ill, and where females are employed in labour that leads to violent exertion and distortions of the body, the growth of the brain may be affected, – its developement [*sic*] impeded, and even the form of the cranium altered.

The other cause was, in Halliday's view, 'the careless inattention in suffering female, as also male, idiots to procreate their species'.[5]

Until the adoption of medical nosologies to categorize the insane, people regarded as 'silly' or 'foolish' (*gwirion* or *twp*) would all be bundled together under broad descriptions. People would say that a person was 'only half-wise' or 'half-witted' (*dim ond yn hanner call*). An analysis of the annual lunacy returns for Denbighshire, for the years 1828–58, indicates that sometimes an individual was labelled and relabelled over time.[6] Following the opening of the Denbigh asylum a clear pattern emerged whereby those who were sent to the asylum were labelled 'lunatics' and those remaining in the community were labelled 'idiots'. The statistics do little more than reflect the methods used to enumerate and categorize people at that time, so should be read as a social construction and not as proof of a biological difference between the Welsh (or Scottish) and the English.

In all of Wales there were in 1828 only thirty-eight insane persons in institutional confinement. Six counties reported that they had no insane persons in confinement, and three others had only one inhabitant in confinement, in either a public or private asylum. Pembrokeshire, the only county at this date to have its own asylum, had fourteen insane persons in confinement, and was thereby quite exceptional. Other than this, Denbighshire had seventeen and Flintshire four insane persons in confinement, either in public or private asylums or licensed houses outside Wales.[7] This suggests a reason why the campaign to establish a joint subscription and public asylum should originate in these two counties. Denbighshire magistrates had the most experience of sending patients to asylums, and ratepayers were aware of the fees being charged by asylums in England.

The uneven pattern that appeared to exist across Britain gave rise to calls for more detailed information to verify regional variations. In 1839 the Poor Law Commission began a series of inquiries and these were followed up by ones from the Home Office and the Lunacy Commission.[8] The case of the island county of Anglesey illustrates the persistence of central government in pursuing information.

The chairman of the Quarter Sessions and the clerk of the peace for Anglesey were bombarded with requests for data on the numbers, distribution, condition and public costs relevant to the maintenance of those of unsound mind within and outside asylums.[9] Both the Metropolitan Lunacy commissioners, who had their powers extended over the provinces in 1842,[10] and the Home Office demanded information regarding publicly funded provision for the insane.[11] Although not explored here, a certain bureaucratic rivalry existed between these two agencies of the state.[12]

In the autumn of 1842 the Metropolitan Lunacy commissioners began carrying out a countrywide survey of madhouses and asylums, while the Home Office issued letters of inquiry in the same year, followed by others in 1843, requesting a return of the number of criminal lunatics under confinement.[13] The returns supplied by provincial magistrates' clerks were invariably brief and tokenistic and did not satisfy the needs of central government, nor of those concerned with lunacy reform. In 1842, possibly as a result of the local representations detailed in the next chapter, the Home Secretary, Sir James Graham, appointed Samuel Hitch to the post of temporary assistant commissioner to the Poor Law Commission to carry out a special enquiry into north Wales.

Medical superintendent of the Gloucester Asylum, Hitch advocated progressive methods in the treatment of the insane.[14] He found that in the six counties of north Wales there were 664 insane persons chargeable to the different parishes as 'lunatic paupers', this giving about one pauper lunatic to every 596 of the whole population. He was unable to calculate the number of insane not counted as paupers, but suggested that, 'from the many I was informed of, I am led to believe that in numerical proportion they are at least equal to their poorer brethren; making a frightful exhibition of the demented amongst our Welch neighbours'.[15] Nineteen of the pauper lunatics were in English lunatic asylums, thirty-two were in Welsh union workhouses and 303 lived with relatives, while a large number, 310, lived with strangers or were ' "farmed out" to these, at various weekly sums, according to the degree of utility they could be of to their respective masters'.[16]

The Poor Law commissioners stated that they knew of 'No county asylum and no licensed house for lunatics in the whole principality of Wales'.[17] They deplored this situation, noting that in England 42 per cent of lunatics chargeable in 1843 were receiving medical treatment in either asylums or licensed houses, but in Wales the figure was only 6.5 per cent.

They considered that one asylum for south Wales and another for north Wales would 'probably answer every purpose', but acknowledged that implementation posed practical difficulties. If the matter was not speedily resolved 'some legislative interference should take place' in order to secure for the lunatic poor of Wales 'the advantages of treatment which they ought to receive'.[18] Thus the lack of asylum provision in Wales fuelled demands for a change in the legislative and administrative framework of lunacy provision. Central government recognized that, without enforcement, a comprehensive system was not likely to emerge across all of England and Wales. The 'dramatic changes' which Andrew Scull has described for England were limited to that country. Whereas in the mid-eighteenth century the overwhelming majority of the insane were still to be found at large in the community, Scull suggests that 'By the mid-nineteenth century . . . virtually no aspect of this traditional response remained intact.'[19] Yet in Wales it remained almost wholly intact.

This begs a number of fundamental questions. Wales does not fit neatly into Scull's periodization. Is it because Wales was simply 'lagging behind' England? Scull argues that it was not industrialization as such, but rather the penetration and dominance of the market that made the change from a community-based to an institutional response necessary.[20] If so, did Wales deviate from the norm because market forces had not sufficiently penetrated into Wales? I have argued elsewhere that Welsh agriculture was already being transformed by market forces.[21] The growth of coastal trade and shipping, the spread of banks, the opening up of mines and quarries, the growth of manufactures, all involved the same market forces that were operative in England. But capitalism creates uneven development. Historically Wales had not had the same growth of towns, or of urban culture, so consequently there was less of a civic tradition.[22] Unlike in England there was not a strong tradition of voluntary subscription hospitals.[23] One reason for the failure to develop institutional provision may have been the very characteristic which William Day, the assistant Poor Law commissioner, had identified – poverty. The market produces wealth, but it also creates inequality, not only class inequalities, but also regional inequalities. It siphons wealth and resources away from the periphery, to concentrate them in the metropolitan areas. Therefore Scull's basic argument may still hold good. In order further to promote a free market in labour and create a larger reserve army of labour, by releasing individuals from the ties of caring for the dependent insane, the market required the assistance of the state. Yet this can only be understood as an underlying structural imperative. It was never articulated as a reason for lunacy reform. The history of institutional care of the insane in Ireland serves to illustrate the critical role of the state in the development of a comprehensive system of public asylums. It was primarily 'the relative freedom of Dublin Castle to govern in a highly interventionist style in the early nineteenth century' that determined the early enforcement of a national system of public asylums under legislation adopted in 1817.[24]

Prior to the introduction of compulsion in England and Wales under the 1845 Act, the foundation of each asylum still rested upon the reformist zeal of those able to extol its merits in moral and therapeutic terms. Each asylum, therefore, was established by a group of activists or local reformers. Although change may have taken place in response to the evolving manpower needs of the capitalist system it seems doubtful whether, without the intervention of the central state, a comprehensive system of public asylums would have been inaugurated. The underlying social conditions varied somewhat from region to region. The gendered structure of the industrial workforce in Wales was one reason why community care of the insane could continue for so long. The developing industries and sources of employment in both south and north Wales created predominantly male occupations. The main employment for women remained that of domestic service. The geographical movement of men, towards the quarries of the north-west and the coalfields and metallurgical industries of the north-east, drew them away from the rural areas. In many parishes of rural Wales this left behind a preponderance of women, available for caring for insane dependants. In Ireland the reverse was true. Females formed the majority of Irish emigrants leaving in search of a better life, whereas the inheritance system encouraged men to stay behind in anticipation of acquiring land. Scheper-Hughes has argued that the economic, social and agrarian system of Ireland led to a higher level of institutionalization and was also the cause of a higher incidence of insanity.[25]

The Report of the Metropolitan Lunacy Commissioners, 1844

In 1844 the Metropolitan Lunacy commissioners announced their own special investigation into the care of the lunatic poor in north Wales. Anticipating the close scrutiny of visiting commissioners, Poor Law doctors became more forthcoming. The correspondence between them and the clerk of the peace in Anglesey illustrates the exchange of information that took place as a prelude to these investigations.

In June 1844 Dr J. S. Davies of Newborough informed the clerk of peace for Anglesey about the number of lunatics in his district, and described their treatment. He named Jonathan Davies, a pauper, of Llangeinwen, who was guided and handcuffed, but who had been under Dr Davies's 'medical' and was now cured. Thomas Evans, of Helynfured, who had never, in Dr Davies's knowledge, been administered any medicine, was frequently unsafe to be at large. Elizabeth Owen, a pauper lunatic from Llangeinwen, he described as being 'full of Hysteria', and one who 'at times does mischief'. [26]

James Roose, medical officer for Amlwch district of Anglesey union, wrote that in his district there were five lunatics but none were dangerous. There was also another lunatic who had been discharged incurable from an asylum. In addition there were four idiots regarded as harmless, and who 'appear to be comfortable'.[27]

W. T. Lewis of Beaumaris, who had examined all thirteen cases of pauper lunatics in his district, felt that they could be categorized under three forms of insanity: 'mania or furious madness; dementia and mental imbecility; and fatuity or annihilation of the powers of the mind which may be either adventitious or connate the latter (connate) constituting the idiotic form of insanity'. He had three cases of mania, four of dementia, two of fatuity and four of idiocy, two of which were complicated with epileptic fits. All of them could 'with propriety' be allowed to be at large, 'in as much as restraint or seclusion *without due precaution or proper judgement* would be rather injurious than otherwise'. All thirteen pauper lunatics were tolerably well taken care of with regard to diet and clothing, although he observed that little or no attention appeared to be given to their general health which 'exerts most material influence on their mental disorder'. With but one exception, none had been given any medical treatment, either physical or moral. It was in vain to expect any amelioration 'in their forlorn and pitiable condition', as long as they were left in the care of persons who were 'quite ignorant of the principles which ought to guide them in the management of the insane'. He supported the suggestion of forming a lunatic asylum for the principality, stating his conviction that 'some of the cases which I have specified above might be at least benefited, if not permanently restored to the possession of their reasoning faculties by removal to an Asylum'.[28] When the clerk of peace asked how many of the patients he thought might be cured by removal to an asylum, Lewis replied that it was quite impossible to state the exact number, but estimated that one half of them would benefit.[29]

This information on the condition of the insane poor in Anglesey suggested that numbers were not sufficient to warrant an asylum. A largely rural population and dispersed settlement patterns meant that the problem of the lunatic poor was not highly visible. For the most part it was possible to make informal arrangements within the locality. There were few towns of any importance, and no middle class of a size likely to provide customers for a private madhouse or contribute to the cost of a public/private asylum. In Anglesey as in Merioneth, the other largely rural county of north-west Wales, there was considerable opposition to the establishment of union workhouses. (Even in the mid-1850s there was still no workhouse on the island, although some parishes in the south of the island formed part of the Bangor and Beaumaris union which opened a workhouse in Bangor in 1844, and others to the south-west formed part of the Caernarfon union.) The ratepayers in either county did not support establishing a pauper lunatic asylum, preferring familial and local contractual arrangements. Also the language was a significant consideration. As the vast majority of the population spoke Welsh, many being monoglot speakers, this meant that only in exceptional circumstances would a pauper lunatic be sent away to an English asylum. The distance of the journey too was prohibitive. When counties faced large bills for the maintenance of pauper lunatics in other counties' asylums, there was an economic argument for establishing one of their own. However, when pauper lunatics could be maintained locally for what the commissioners in lunacy described as 'a pittance', there was no financial pressure to seek a more rational system. Therefore, there was little impetus from within Anglesey, or indeed the other western counties of north Wales, to promote the establishment of a county lunatic asylum. Not, that is, without central government legislation making it a legal obligation on county magistrates to provide a public asylum.

As information was fed back to London it began to paint a bleak picture of conditions in Wales, and in July 1844 Lord Ashley expressed the concerns of reformers in a speech to Parliament, when he spoke of the need to investigate: 'If they went to the Principality, they would find that they were too often treated as no man of feeling would treat his dog; that they were kept in outhouses – chained – wallowing in filth, and without firing, for years.'[30] One of the main outcomes of the 1844 report was the ammunition it gave to those parliamentarians concerned to promote new legislation making it compulsory for all counties to cater for their lunatic poor. Some of the most powerful and damaging information used to persuade Parliament of the necessity of introducing mandatory legislation to supersede the purely enabling legislation of the 1808 Act, was drawn from the *Supplemental Report* on Wales.

Findings of the Investigation

The Metropolitan Lunacy commissioners found a clear pattern – dominated by domestic and family care, with arrangements for boarding out in cases where family care was unavailable or inappropriate. In many instances officials recognized that the care was satisfactory. Hugh Ellis, of Denbigh, was said to be 'comfortably boarded with a relation', and Richard Jones was apparently 'well–clothed and kindly treated'.[31] It seems likely that many other instances of satisfactory arrangements were not brought to the attention of the lunacy commissioners. The report may therefore have a built-in bias towards highlighting problem cases and emphasizing the deficiencies of the system.

Where the care of pauper lunatics was contracted out to small farmers or tradesmen, the Poor Law allowance was usually paid to the male house-holder, though in many cases the responsibility devolved to the wife. This was clearly so with Catherine Williams, 'consigned to the care of a small farmer, named Edward Gray', at Bryniadwn, Llandegfan, near Beaumaris. The parish had been paying up to to 7*s*. 6*d*. weekly for her care; when the vestry proposed sending the pauper to Haydock Lodge Asylum, 'Edward Gray's wife consented, on the part of her husband . . . to a reduction of the weekly charge to 5*s*.'. Ellen Davies, described as 'a harmless idiot' of sixty-six years of age was also farmed out with the Grays at 2*s*. 9*d*. per week, besides clothing. Such a system could work effectively, offering security and a home to the afflicted sufferers, whilst simultaneously securing a basic income to the carers. In the case of Edward Gray's home, the visiting commissioners noted that 'Both these women appeared to be fairly accommodated; and to be treated with kindness'.[32]

The greatest problems arose when a 'lunatic' was not manageable. If they physically attacked or threatened others in the family or neighbours then some practical solution had to be found as a matter of urgency. The commissioners' evidence suggests that the management of violent and dangerous lunatics presented common problems often leading to the adoption of similar rudimentary solutions. Hamilton Owen Roberts, for many years a surgeon in Caernarfonshire, had previously investigated cases of pauper lunatics in the slate-quarrying districts of Llandegai and Llanllechid. He gave evidence that, upon the first symptoms of violence appearing, the insane would be 'tied down with cords', and that there was never any attempt 'at medical or moral treatment'.[33]

Physical restraint seems to have been commonly employed throughout north Wales. When visiting the Llŷn Peninsula, the commissioners heard evidence concerning Thomas Parry of Edern, near Porthdinllaen, who, dirty and badly clothed, wandered about the village with 'his legs chained, and occasionally handcuffed'.[34] They also heard of Griffith Williams of Llanbedrog, who on becoming 'furiously maniacal . . . was tied down with cords and confined by a strait jacket', having attempted to cut his own throat. Previously 'a dangerous character and addicted to fighting', he was subject to epileptic fits, rendering him liable to assault people indiscriminately. He often threatened to kill them, saying that 'being mad he was not responsible'.[35]

At Bangor, Dr O. O. Roberts, who was to become deeply involved in the asylum campaign, reported on a number of cases, including that of John Jones, who was then being cared for by an eighty-three-year-old woman, Grace Jones, who 'tends him kindly'. John Jones was by this time himself an elderly man, but in former days he had been 'violent and dangerous, and confined in a place adjoining a cow-house, upon a farm near Bangor . . . and fed through a hole in the wall'.[36]

Physical restraint was not regarded as something that had to be hidden from view. At Ruthin, Robert Jones, described as 'a dangerous Idiot', was allowed out into the street near his father's house, 'with his legs fettered by a strap, and his arms and hands secured by a strong web, something similar to cheese-filleting'.[37]

When the family was unable to cope boarding arrangements were often made with a neighbour, usually another pauper in receipt of relief, in return for a weekly payment. In Tremadog, Caernarfonshire, a poor woman, Mary James, was paid 9*d.* a week to bake and wash for her neighbour Griffith Pritchard of Pwllglenlas and his son Robert, who had been 'attacked with insanity twelve years ago, after a hard day's work in the hayfield'. Occasion- ally Robert, who 'was mute, and apparently fatuous', would become violent and have to be restrained. Mary James kept a straight waistcoat 'ready to employ as occasion requires'.[38]

Similar cases were reported across the five counties of north Wales, but more especially in the three western counties. David Davies, of Corwen, Merioneth, was 'very troublesome'. The Poor Law guardians employed another pauper 'to watch him'. At one time he became very violent, and was for three weeks under restraint 'day and night'.[39] In many instances neighbours would be called upon to assist. David Williams, of Llanrwst, aged forty-four, was boarded with his mother. He was at times very violent, and neighbours would sometimes be called in to protect the mother from his violence.[40]

With the development of a system of law enforcement, constables were often requested to control violent lunatics. Zechariah Williams was a former sailor who was lodged with his father and, according to his brother, he was 'harmless and inoffensive'. But in the opinion of the local doctor, and clerk of the guardians, and the local police, he was quarrelsome and violent. When the commissioners in lunacy visited Bangor in July 1844, they learnt that on the previous night he had been found fighting in the street. Due to his persistent violence, he was constantly being watched by the police, as 'a necessary precaution'.[41]

Sometimes police interceded in instances of domestic violence. William Lewis was a stonemason who had become insane after an injury to the head. He occasionally became very violent, and his daughter would call on the local policeman, who once found William Lewis brandishing a poker and 'threatening to knock out the brains of anyone who entered the house'. The doctor too was called, and as a form of treatment her father was copiously bled. Occasionally William would be tied down to the bed. He had probably suffered a serious brain injury, for he was said to be of 'filthy habits, and insensible to the calls of nature'.[42] In order to sustain home care in such a difficult case, outside professional help was of material importance.

Dealing with the mentally ill or handicapped during a difficult phase presented real problems of management, and carers adopted a variety of strategies. If the patient was male and of strong physique, handling him could be challenging, and sometimes beyond the strength of the immediate family. One solution was to recruit someone capable of overpowering the lunatic. Richard Parry of St Asaph was described as athletic, formerly a farm labourer, epileptic and 'decidedly insane'. He was admitted to the workhouse in December 1841 but previous to that he suffered from 'frequent paroxysms of furious Mania', and used to be frequently restrained. He had twice, for short periods, been placed under the care of Samuel Davies at Abergele, 'a powerful man . . . of somewhat indifferent character', who was the 'only person in the place who would take charge of him'. For this Samuel Davies allowed a guinea a week by the parish – a considerable sum, when compared to the 2–3*s*. usually paid for the care of a lunatic. It was said that Samuel Davies treated him harshly. At one time Richard Parry was placed in the Chester Asylum, but after a few months he was returned to the workhouse in Abergele. While there he was employed, and 'kept on a low diet', and proved generally harmless. However, he could still prove a danger to other inmates, and during a dispute with one 'feeble old man, he lifted him up and placed him upon the stove in the Day-room'.[43]

One alternative to physical domination was to reduce the bodily strength of the insane person. Keeping the patient low by restricting diet was often resorted to and John Edwards of Ruthin was 'Subdued by short diet occasionally'.[44] Alternatively, Robert Jones, of Tremadog, was 'Kept low by medicine'.[45]

A lunatic committing a serious assault might appear in court and be sentenced to prison. Richard Williams of Beaumaris had been sent to the Liverpool Asylum following a violent assault, but he had escaped from there some years previously, after which he had committed an 'aggravated assault upon a child'. For this he had been given twelve months imprisonment. Following release, he began to drink heavily, again became violent, and was returned to prison having breached sureties of good behaviour. However, the surgeon inspecting the prison declared him insane, and therefore unfit to be so detained. Hence in June 1844 he was transferred to the newly opened Haydock Lodge Asylum in Lancashire.[46]

When violence forced families to seek outside help, the problem became exposed to public view. Others remained within the domestic sphere. A practical difficulty, which could affect the household budget, was that the insane sometimes had insatiable appetites. For those living in poverty, and indeed for a large proportion of the Welsh rural population in the nineteenth century, food was a scarce commodity. The burden placed on a family, when required to find extra food to satisfy the cravings of a hungry, dependent lunatic, added to the strains of caring for the mentally ill. Hugh Roberts, aged twenty-four, of Holywell, described as an epileptic idiot, lived with his father who received support of 4*s.* a week from the parish. The son was of 'a robust frame, and of a ravenous appetite', which could rarely be satisfied, so that he was always 'restless, moaning, and craving for food'.[47] Ann Thomas, of St Asaph, who was confined in a dark and fetid room, complained of not having sufficient food. Her daughter told the investigating clergyman that her mother would 'eat every hour of the day', and when he inquired what food was available for her, she pointed to the grate and said 'there is meat for her, sir, now on the fire'. He was shown a small tin, containing about half a pint of buttermilk warming on the bars of the grate. [48]

Insane relatives needed to be carefully watched to guard them from danger. Emma Jones of Denbigh, a twenty-five-year-old woman described as having a 'disordered intellect', had been subject to epileptic fits since she was four years old. On the approach of a fit she would become very trouble-some, and dangerous to herself. She required constant watching, 'amongst other things to prevent her from falling into the fire'. The whole family, including Emma and her father, and her sister and her husband, all slept together in one room.[49]

Overall, the outstanding impression which the commissioners took away from their expedition to Wales was 'the reluctance which we have generally found exhibited by the poorer classes in Wales to part with their Insane relations, however troublesome and dangerous, and however disgusting their habits'.[50] A woman in Caernarfon said that it would 'break her heart' to part with her idiot sister.[51] Even the father and sisters of Hugh Roberts, the ravenous epileptic, who was of 'filthy habits, and insensible to the calls of nature', said on being asked that 'they would not part with him'.[52]

The high level of dependence on domestic solutions impressed the visiting commissioners. Many of the insane paupers to whom their attention was drawn were viewed by neighbours and occasionally by members of their family as 'threats' to the safety of those around them. Yet it was not this aspect which caught the imagination of the commissioners so much as the vulnerability of the insane themselves and the isolated cases of mistreatment. It was the picture of pauper lunatics as 'victims' of cruelty and physical restraint, of starvation and abuse, which fired the commissioners with indignation, and was to act as a powerful catalyst of public opinion, inspiring both the founding of the Denbigh asylum and reform of the law.

'Instances of Atrocious Cruelty'

It was on their return journey, having already visited the north coast, Anglesey and the Llŷn peninsula, that the commissioners reached Ruthin where they came across the one case which was to serve their purpose best. They heard about this woman from a relieving officer and from a surgeon of the union, who described her condition as 'filthy and disgusting'. They reported that 'some provisions placed by her side remained untouched, and near them were a chamber utensil and bowls, full of feculent matter'.[53] This was just the sort of unsavoury detail the investigating team were seeking, and two of the commissioners conducting inquiries in north Wales, Lutwidge and Waterfield, made arrangements to visit this 'poor creature'. So it was that, between 8 and 9 o'clock one summer evening, they arrived at the cottage, accompanied by Dr Richard Lloyd Williams of Denbigh, who acted as interpreter. Their report graphically conveys their horror at what they witnessed. This one case, more than all of the others, had the effect of exciting moral outrage, and served as a fine 'exemplary case' which was then used to press for reform of the entire system. The final published report brings the scene vividly to life, over a century and a half later. The style and imagery conjure up the atmosphere so powerfully that the reader virtually enters the 'loathsome chamber' alongside the commissioners, inhales the smells of stale urine and cringes at the sight of the woman's frightful distortions. That, certainly, was the writers' intention:

In a dark and offensive room, over a blacksmith's forge, upon opening a bolted door, we discovered the miserable object of our search. The only window was closed up by boards, between which little air could find admission, and only a feeble glimmering of light.

In the middle of this loathsome chamber was Mary Jones, the Lunatic, on a foul pallet of chaff or straw; and here she had been confined for a period of fifteen years and upwards. She was seated in a bent and crouching posture, on her bed of nauseous and disgusting filth. Near to her person, and just within her reach, was a cup into which she was accustomed to pass her excretions, which she emptied, from time to time, into a chamber utensil. This last vessel contained a quantity of feculent matter, the accumulation of several days. By her side were the remnants of some food, of which she had partaken. Within a few feet of the pallet, which was on the floor, stood a large earthen jar, nearly full of fetid urine, the produce of the three other persons in the cottage. It had, as stated by the mother, been placed there in order that it might, from the warmth of the room, undergo a more speedy decomposition, for the purpose of being used in dyeing wool. The stagnant and suffocating atmosphere, and the nauseous effluvia which infected it, were almost intolerable.

Long and close confinement had produced in Mary Jones's person the most frightful distortions. The chest bone protruded forwards five or six inches beyond its natural place; and there was an excoriation of the parts below. The legs were bent backwards, and the knee-joints were fixed and immovable. The ankles and feet also were greatly twisted and deformed.

She was emaciated in the last degree, her pulse was feeble and quick, and her countenance, still pleasing, was piercingly anxious, and marked by an expression of despair. Her garments were loathsome; and from her person was emitted a most offensive odour.[54]

The olfactory imagination was marshalled to the aid of the reformer.

The commissioners interviewed Mary's mother, and learned that she had first been 'attacked with insanity at twenty-one, when a servant in the family of the late Clerk of the Peace'. At that time she was still as 'straight as an arrow' and had no signs of deformity. Mary had at one time been treated as an outpatient at the Denbigh Dispensary, but for the last fifteen years she had occupied the small chamber above the forge. The living quarters of the rest of the family were in the other half of the building. (The building remains practically unchanged, except that the forge is now a pottery.) For the first five years of occupying the loft Mary had been allowed to go down-stairs during the day, but for the past ten years she had been entirely confined to the chamber. During nearly the whole of that time the window had been boarded up. What puzzled and perplexed the commissioners was that 'her pitiable situation appears to have been veiled in mysterious secrecy', despite the fact that 'her habitation was in close proximity to the church, and contiguous to the public road'.[55]

On 5 August, following his visit with the commissioners, Dr Lloyd Williams contacted the dean of St Asaph, and requested that he accompany both himself and Dr Cumming on a further visit to Mary Jones so as 'to take some steps for her relief'. The dean accordingly rode over that very morning. The room was as described by the commissioners, although the 'offensive' items had been removed. They questioned Mary Jones, and the answers that she gave were 'perfectly rational'. The three men settled upon the option of admitting her to the Denbigh Dispensary, since they decided that 'it would be dreadful either to leave her where she is, or to send her to an English Asylum, where the poor object could not express her wants'.[56] In order to send her to the Infirmary it was necessary for them to affirm that she 'was not insane' since the rules of the institution forbade admitting a patient who was a lunatic, or of unsound mind, a rule common to most voluntary hospitals. This case neatly exposed the full absurdity of the lack of appropriate provision for the lunatic poor, who could not be treated in Wales, in their own language, and so were left to languish in filthy and fetid conditions. Dr Richard Lloyd Williams returned again to see Mary Jones, as it had been arranged that the local squire would send his caravan to transport her to Denbigh. But the day was wet, and the vehicle had not arrived, and so the doctor, or his son, drew a rough sketch of Mary, which they forwarded to the commissioners. Later on she was admitted to the Infirmary, where she spent the night 'cheerful and comfortable'.[57] The rescue had been accomplished.

Subsequently Dr Richard Lloyd Williams uncovered two other 'atrocious cases'. One was a man, Peter Powell, whom he found 'in a wretched shed, on a filthy straw pallet'. The other, in a 'still more deplorable state', was a woman, Anne Hughes of Rhyd Issa, near Meliden, who had been bed-ridden and insane for upward of twenty years, and was confined in a 'sort of trough' in an outdoor shed.[58] Dr Richard Lloyd Williams expressed his opinion that 'Hers was also a curable case at its onset'. He went on to point out the anomaly that both were 'put down as Idiots' in the returns, but said that he regarded them rather as cases of 'neglected Insanity'. (This supports the proposition that it was only the mediation of medical men with an interest in psychiatry that led to patients previously labelled as idiot becoming recategorized as insane.) Lloyd Williams, who had for the past two years or more 'worked tirelessly' for the cause of establishing a lunatic asylum at Denbigh, went on to praise the work of the commissioners and express his appreciation of their intervention: 'Your happy discovery of Mary Jones will, I doubt not, lead to more vigilant inquiry, and I feel confident that many deeds of darkness and of atrocity will come to light.'[59] This sense of missionary endeavour was central to the 'heroic' attempts to establish a lunatic asylum in north Wales and to reform the morals of the native-speaking Welsh. The unusual grouping of churchmen and medical men, squirearchy and Nonconformist radicals, which finally brought about a revolution in care and treatment of the insane, is the subject of the next chapter.

The proceedings of the 'special investigation' indicate an element of reciprocity in the relationship between the doctors and churchmen in north Wales, who were campaigning for the establishment of a Welsh asylum, and the Evangelical reformers at the Lunacy Commission in London. The Metropolitan commissioners in lunacy were 'pointed in the right direction' and then could draw attention to the plight of the 'poor lunatic' in Wales. For south Wales, where such a fruitful coincidence of interests did not emerge, the commission's activities did not generate evidence of the same scale. In June 1845 Lord Ashley (later Lord Shaftesbury) presented a Bill to the House of Commons to make it a requirement on all counties, either singly or in union with another county or borough, to provide a lunatic asylum. During his speech in favour of the Bill he cited the case of Mary Jones and told the House that, on the authority of Dr Williams of Denbigh, 'she must at one time have been fully capable of cure'.[60]

Ashley employed examples from Wales to press home the need for a reform of the legislation. It is unlikely that he was expressing anti-Welsh sentiments, for he had previously spent a summer in Aberystwyth learning the Welsh language, at the end of which, in his own words, the people 'held a great meeting at which I was created both a Bard and a Druid'.[61] His eloquent pleas concerning the condition of Welsh lunatics seem to have swayed the views of his listeners, and Parliament voted overwhelmingly in favour of the new legislation.

Parliament also accepted that it was necessary to establish a national inspectorate, and so the Metropolitan Lunacy Commission was abolished and the Lunacy Commission was created. The new commission had a wider remit and greater powers, and was to supervise, monitor and advise the chain of county asylums throughout England and Wales. Lord Shaftesbury was to remain its chairman until his death in 1885.[62]

✳

CHAPTER THREE

The Founding of the North Wales Lunatic Asylum

By the beginning of the nineteenth century charitable institutions had been established in a number of English cities to provide care for the insane poor. These voluntary efforts embodied the notion that the care of the insane was a public duty and not merely the private responsibility of the family. The idea that it was the state's duty to provide care for the insane poor began to take root early in the nineteenth century. In 1807 Sir George Onesiphorus Paul, the high sheriff of Gloucestershire and active prison reformer, presented a petition to Parliament highlighting the plight of the criminal lunatic and emphasizing the inadequate provision for the insane.[1] A Parliamentary Select Committee, under the general direction of George Rose and Charles Watkin Williams Wynn, MP for Montgomeryshire, was appointed to look into the question.[2] Its report advocated state intervention. The ensuing County Asylums Act of 1808 was permissive, enabling county magistrates to raise a rate for the purpose of establishing a county lunatic asylum.[3] It became known as Wynn's Act. The first two county asylums to be built under its terms were Bedford and Nottingham, both opened in 1812.[4]

There is no evidence of any charitable institutions being established in Wales, but in 1810 an attempt was made to found a public asylum. An advertisement was placed in the Chester papers giving notice of a meeting of a committee of magistrates of Denbighshire and Flintshire to treat with the county of Merioneth for building a joint counties lunatic asylum.[5] Wynn wrote to the clerk of Denbighshire Quarter Sessions informing him that Montgomeryshire magistrates had similarly appointed such a committee. He endorsed their efforts and expressed his opinion that a union of the counties of north Wales would be 'highly desirable'.[6] The obstacles to reaching a collective agreement between counties were considerable, and there was little interest in the scheme. In the absence of any state compulsion justices of the peace were not likely to commit the large expenditure. Transport facilities were poor so that the idea of a central institution for north Wales did not appeal to the western counties, which still favoured domestic arrangements. The result was that another thirty years passed without any serious endeavour to establish a public asylum. By 1845 only sixteen of the forty counties in England had made any provision, and in Wales where there were twelve counties only the Pembrokeshire asylum had been established.[7]

When, in 1841, a further attempt was made to found a joint counties asylum for north Wales the initial response was again discouraging. Twelve months after a committee of campaigners began seeking support from county magistrates the *Carnarvon and Denbigh Herald* reported that, despite 'the justice, the humanity, and the sound policy, (as far as even financial economy is concerned), of the undertaking', the attempt 'to get the adjacent counties to act in unison, has failed'.[8] The committee, comprising 'several gentlemen of the County of Denbigh', issued a circular to the chairmen of Quarter Sessions and the lord lieutenants of the five counties of north Wales proposing the establishment of an asylum. The response, 'refusals from some quarters and apathy from others', was disappointing. When presented with proposals to build an asylum at an estimated cost of some £22,000 magistrates complained that 'the debt is already oppressive and the very great depression throughout the county did not warrant the Magistrates to entertain them'.[9]

Determined to press forward, the committee wrote to the Home Secretary, who informed them that it was proposed 'to introduce some legislative enactments to provide for the remedial treatment and further care of the insane poor'.[10] Fortified by this assurance, the committee continued to campaign. In a letter to the Poor Law commissioners the chairman of the Denbigh magistrates pointed out that currently little attention was paid to the probability of recovery of those recently or temporarily insane, 'whilst those afflicted from their birth, or of long standing, are left objects of fear and terror to their friends; or wander abroad, frightful and dangerous to the sensitive, seeking food and commiseration from the public; or insane perishing with cold, hunger and want of shelter'.[11] Whether these appeals to central government influenced Sir James Graham to appoint Samuel Hitch to investigate north Wales on behalf of the Poor Law Commission is not clear, but certainly the correspondence served to bring the situation in the region to the attention of both the Poor Law Commission and the Home Secretary.[12]

Following the completion of his survey of north Wales Samuel Hitch wrote a letter to *The Times* in October 1842, calling for public support for the establishment of an asylum in Wales to provide humanitarian care for Welsh-speaking lunatics. *The Times* played an active role in advancing lunacy reform and had recently promoted John Connolly, the medical superintendent of the new Middlesex Asylum at Hanwell, to the status of a national celebrity.[13] Hitch's survey indicated the overwhelming reliance upon domestic arrangements for care of the insane in Wales and the lack of asylum provision or facilities for curative treatment. He emphasized the disadvantage suffered by Welsh-speaking lunatics sent to English establishment, describing how recently he had observed two cases in his asylum at Gloucester, neither of whom spoke or understood English. They had 'derived more comfort and made more progress towards recovery through an occasional conversation with a Welch clergyman, who conveyed to them what were my wishes towards them, than by all the other means which are placed at my command'.[14] He declared that the incarceration of Welsh lunatics in English asylums amounted to a form of abuse:

> So few of the lower class of the Welch . . . speak English . . . whilst both the officers and servants of our English asylums, and the English public too, are equally ignorant of the Welch language, – that when the poor Welchman is sent to an English asylum he is submitted to the most refined of modern cruelties, by being doomed to an imprisonment amongst strange people, and an association with his fellow men, whom he is prohibited from holding communion with. Nothing can exceed his misery: himself unable to communicate, or to receive communication, harassed by wants which he cannot make known, and appealed to by sounds which he cannot comprehend, he becomes irritable and irritated; and it is proverbial in our English asylums that the 'Welchman is the most turbulent patient wherever he happens to become an inmate'.[15]

The Welsh patient could not be 'approached by conversation', and therefore was denied the 'personal communion with educated minds' which Hitch considered to be one of the main benefits of asylum care. It was no surprise, therefore, that 'the poor Welchman, after having undergone this species of solitary confinement in our English asylums, should leave it at least no better, and often worse, than when he entered it'.[16]

The campaign to provide therapeutic care for the insane 'Welchman' in his own language was presented as a heroic cause, and as a struggle against injustice. It therefore seems a little ironic that some of the main benefactors were English-speaking landowners and churchmen who in other contexts were unsympathetic to the Welsh language. (The medical practitioners associated with the project were mainly Welsh-speaking, however, and some took an active pride in their native language.) The unlikely alliance of personalities involved in this campaign to establish an asylum in north Wales therefore begs attention.

Magistrates, Landowners and Subscribers

In conjunction with the publication of Samuel Hitch's letter, a determined attempt was made to establish a founding committee. Appraised of the difficulties of persuading all of the counties of north Wales to act in concert, the committee adopted the strategy of launching a subscription account. The first official gathering took place in the boardroom of the Denbigh General Infirmary, in October 1842, attended by local landowners, doctors, Anglican clergy including the dean of St Asaph, members of the town council and of the magistracy.[17] Motions were adopted resolving upon the need for an asylum. John Heaton of Plas Heaton, chairman of the Denbighshire magistrates, presided. Joseph Ablett of Llanbedr Hall, called for the establishment of a 'Hospital for the Insane . . . with a view to relieving this – the most grievous calamity that can befall humanity'.[18] Reference was repeatedly made to the establishment of a 'Hospital for the Insane'. A meeting of the Royal Medico-Psychological Association held in Gloucester the previous year (July 1841) had resolved to abandon the term 'lunatic' and 'Lunatic Asylum', except for legal purposes, and substitute the term 'Insane Person' or 'Hospital for the Insane'. The aim of this was to remove the stigma attached to the term 'lunacy', so that the terminology followed by the advocates of a Welsh subscription asylum, or rather 'hospital', reflected the most advanced thinking of the day.[19]

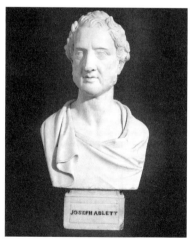

2. *Bust of Joseph Ablett. In all probability*
this is by John Gibson, the Welsh sculptor
whose studio was in Rome. Crown copyright:
Royal Commission on the Ancient and
Historical Monuments of Wales

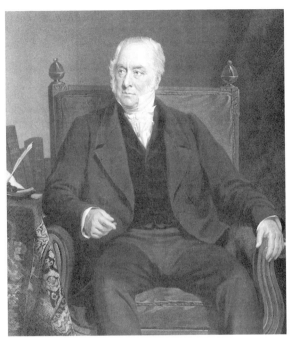

3. Portrait of John Heaton of Plas Heaton, chairman of the subscribers to the Denbigh asylum and chairman of the Denbighshire magistrates. Lithograph engraved by Edward McInnes and printed by E. W. Eddis. Plas Heaton MSS, Denbighshire Record Office

Dr Richard Lloyd Williams proposed an institution to be staffed by Welsh medical officers and attendants, 'acquainted with the only language through which any soothing influence can be conveyed to calm the horrors of his excited mind – to dispel the delusions, which have temporally driven reason from its seat, or to test the returning consciousness, by aiding his Memory and reflection'.[20]

Dr George Cumming pointed out in Benthamite terms the economic rationale of the proposition, and held that a weekly sum of 5s. a head could be realized if the counties contributed towards the cost of running their own asylum, as opposed to sending pauper lunatics away to England. The saving could be further increased if early treatment were provided to avoid the heavy expenses associated with the long-term care of neglected cases.[21] Dr John Williams referred to the powerful impact of the New Poor Law in bringing many cases to light, which 'heretofore had been kept secret' and to the clause of the 1834 Act that rendered the detention of any dangerous lunatic in a workhouse for more than fourteen days a misdemeanour. He urged the counties to action before it became compulsory by statute, in order to remove 'what cannot be deemed but a blot, upon the humanity of the Principality'.[22] The chairman was instructed to circulate all of the lieutenants of counties and chairmen of Quarter Sessions in north Wales with a copy of the resolutions. At the close it was triumphantly announced that a 'munificent offer' had been received from an anonymous benefactor ready to donate about twenty acres of land 'in a very eligible spot in the immediate vicinity of Denbigh'.[23]

The 'anonymous benefactor' was a local landowner, Joseph Ablett of Llanbedr Hall near Ruthin. He enjoyed the life of a country gentleman, directing his household along paternalistic lines. Inscribed on a slate tablet mounted in the hall was a list of fines to which the servants would be subjected – 6*d.* for taking the Lord's name in vain, 3*d.* for cursing or swearing, 2*d.* for 'asking for meat and then to leave it', and then, as a sanction against his servants speaking their own native language, the following warning: 'No Welsh to be Spoken in this Hall' on pain of a fine of 1*d.*! Ablett achieved some notoriety in the neighbourhood for refusing to grant the Nonconformists of the Llanbedr district the site for a chapel. He expected his tenants to attend the parish church. However, after local protests, he finally relinquished a small parcel of land for the Methodists to build a place of worship.[24]

His philanthropy extended to supporting artistic and literary ventures and Walter Savage Landor was a frequent guest. The two friends once visited Southey and Wordsworth in the Lake District. Robert Southey was a close friend of Charles Watkin Williams Wynn, the MP for Montgomeryshire and promoter of lunacy reform.[25] Not only Wynn, but other lunacy commissioners, including Shaftesbury and Proctor, were influenced by Southey's romantic conservatism and shared his belief in the ideal of paternalism.[26] Robert Southey's younger brother Henry held the post of Lord Chancellor's medical visitor in lunacy, being one of Lord Brougham's protégés.[27] Such interconnections in the social and cultural milieux within which some of the founders of the asylum moved are relevant to an appreciation of how local, regional and national elites functioned to promote social reform.

When Landor visited Llanbedr Hall in 1843 Ablett enlisted him to pen a public appeal for the asylum fund. This appeared in *The Examiner* in August, and was reprinted a week later on the front page of the *Carnarvon and Denbigh Herald*. 'Wales is the only country in Europe', Landor began, 'where there is no asylum for lunatics.' Referring to the 'munificent humanity' of Mr Ablett, in donating land on which to build an asylum for 'these poor creatures', he went on to substantiate his argument with figures revealed by the 'accurate investigation of Dr Hitch'. If the proportion of pauper insane discovered by Dr Hitch should be matched by the same proportion of non-paupers, he argued, then there must in Wales be at least one insane in every 200 persons. 'No other country on the whole earth exhibits so appalling a multitude', claimed Landor.

> And yet no asylum has been erected for the sufferers. Even mismanaged, insulted, degraded, distracted Ireland, has prepared this ultimate place of refuge for the most unfortunate of her unfortunate children. The rich even there, where the rich have always been considered as having the fewest and feeblest sympathies with the poor, have provided, at least against this one calamity.[28]

Thus was Wales portrayed as inferior even to Ireland!

Ablett's early commitment to donate land was undoubtedly a key factor in the success of the campaign to establish an asylum, and the property was formally transferred to the trustees in 1844.[29]

Anglican Prelates

Most Denbighshire parishes lie within the see of St Asaph, and its dean since 1826, Charles Scott Luxmoore, was the most prestigious member of the Anglican clergy to play a role in the campaign. From a wealthy family, Luxmoore had extensive social and family connections with members of the church movements associated with Oxford – both the Evangelicals and Tractarians. Luxmoore's younger brother married the sister of E. B. Pusey,[30] and through this connection he was related to Lord Shaftesbury.

He was able to offer the committee considerable experience of asylum administration. His father had been involved with the Hereford Infirmary when that voluntary hospital decided to open a special lunatic ward and later in 1791 to erect a separate purpose-built asylum. John Nash was appointed architect and the complicated financial and contractual problems that ensued must have acted as a salutary lesson to the younger Luxmoore of the dangers inherent in such a major capital enterprise.[31]

Luxmoore continued to retain his livings in Herefordshire and to serve as a visitor to the Hereford Lunatic Asylum. In this capacity in 1838 he dealt with a serious complaint concerning the ill-treatment of an inmate. This led to a report which was critical of the management and raised fundamental questions about the nature of the asylum. If it was a curative institution then punishment had no role to play.

> Either the unfortunate patients here confined are responsible or they are not – If *they are* surely a Lunatic Asylum is not a fit place for responsible beings – If they are not, which they assume from their being in the asylum, however necessary restraint gloves or the belt, or the waistcoat or even the

manacles and fetters may be; yet the idea of punishing an irresponsible being is quite abhorrent from every proper feeling.[32]

Hence it is clear that Luxmoore committed himself to the North Wales Asylum campaign when possessed of a mature appreciation of the hazards of running such an institution and the onerous responsibility entailed in becoming a 'visitor'. He was again to play a role in investigations into the Hereford Asylum in 1846, at a time when the campaign to establish the Denbigh asylum was itself approaching a crisis.[33]

Luxmoore already knew of the work of Samuel Hitch. In 1839 Luxmoore had accompanied the high sheriff of Herefordshire on a visit to the Gloucester Asylum, whereupon they expressed their 'unqualified admiration at the state and management of the Institution'.[34] The dean judged the system at Gloucester to be 'really practical, and capable of being varied upon any of those occasions which so painful a malady may require'.[35] Gloucester was to become the model for the North Wales Lunatic Asylum at Denbigh.

Luxmoore abhorred the rough and ready treatment that he saw meted out to the insane in north Wales, and on occasion interceded on behalf of individual lunatics who were kept in restraint. In 1841 he intervened in the case of pauper lunatic Evan Lewis, left to wander about the streets of Abergele in a miserable condition, handcuffed and leg-locked. Luxmoore secured his removal to Chester Asylum, and in this and other ways attempted to reform the moral landscape of his parishioners.[36] Occasionally Luxmoore wrote to the north Wales press under the pseudonym 'Homo' in support of the campaign to build the asylum.[37]

The dean was supported in his endeavours by his colleague the Revd William Hicks Owen. He too corresponded with the newspapers, under the pen-name of 'Clericus'. In 1839 he took a leading role in securing the conviction of a farmer in his parish for the cruel treatment of his mentally ill wife, Ann Thomas. Owen had seen the woman locked in a room, where she sat 'cowering, trembling, and moaning loudly on the floor, surrounded by filth' and fastened to a chain driven into the wall.[38]

Luxmoore and Owen were public champions of Anglican enlightenment and paternalism, but throughout north Wales other members of the established church provided a solid bloc of support for the asylum campaign, regarding this social action as a natural extension of their moral authority. The traditional pastoral role of the clergy in raising alms for needy cases during church services meant that they could claim to have a legitimate concern for the welfare of the sick and the suffering.

These clergymen tended to support the reformists' view of lunacy, as a condition that could be ameliorated and was subject to cure. They also saw themselves as battling against the remnants of superstition concerning the influence of the spirit world, and this informed their intervention on a number of occasions. An example occurred in 1844 when the Revd Philips, the vicar of Bettws, took the Metropolitan Lunacy commissioners to visit a cottage at Pengwern:

> In one bed was the poor creature in a maniacal state, and in another, in the same room, her sick husband. She had been cheated and robbed by a fortune-telling gipsy, under pretence of curing her husband, and transferring a supposed curse from him to other parties. Compunction, and disappointment at the failure of the charm, and loss of property, had produced a shock which suddenly deprived her of reason. So gross were the ignorance and superstition of the villagers, that they all believed her to have been bewitched by the gipsy woman.[39]

Soon after the visit the woman, Grace Williams, became very violent and 'for want of a Lunatic Asylum, was sent to the Denbigh Infirmary'. The commissioners received accounts of her progress thereafter from Dr Lloyd Williams, who assured them that she 'had become tranquil, and her delusions were fast vanishing'.[40] This intervention was seen as proof of the efficacy of humane, progressive treatment. The metropolitan commissioners cited this case as a clear indication of the 'urgent necessity for an Asylum'.[41]

Dr Richard Lloyd Williams and the Role of Medical Men

The medical men who became members of the founding group of the Denbigh asylum were associated with the Denbigh Infirmary, the voluntary hospital originally founded as the Denbighshire General Dispensary in 1807. Despite a clause, common to voluntary hospitals, forbidding admission of those of unsound mind, both Mary Jones and Grace Williams were finally admitted to the infirmary, due to the doctors' intercession. The two doctors who took the most active lead in establishing the asylum held offices at the infirmary. Dr George Cumming was described as 'Founder of and Senior Physician to the Denbighshire Infirmary and General Dispensary'. He was much interested in therapeutic innovations, including the use of the Turkish bath.[42] Dr Richard Lloyd Williams was consulting surgeon to the Denbighshire Infirmary and General Dispensary.[43] The meetings to establish the asylum were all held in the boardroom of the Denbigh Infirmary. This close connection with an existing voluntary hospital mirrors the establishment of both the Hereford and Gloucester asylums.[44]

Dr Richard Lloyd Williams, the most energetic and influential medical advocate of asylum care for the insane in north Wales, was born in 1791, at Penmachno, and was distantly related to Charles Watkin Williams Wynn.[45] Williams trained at St Bartholemew's Hospital and became a member of the

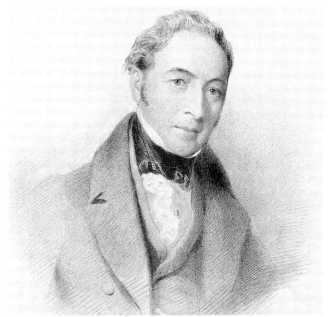

*4. Portrait of Richard Lloyd Williams, MD, first secretary of the subscribers to
the Denbigh asylum and first visiting physician to the asylum. Stipple engraving
by J. Posselwhite, 1848, after H. W. Phillips. R. Burgess,* Portraits of Doctors
and Scientists in the Wellcome Institute, *London, 1973, no. 3189.1.
Reproduced by kind permission of the Wellcome Institute Library, London.*

Royal College of Surgeons in 1813. He returned to establish a practice in
Denbigh, probably in about 1815, and obtained an MD from the University of
St Andrews in 1822. When the North Wales Lunatic Asylum was finally
opened in 1848, he was appointed the first visiting physician. In 1851 he was
elected president of the north Wales branch of the British Medical Association, the newly formed professional body that played such a crucial role in
raising the status and consolidating the power of medical practitioners.

Undoubtedly his involvement with the campaign contributed significantly to his standing as a doctor, and to the development of his career. He
was elected mayor of Denbigh in 1846 and again in 1847, so that he held
office in 1848 when the asylum opened.[46] His commitment to the cause of
the insane also consolidated many of his social connections, and improved
the prospects of his large family. It was a key move in his personal career
trajectory and at the same time contributed to the larger project of claiming
for the medical profession sole legitimacy for treating insanity.[47]

His death in 1862, aged seventy, was recorded by the *Baner ac Amserau
Cymru*, in a brief notice which stressed his humanitarian treatment of the poor:

Galerir amdano gan berthnasau a chyfeillion lliosog, a chaiff y tlodion golled ddirffawr, trwy golli un o'u cynorthwywyr mwyaf haelionus. Yr oedd yn hynod am ei ddyngarwch a'i diriondeb at bawb mewn adfyd a chaledi; ac yn hynod o ffydlawn am lawer o flynyddoedd yn weinyddu i dlodion afiach yn rhad yn ysbytty Dinbych. Dioddefodd gystudd maith gydag amynedd Cristionogol, a gobeithiwn 'fod marw yn elw iddo'.[48]

At the first meeting of the subscribers to the asylum, Dr Richard Lloyd Williams was elected to the post of secretary, and his brother-in-law, John Heaton, was elected chairman. From a long-established family of Henllan, near Denbigh, Heaton was educated at Eton and Cambridge. A staunch Whig, he was chairman of the Quarter Sessions of Denbighshire for eighteen years, and a magistrate for over forty. He was elected chairman of the North Wales Asylum when it opened in 1848.[49] Others on the subscribers' committee included R. B. Clough (whose wife, a cousin, was an aunt of the poet, A. H. Clough, and of Jemima, pioneer of women's higher education); also J. H. Clough of Castle House, Denbigh, whose son-in-law John Williams Ellis, of the Glasfryn and Brondanw estates in north-west Wales, also played a leading role in the campaign for the asylum.[50]

These biographical portraits show the extent to which the impetus for the asylum venture came from a small oligarchy connected by religious and family ties. As a result, the subscribers to the asylum could from the outset not only rely on the support of justices of the peace in Denbighshire but also exploit valuable channels of communication to other centres of power, both governmental and intellectual, regional and national.

The precise location of the asylum reflected the territorial base of this particular constellation of interests and alliances between the landowners, clergy and an influential professional elite. Nestling in the Vale of Clwyd, Denbigh was a substantial and thriving market town. Located on an important commercial route stretching from London to Ireland, it had a number of coaching inns, although the railway line did not reach the town until 1862. It had no major industry, but had important tanneries, a limestone quarry, printers, millers and some clothing manufacturers, and had long been a commercial centre.[51]

The town boasted a solid and stable municipal administration.[52] During the decade in which the asylum was built the town was investing in a new town hall, a market hall and two new schools, one of which was the earliest non-denominational school in north Wales. This strong civic structure helps to explain why the asylum had its roots in Denbigh. Probably no other town in the region could have provided the social capital, comprising experience, confidence and support which enabled the founders to pursue this venture to a successful conclusion despite formidable difficulties. Only the energetic endeavours of the subscribers succeeded in sustaining the financial commitment and cementing an alliance of five counties. In the absence of any comparable group of enthusiasts in south-west Wales, little progress was made there. There were endless arguments over the projected site and ultimately the Home Secretary had to intercede before the Joint Counties Asylum in Carmarthen was finally opened in 1865.[53]

Campaigning for the Asylum

In the efforts to rally support to the cause of a joint counties asylum for north Wales sections of the press were to play a crucial role. The *Carnarvon and Denbigh Herald* pledged itself to 'devote the agency of a free and unfettered press to shew [*sic*] the glaring necessity of a Welsh Asylum for Welsh Lunatics'. The editors appealed to the nationalistic sentiment of their readers, by declaring: 'We trust that the gentry of North Wales generally will endeavour to remove what is in itself a national disgrace. Our Saxon neighbours are surprised at our apparent indifference on such a point.'[54] By cajoling its readers, exposing cases of neglect and encouraging subscribers to emulate the example of others, the newspaper was to engage the concern of a wider 'public'.

While the *Carnarvon and Denbigh Herald* was a strenuous advocate of the need for an asylum, the *North Wales Chronicle* initially voiced opposition. This newspaper was one of the oldest examples of the Tory press in Wales, originating in Boston's *North Wales Gazette* of January 1808,[55] and as such it represented the interests of a reactionary section of the landowning elite in consistently opposing increased public expenditure. Although it reprinted Hitch's letter from *The Times*, it also promoted the position taken by Caernarfonshire magistrates, who repudiated the need for an asylum. The findings of their clerk, Mr Poole, were substantially at variance with those of Hitch for, 'much to the satisfaction of the bench', Poole maintained that the number of lunatics was very small, and that 'not more than the proportion of one in each parish, and in some parishes not even one' lunatic could be found.[56] For the newspaper's editorial writer the whole question

> resolves itself into this. If North Wales contains madmen enough to people an asylum, and that the comfort . . . will be best provided for there, the asylum ought to be proceeded with forthwith – if, on the contrary, there is no such exigence in the case, then would the North Walians be madmen to charge themselves with the support of a prison-house, on the portals of which Dante's inscription 'Ye who enter here, leave hope behind' might with great truthfulness be placed.

Far from being a stain on the humanity of the people of north Wales, the paper argued, the absence of an asylum might indeed reflect well upon the society. 'From some inklings which have from time to time transpired of the barbarous treatment which lunatics receive in many of the English asylums, we should deem it a credit rather than a reproach to North Wales that no such institution has been founded here.'[57] The newspaper followed up this editorial with a report giving detailed evidence from Poole's report, which showed that, of the total parishes in Caernarfonshire, only thirty-five out of the seventy-three had any lunatics or idiots within their bounds. The total number of lunatics and idiots reported was only ninety-seven, and of these only six were deemed to be 'dangerous'. Furthermore, argued the newspaper, care at home and within the local community was much to be preferred. For, 'in cases of mental aberration unaccompanied with a predisposition to violence . . . the confinement and discipline of an Asylum is not recommended by the medical profession. On the contrary', argued the newspaper, 'comfort if not cure, is considered to be more attainable in the society of friends and by moderate exercise in the open air and among scenes and localities to which the patient is accustomed.'[58] In this way the *North Wales Chronicle* questioned the need for institutional care of the insane. The same edition of the newspaper, however, contained a letter from 'Clericus' of St Asaph (W. H. Owen), referring to the cruel mode of treatment of the insane in north Wales.[59] The notion that those not confined in an asylum were enjoying 'liberty and the society of friends' was challenged by such evidence. A fortnight later the newspaper published a similar letter, signed 'Homo' (Luxmoore).[60] So, although in its editorials the newspaper at first supported conservative opinion, it did allow a voice to more enlightened viewpoints and subsequently swung around in support of the campaign.[61]

In the face of adversity in 1842 the founders had concluded that the only way forward 'must be by applying for the generous support of the public, to enable the Committee, by Voluntary Contributions, to provide the means required' to build an asylum.[62] The *Carnarvon and Denbigh Herald* was now to play a vital role in the campaign through its publication of the names of subscribers.

When a subscription account was opened Dr Richard Lloyd Williams proposed forming local committees in various towns to raise funds. J. H. Clough, who replaced Dr R. Lloyd Williams as treasurer when the latter found the duties too onerous, made use of his extensive social connections to promote the cause, and immediately sent a letter to the Lord Chamberlain, seeking advice on obtaining the patronage of the prince of Wales.[63] This resulted in a subscription of 100 guineas from the prince and a £50 subscription each from Queen Victoria and Prince Albert, which was received 'with a warmth of feeling peculiar to Welshmen'.[64] This stamp of royal approval proved a stimulus to renewed efforts. In early 1843 the founders launched a series of newspaper advertisements calling for donations, including ones in *The Times* and the *Morning Chronicle*, and Dr Hitch was requested to have advertisements placed in the Gloucester papers. It was further resolved that 'an address from Dr. Hitch to the lower Classes' be printed in the Chester and north Wales papers as well as in the Liverpool papers, and that 'several copies be printed for general Circulation', with a view to collecting small sums.[65]

At the beginning of February a new form of fundraising was adopted through the issuing of cards for small collections, priced at 5*s.*, 2*s.* 6*d.*, 1*s.* and 6*d.*[66] The collection activities provided a role for middle- and upper-class women to help in support of the asylum, at a time when women were generally excluded from public life, and hence absent from the committee.

Circulars were sent to all the clergy in the diocese of St Asaph inviting their cooperation in support of the subscription account.[67] However, members of the Church of England were in a minority amongst the population in north Wales, and so an important decision was taken to broaden the denominational basis of support. In March it was resolved to 'Solicit the attendance of Mr Reece, Mr Parry and Mr Ffoulkes, influential persons resident in this town and connected with the different Congregations of Dissenters in order to suggest a Co-operation with us to solicit subscriptions wherever their and our influence extended throughout North Wales'.[68] The Anglican clergy appear to have acknowledged that only an interdenominational approach could guarantee success. In April, 'Mr Gee undertook to request the attendance of those persons who collect for the Bible Society, to arrange for a general collection from house to house'.[69] The influential Methodist, Thomas Gee, who by this time had established himself as a successful printer and publisher in the town of Denbigh,[70] thereby appears to have given official Nonconformist sanction to the campaign.

In February 1843 the *Carnarvon and Denbigh Herald* published a 'Letter from a Poor Welshman', urging everyone in north Wales to donate a penny 'towards this great act of benevolence', by which means he calculated a sum of £1,647. 17*s.* 2*d.* would be raised. Readers were reminded that it was for the good of all, for: 'If it should then please providence to afflict any members of our families with this sad and increasing disease, we should be sure that a home and a protection was afforded them towards which we had lent a helping hand.'[71]

The successful collections reported by the paper were indicative of lower-class support for the asylum.[72] Many friendly societies and workingmen's clubs specifically excluded giving sickness benefit to members afflicted with insanity, since it often led to long-term claims, with the potential to bankrupt the societies. This rendered any form of mental illness a serious concern for workmen and their families. The Conway Friendly Society voted a donation of 5 guineas from its funds towards the asylum collection and the Oddfellows of Bethesda planned to raise a similar sum.[73]

The *Carnarvon and Denbigh Herald* reported that 'The colliers and miners of Mostyn and Flintshire generally have nobly responded', and that

'Forty of fifty workmen at Kinmel Park have contributed, few less than sixpence, and many with a promise to give the same quarterly'. The newspaper congratulated Lady Erskine on the 'great pains she has taken in promoting the distribution of circulars explanatory of the institution, and thereby creating for it an interest in the good sense and good feeling of the people'.[74] The reform of manners and the promotion of good feeling and cooperation between the classes in aid of a common need were essential aspects of the cause. Insanity transcended class and could visit all, from the highest to the lowest in society.

✴

CHAPTER FOUR

Building the Asylum

In February 1843, heartened by their early fundraising efforts, the committee began to explore the availability of building materials on land near the Ablett fields.[1] Dr Hitch offered to provide hospital plans and estimates free of charge, with the assistance of Thomas Fulljames, architect and county surveyor for Gloucestershire.[2] In 1831 Fulljames had designed an extension to the Gloucester Asylum.[3] The prospect of legislation requiring each county to erect an asylum held out the promise of a potentially lucrative source of business for architects. Fulljames was later to design a series of other asylums, including the Pen-y-Fal asylum at Abergavenny and the Worcestershire Asylum. He gained a number of contracts for public buildings in Denbighshire, including the market hall in Denbigh.[4] A second architect, Mr Penson, the county surveyor for Denbighshire, who had a practice in Wrexham, also offered to submit designs.[5] Thomas Fulljames was a close friend of Samuel Hitch, and later Hitch would advise Fulljames on the health of his father whom he had placed in a private madhouse.[6] It was presumably no coincidence that the eldest son of Dr Richard Lloyd Williams became apprenticed to Thomas Fulljames. In May 1843 Hitch and Fulljames visited Denbigh and inspected the site and approved the quality of the materials.[7]

Meetings of the subscribers were well attended, and there now appeared to be the possibility of support from the magistrates of the four counties of Denbighshire, Flintshire, Anglesey and Caernarfonshire.[8] Representatives from Montgomeryshire made contact and suggested they would prefer to ally with Denbighshire, rather than with Shropshire.[9] Subscribers still had to consider whether to commence the building work in advance of an agreement between the counties. Dr Hitch wrote to them recommending that they 'form their road and make their fences and plant immediately to employ the poor during the Winter'.[10] The committee assented, requesting of Fulljames that he 'accommodate the building plan for 200 patients'.[11] The continuing uncertainty made the decision-making process an extremely difficult one. Should they estimate for the needs of one county, two counties, or even five or six counties? An ingenious solution was to request Fulljames to prepare a plan adaptable to different scenarios. He devised one that would provide a central core of accommodation and facilities, with wings to the north and south for the third-class or pauper patients. These could either be taken to three stories in height at the far end, to provide accommodation for 200 patients, or less to provide for 120 or 160 patients.[12]

When Fulljames came to inspect the work initiated over the winter he called an immediate halt, feeling it was not being carried out in strict conformity with his plans, and demanded a suitable clerk of works be found to supervise the work. The committee asked Fulljames to prepare a lithograph of the plan of elevation of the asylum.[13] This had been received by the time of the next meeting, and the committee members requested that as many more copies be struck off as the stone would supply, to be sold at 5s. each together with accompanying plans (see p. 6).[14]

The committee requested that Fulljames supply them with an estimate of the total cost of construction, and meanwhile authorized him to make a contract for the brickmaking.[15] They also instructed the builders to complete the work to ground level, as proposed by Fulljames. This would give the foundations time to settle and mean that construction could be commenced in the spring, the work 'carried up together evenly', and the roof completed before the winter of 1845.[16]

By the late summer of 1844 news was emerging of the findings of the metropolitan lunacy commissioners, and the prospect of imminent legislation gave a fresh impetus to negotiations for an alliance between the counties. In August 1844 a meeting was held between the subscribers and magistrates of Denbigh, Flint and Anglesey to consider the method of apportioning cost between the five counties, but uncertainties about the future arrangements abounded.[17] Rumours had reached Denbigh that Anglesey magistrates were reconsidering their position and that Caernarfonshire and Merionethshire had formed their own committee for establishing a separate asylum. Disappointingly, the Anglesey magistrates proposed that they collaborate, but only in the erection of an asylum for 120 patients, at a cost of £11,371, and only on condition that the magistrates of Caernarfon and Merioneth join in with the scheme. The others present wanted accommodation for 160 and so the meeting adjourned without any agreement being reached.

This placed the subscribers in a dilemma. Should they proceed with the building at all? A special meeting of all the subscribers was called for 31 August 1844, where the committee informed the general body that 'all their efforts to induce the six counties of North Wales to unite in the good work of erecting an Hospital for the Insane have failed'. Plans and estimates had been prepared and considered both by the committee and by two of the commissioners in lunacy, whose approval had been obtained.[18] The counties of Denbigh and Flint had expressed their willingness to contribute to an asylum for 120 patients, in conjunction with the subscribers, and so, considering 'the many lamentable cases of Lunacy which have very recently been brought to light, and the cruelty of delay in providing remedial means for this afflicted class', the committee recommended that the building work proceed.[19]

By May 1845 the building was advanced to the level of the first floor. Meanwhile, bills were pouring in, and the account book shows that the majority of transactions were items of expenditure. The £5,000 which the subscribers had raised was disappearing fast.

In February 1845 a legal agreement was signed uniting the counties of Denbigh and Flint and the subscribers 'for aiding in erecting an Asylum for the reception of Insane persons in or near to the Town of Denbigh pursuant to the Statute of the 9th Geo. 4th Cap.40', prepared under the terms of the County Asylums Act of 1808.[20] The two counties appeared to have successfully united with the subscribers. Then, at the March Quarter Sessions in Mold, the Flint magistrates added a proviso that the contribution of Flint should not exceed £3,600, their estimated apportionment of the building works, and that they would only contribute £900 to the cost of furniture, fixtures and architects' expenses. This was an attempt to tie the hands of the committee of founders and was undoubtedly motivated by some resentment about the costs.[21] Since the agreement had been rendered invalid no progress could be made in securing public funds.

For all the small sums collected by the subscribers, the way in which capital funds really accrued was through the more substantial donations. By the summer of 1844 almost £4,000 had been collected, but by the spring of 1845 donations began to slow to a mere trickle.[22] There seems to have been a drive to solicit gifts during the autumn of 1845, but the momentum had gone out of the campaign, and by this time the committee was heavily indebted and the asylum in an advanced stage of construction.

By July 1845 Fulljames was clearly becoming uneasy about the financial viability of the project, as indicated by his next inspection report:

> I am aware that the Funds of the Subscribers will shortly be exhausted and I therefore feel it my duty to state, that if some arrangement is not made by which we may safely calculate upon a further available fund of from 4 to £5,000, the consequences will be a serious increase of expense ultimately as the works will be retarded – the buildings left in a comparatively unprotected state during the winter, and a good set of workmen obliged to be discharged, and with the additionally unfavourable prospect of increased expence of everything during the next Summer owing to the heavy Railway Works in progress throughout this part of the Country, and the consequent demand for labour.[23]

Flintshire magistrates' financial obduracy had created a stalemate situation. It was agreed to mortgage the asylum site in order to raise a sum of £2,500.[24] With the deeds held as security, the North and South Wales Bank continued to transact the business, and work went ahead throughout the winter. Rather worryingly, the attendance at committee meetings became 'very thin'.

On 1 May 1846 the agreement between the justices of the peace for the counties of Denbigh and Flint to form an alliance with the subscribers was concluded, the share of the costs apportioned and visitors to the asylum were appointed. In compliance with the statutory requirements, the 'hospital for the insane' proposed by the subscribers is henceforth referred to as a 'Lunatic Asylum'. It was now anticipated that it would be possible to raise the capital funding required to complete the project. By this time the North and South Wales Bank had made advances upon the mortgage of £5,000.[25]

In July 1846, the counties of Denbigh and Flint made an application to obtain a loan from the Exchequer Loan Office, but its progress could not be expedited until the next Quarter Sessions on 20 October. At a committee meeting held on 17 August representatives were 'strongly impressed with the necessity of an *immediate Loan* to replace a large amount obtained from the Bank, on the faith of replacing it on the first week in September, 1846, and for which they had personally become responsible'. It was resolved that a memorial to the Loan Office be drawn up.[26]

Legal Difficulties Emerge

At this critical juncture it transpired that the agreement between the justices of the counties of Denbigh and Flint and the subscribers fell outside of the terms of the Act under which it had been originally drawn up.[27] The original agreement dated back to 1844, and was therefore drafted under the terms of the Act of 9th Geo 4th Cap 40. The decision to build had likewise been taken in 1844. An agreement was then entered into between the counties of Denbigh, Flint and the subscribers in February of 1845, 'but in consequence of the order of Sessions for the County of Flint being erroneously based upon a fixed sum instead of the proportion according to the population as directed by the Act – it became necessary to enter into a fresh agreement'.[28]

The Public Works Loan Office obtained a legal opinion that the agreement was deficient. The 1808 Act allowed for a joint agreement between more than one county to erect an asylum, or for an alliance of one county with subscribers if an asylum was already constructed. It did not allow for an alliance between more than one county and subscribers, nor did it allow for a county and subscribers jointly to erect an asylum. The terms of the 1845 Act had stated that any asylum commenced under the old Act of

1808 should still come under the terms of that Act, and not be subject to the regulations of the new Act. The Denbigh asylum, more than halfway to construction, thereby fell outside of both Acts. It was an extremely complicated legal situation, which meant that no public funds could be secured for a project that was not lawfully constituted.[29]

The committee faced its most serious crisis, one endangering the whole endeavour. Meanwhile Fulljames continued to make regular site visits, and a large workforce was employed on construction. By November 1846 the front range of buildings were all structurally completed and roofed over. On the north range of buildings, the plasterers and joiners were at work, and on the female north wing the roofs were slated and secured. The wash house and laundry were being constructed, and the boilers were installed. The only outstanding issues to be resolved concerned gas and water supplies.[30]

The swift progress of the building works only generated more bills. The Public Work Loan Office remained adamant that it could not exceed the law and even pointed to further defects in the agreement between the parties involved. The current committee was not constituted in strict accordance with the terms of the Act. Quite clearly, no public funds were likely to be forthcoming in the immediate future.[31]

The founders therefore had to seek funds urgently on the open market. An approach to the Royal Exchange Assurance in London foundered due to excessive interest demands.[32] Eventually the North and South Wales Bank agreed to 'extend their indulgence . . . for a period of three months longer in order to afford time to make their permanent arrangements'. The committee had until 7 December 1846 to resolve the problem.

At this low point in the proceedings, news arrived that Anglesey and Caernarfon wished to join the union and would contribute towards the costs.[33] What had brought about this last minute change of mind?

The Scandal of Haydock Lodge

The answer is to be found in the scandal concerning the Haydock Lodge Asylum in Lancashire, a private licensed house to which Anglesey magistrates had begun sending their lunatic poor. The reason why this should have had such an impact on the political situation in north Wales requires some explanation. It also requires the introduction of one more key figure in the founding of the North Wales Lunatic Asylum.

Dr O. O. Roberts, who grew up in Eglwysbach, has been variously described as a 'doughty old Radical' or as 'the quasi-revolutionary extremist of Bangor'.[34] After studying medicine at Edinburgh and Dublin, he served as a house pupil, then as apothecary, at the Royal Hospital, Chester, where he trained under the senior physician Dr William Thackeray.[35] A cousin of the novelist Thackeray made a great impression on him not only as a doctor, but for his philanthropy.[36] In 1815 Roberts moved to practise in Llanrwst, then in Caernarfon, and from 1836 in Bangor.

Roberts was fired with a strong sense of social justice. During the early 1830s he took a leading role in the anti-tithe campaigns and published pamphlets showing how money extorted from farmers was underwriting the luxurious lifestyles of the bishops of Bangor and St Asaph. By the 1840s he was attacking the operation of the New Poor Law, and writing on such diverse subjects as education, agricultural economy and drainage. Both he and his brother were contributors to a Welsh version of *Figaro*, a radical newspaper. Clearly he was a lively polemicist and a seasoned agitator. His nomination in 1844 as a Bangor area fundraiser for the North Wales Asylum appeal therefore appears remarkable. It indicates that a shared concern for the humane treatment of the insane could overcome deep-running antagonisms between churchmen and Nonconformists, landlords and tenants, radicals and Tories.

It was at this point in his campaigning career that Roberts was to play a more substantial role in the foundation of the Denbigh asylum than solely as a fundraiser. Caernarfonshire and Anglesey had decided not to commit themselves to the north Wales venture on the grounds that a new asylum had opened which could cater for Welsh pauper lunatics. This was Haydock Lodge Asylum, Lancashire, opened in 1844.

Haydock Lodge was a private madhouse owned by George Coode, an assistant secretary to the Poor Law commissioners, and managed by a former assistant commissioner, Charles Mott. A subsequent inquiry carried out by the lunacy commissioners in 1846 identified the north Wales market as critical in Coode's decision to embark on this business venture. It noted that, throughout north Wales,

> there was no County Asylum or Licensed House and it had lately become known through the Local enquiries of the Metropolitan Commissioners in Lunacy that the Insane Poor of the Principality were in some places kept in a neglected and miserable state and occasionally chained and imprisoned in hovels and out-houses . . . Under these circumstances it was thought a most fortunate occurrence that a new Lunatic Asylum should be opened at Haydock.[37]

Demand proved even higher than anticipated and patient numbers grew, from between sixty and seventy in 1844 to nearly 500 in 1846. Such a rapid expansion was likely to generate problems in any institution but, as subsequent inquiries were to establish, the management of Haydock Lodge left much to be desired.

In 1844 Dr O. O. Roberts recommended that a patient of his, Evan Richards, vicar of Llanwnda and Llanfaglen, be sent to Haydock Lodge.

The family of Revd Richards had been concerned about his 'loss of mental power'.[38] Roberts believed Haydock Lodge to be 'conducted like Hanwell or Gloucester'.[39] Later Roberts said that he usually received a report every five to six weeks on the progress of the numerous patients he sent there. He heard nothing disadvantageous about the asylum until towards the end of 1845. Then in 1845 a patient, whom he considered a 'dangerous lunatic', escaped from the asylum and returned home. Roberts became alarmed when he heard that Mott had claimed that the man had 'been cured'. The patient, who had suffered 'a fracture of the brain by a blast firing on him', proved to be very dangerous, and his family were afraid that he might commit murder, for he 'had taken a notion that nothing would cure him unless he could wash his hands in the hearts blood of two Milk Women'.[40] Roberts threatened to prosecute the parish authorities for allowing him to remain at large. As a result of this and letters of complaint to Mott, someone was sent from Haydock Lodge to collect the patient.

More disturbing news arrived when a young boy was fetched home from Haydock Lodge by his parents. This boy told stories of negligence and wilful abuse to patients, and how the Revd Evan Richards was whipped, beaten, showered in cold water and left naked. By this time Roberts knew that two nurses, whom he had recommended to Mott, had been dismissed. The fact that these nurses would be able to communicate with Welsh-speaking patients had been seen as a strong advantage in sending patients to Haydock Lodge. Rumours were now circulating about the circumstances of their dismissal and allegations of misconduct that had been made against them. Roberts advised the wife of Evan Richards immediately to send a relative to fetch her husband from Haydock Lodge. As soon as her husband arrived home on 5 January 1846, Roberts visited him and

> was shocked to find, upon a personal examination, the clearest proofs of shameful neglect and cruel treatment. That his body was covered with bruises, scars, and discolourations. That one of his toes was severely crushed. That one of his ears was as if it had been all but pulled off, and that his clothes were filthy and disgusting in the extreme.[41]

At the time that these stories came to light, Roberts was engaged in confrontation with Bangor officials of the Poor Law for failing to make any provision for an elderly pauper who, Roberts claimed, died of starvation in consequence of neglect. At the inquest, a coroner's jury recorded a unanimous verdict that the parochial authorities had grossly neglected their duties. In a letter to the *Carnarvon and Denbigh Herald* Roberts cited other examples of neglect, including the case of Griffith Jones, a lunatic in the parish of Bangor, who had been kept locked in a darkened stench-ridden room and was found to be 'one living mass of vermin'.[42] To discover, at the very time that he was publicizing these instances of cruelty and neglect in his locality, that patients referred by him for treatment at a distant asylum were being subjected to cruel and callous treatment was a salutary experience.

Roberts immediately wrote a letter of complaint to the lunacy commissioners concerning Haydock Lodge, but following standard practice they merely referred the matter to the local visiting magistrates.[43] The magistrates' brief inquiry in 1846 entirely acquitted the keepers of any malpractice. Not satisfied, Roberts now joined forces with the Denbigh practitioner, Dr Richard Lloyd Williams.[44] They wrote to the lunacy commissioners in May 1846 requesting an official investigation, but the commissioners still felt that the matter could be adequately dealt with internally. The keepers named in the allegations had been dismissed, and the commissioners were satisfied that attempts were being made to reform the establishment. Not satisfied with this placatory stance, Dr Roberts presented a petition to Parliament calling for a full inquiry. By this time Roberts surmised that friends in high places were providing the ex-Poor Law officials some protection. When he heard rumours of a potential link between Charles Mott and Sir James Graham, it was easy for him to suspect a conspiracy. The suggestion was that, after his Poor Law appointment came to an end, Mott had found employment on a journal which allegedly received the patronage of Sir James Graham.[45]

This was a matter for Parliament, and Roberts approached the MP for Anglesey, William Owen Stanley, a staunch defender of political and religious freedoms.[46] Once alerted, Stanley challenged Sir James Graham to produce evidence of any minute or correspondence of the Poor Law commissioners concerning the affair. Sir James categorically denied any link with Mott. However, it did transpire that there was truth in another allegation, which was that Mott served as a Poor Law auditor in a district adjacent to the asylum. This appointment was made not by the commissioners, but by the boards of guardians of the district.[47] Nonetheless, this clearly represented a potential conflict of interest. Roberts's chief allegation, that the Haydock Lodge asylum 'was established as a joint speculation by parties directly and officially connected with the Poor Law Commission', did not reflect well upon the commission. Coode was asked to resign, and Mott relinquished his position at Haydock Lodge in August 1846. Both men ultimately suffered bankruptcy.[48]

The Haydock Lodge affair had extensive repercussions in north Wales, for it brought about a significant realignment of policy by the magistrates of the north-west. As predicted, the 1845 Act required every county to make provision for its pauper lunatics, and the clerk of peace in Caernarfonshire issued a notice to the next Quarter Sessions that a committee be appointed to consider the options.[49] The magistrates voted to 'conjoin with the counties of Anglesey and Merioneth, for the purpose of erecting an asylum for the reception of pauper lunatics'.[50] Caernarfonshire still did not wish to support an asylum located in Denbighshire, but hoped to erect one inside its own county boundaries that would also cater for the two neighbouring counties in the west. Magistrates in Anglesey and Merioneth, however, remained reluctant to commit themselves to the cost and little further progress was made.[51]

In the mean time, Poor Law unions in both Anglesey and Caernarfonshire had been regularly sending their pauper insane to Haydock Lodge. However, with the publicity attached to the scandal there was a groundswell of opinion in support of a joint counties asylum at Denbigh.[52]

Finally, in October 1846, the Anglesey justices affirmed the proposal to unite with the counties of Denbigh and Flint and the subscribers, and placed no restriction on the sum required. Not only was this heartening news for the committee, but within a few days the secretary of the founders received a letter from the clerk of the peace in Caernarfonshire asking if it was too late for them to join. This sudden turnaround followed the receipt of a letter from the justices of Anglesey, notifying the magistrates of Caernarfon that their previous resolution of August 1845 to appoint a committee 'to treat with the County of Carnarvon in the matter of a Lunatic Asylum be rescinded'. On receiving a positive response Caernarfonshire voted to join the alliance for the Denbigh asylum, although only on condition that the difficulties which had arisen with regard to securing public funds be resolved.[53]

It was soon made perfectly clear that no public loan would be forthcoming without an amendment of the Act, allowing for the particular circumstances of the Denbigh scheme. A memorial to the Home Secretary Sir George Grey, personally presented by Charles Watkin Wynne, received a further rebuff, for the answer simply stated that 'Sir George Grey does not see how Government can afford assistance in this case and interfere in anyway otherwise than as the Act directs'.

While these difficulties were impeding progress on the financial and legal front, the building work went on. The joining of two additional counties meant that the projected accommodation for 120 patients was now likely to be insufficient, and it was agreed to adopt the plan for 200 patients. This was only just in time, for the work had reached the stage where the angular buildings designed for the extended accommodation had begun to be roofed over, necessitating some alterations. This decision, of course, involved a further increase in the financial commitment.

Desperate attempts were made during the year 1846 to raise money, and Mr Peers finally succeeded in obtaining the sum of £3,400 upon security of promissory notes from a number of gentlemen. The names are left blank in the minute book, suggesting that these were probably personal loans. The

London money market was scoured for funds but, as accountants acting on the founders' behalf discovered, 'The Railway Debentures seem to have sucked up all the money in the Country.'[54]

Negotiations began for an amendment to the Act of Parliament which, if accomplished, would release state finance. The arrangements for drafting an amendment took a considerable time and the worries over the financial situation continued. But, with an agreement between the magistrates of the various counties under way, Mr Peers, the clerk of peace for Denbighshire, increasingly assumed responsibility for the financial negotiations. In fact, by this time the number of counties was five, for in February 1847 the justices of Merioneth had requested membership.[55]

The Bill to amend the Act was rejected at its first reading in the House of Commons in June, but the Attorney General introduced another Bill with the Lords Amendments, and this was passed in August 1847, presumably removing 'every difficulty the Committee had to contend against'.[56]

Not quite, for there was continued prevarication on the part of the magistrates of Caernarfon and Merioneth, before an ultimatum from the counties of Denbigh and Flint forced them to sign the final agreement. This at last satisfied the requirements of the Exchequer Loan Office and public funds were finally released. This meant that the financial difficulties continued almost until the completion of the building work.

Considering the enormous problems surrounding the project, the achievement was the more remarkable. The final cost of the building, together with fittings, was £23,195. 3s. 6d. Besides the belated adoption of the plan for the larger building to accommodate 200 patients, other additional work had been carried out. The main increase in expenditure was caused by interest charges and by the inflation in the cost of labour and materials, which resulted from the enormous competition during the years 1845–8, especially from railway projects in the region. It had been necessary to bring in workmen from great distances. The architect estimated that all of this had added 20 per cent to the total expenditure. Fulljames expressed his appreciation of the careful 'management, attention and zeal' of the clerk of works, Mr Hawkes. He was 'confident if this building had been erected by contract, it would have cost from £7,000 to £8,000 more, and the work have been of a greatly inferior character'. Throughout the project, and despite the catalogue of uncertainties that beset it, Fulljames's professional advice seems to have been admirably sound.

Appointing Key Staff

Some steps had already been taken to recruit suitable staff when, in anticipation of the completion of the asylum, Dr Richard Lloyd Williams wrote to

Dr Conolly, the renowned superintendent of the Hanwell Asylum, asking him to recommend a suitable candidate for the post of medical officer.[57] A suggested candidate was approached but declined the invitation. In the summer of 1847, the committee had the confidence to elect a medical officer, Mr George Turner Jones, who had formerly been employed as surgeon to the Liverpool North Dispensary.[58] It was proposed to send Mr Jones for 'Instruction to the Gloucester Institution'.[59] Other key appointments were made. On the recommendation of Dr Williams, Mrs Nichols of Ruthin was selected as matron, on condition that she attend the Gloucester Asylum for instruction and be approved by Dr Hitch. At the same time, Mr Robinson, inspector of the police in Ruthin, became head keeper and his wife was made attendant at the lodge and they too were sent to Gloucester. The appointment of a police inspector clearly affirmed the custodial nature of the institution. Sending all these new staff for training to Gloucester, where they gained experience in the practicalities of running an asylum, and assimilated the philosophical principles of moral treatment of the insane, was a well-conceived plan. The staff also had time to see whether the work suited them. After the trial, Mrs Nichols feared that the responsibility was more than she dared undertake, and so Mrs Shaw, whom the committee had previously considered too advanced in years to be elected, was appointed matron.[60] She proved to be a most efficient officer. This investment in training imbued in the staff the high standard of care, strict discipline and careful financial management that were hallmarks of the regime from the outset. This is best appreciated when compared to the experience at some other asylums, where staff problems beset the institutions from their earliest days. The joint counties asylum at Carmarthen, for instance, had to replace all of its key staff after the first year of operation.[61]

Having completed their apprenticeship in Gloucester, the newly appointed officers returned to the asylum which was virtually complete. Mr Robinson took responsibility for all of the administration and book-keeping; George Turner Jones began to instruct his attendants and made preparations to admit the first patients. The asylum was ready to open.

✳

CHAPTER FIVE
Operating the Asylum

Constitutional Issues

As the asylum approached completion, the visitors consulted with the lunacy commissioners, perused the rules and regulations of Gloucester, Chester and Liverpool asylums, and drew up a constitution. The rule book, specifying the roles and responsibilities of the committees and staff, provides an insight into the official organization of the institution. Similarly, some of the disciplinary decisions taken by management to enforce the regulations reveal a little of the 'underside' of this 'total institution'.[1]

Categories of Patient

The intention was to offer accommodation for three separate classes of patients. Superior rooms at the front of the asylum were designed to accommodate twelve first-class patients, six male and six female persons 'whose habits and means may require the comforts resembling those provided in a gentleman's family'. They were to be admitted at the discretion of the house committee and charged at prices 'adapted to their situations in life'.[2] There were to be no national, linguistic or residential requirements, but in the case of second-class patients priority was to be given to 'such as are connected by birth or residence with North Wales'. A maximum of ten of each sex were to be admitted and charges, whilst always to be fixed above those of the parochial class, might vary along a scale according to the means of the patient or their family. The largest body of patients would be third-class or 'parochial patients'. The five counties funded the public provision jointly, and so a quota system became necessary to allocate a proportion of the beds to each county. Initially, in order to facilitate the speedy take-up of beds and make the institution financially viable, patients could be sent from any of the Poor Law Unions of the united counties.

The Committee of Visitors

The committee of visitors oversaw the conduct of the asylum and comprised representatives of the subscribers and magistrates elected from each of the counties. The committee of visitors held the ultimate statutory and financial responsibility for the asylum, it being a legal requirement that they were to inspect the asylum 'and see every Lunatic therein' at least once in every three months, and to record in the visitors' book their opinion as to the condition of the asylum, and all of its inmates. They were responsible for the appointment of all senior members of staff.

The House Committee

The house committee of twelve was to oversee the weekly running of the asylum. At least one member of the house committee was to visit each week, and at least three were to visit monthly to see all of the patients, to record their inspection and examine all orders, certificates and notices. The committee was to take responsibility for hiring and discharge of attendants and servants, taking into consideration the reports and recommendations of the resident medical officer.

The Visiting Physician

The visiting physician was required to attend the asylum on at least two days of each week, and be prepared to see patients at other times should the necessity arise. He was expected to consult with and advise the resident medical officer on both the general management of the patients and specific treatments, and to keep a proper record of his consultations in a designated journal.[3]

Dr Richard Lloyd Williams, having vigorously promoted the cause of the asylum, was appointed the first visiting physician, a post he continued to hold until shortly before his death in 1862. His influence upon shaping the character of the institution during its early years was profound.

The Resident Medical Officer

The resident medical officer was to be a full-time salaried officer of the asylum, who should 'never absent himself for one night or more, without the previous written consent of one of the committee of visitors; and then only on condition of his providing a person properly qualified to reside in the

Asylum, and perform his duty during his absence'.[4] He was forbidden from 'engaging in any professional or other business or employment'. Directly answerable to the committee of visitors, he was required to present an annual report, detailing the number of admissions, removals and discharges. In conjunction with the visiting physician he was to report on the general condition of patients. His duties were onerous since he was responsible both for the general management of the asylum and for the direction of the medical, surgical and moral treatment of the patients.

George Turner Jones was twenty-eight years of age when he was appointed resident medical officer and he worked at the asylum for the next twenty-five years.[5] In 1853 his salary was raised from £37. 10s. per half year, to £50 per half year. In 1862, following the death of Dr Richard Lloyd Williams, the decision was taken not to appoint another visiting physician, but to promote Dr Jones to the position of 'medical superintendent'. A separate residence was then provided for him in the hospital grounds, and his salary was increased to £350 per annum. At this point a full-time assistant medical officer, Edward Robert Barker, was also appointed.[6]

The Matron

The matron was to be responsible for the female side of the asylum, 'under the control of the Committee of Visitors and of the Superintendent'. She herself was to have 'control over the female attendants and servants, in common with the resident Medical Officer'. Thus, although in regard to the female staff her power was equal to that of the male medical officer, in regard to the overall management of the asylum her position was clearly subordinate. She was to see all of the female patients at least twice a day and had responsibility for the domestic management of the asylum. She was expected to enforce the norms and expectations of her sex, and the rule book explicitly stated that she must 'use her best endeavours to induce the female patients to occupy themselves in needle and household work, and other fit employments'.[7] She had a crucial role to play in regulating the gendered boundaries of the asylum, and in setting the general tone and standard of the institution. The first matron to take up post, Mrs Shaw, held her position until retirement in 1862.

Clerk and Steward

The general, non-medical management of the asylum was the responsibility of the clerk and steward. In the Denbigh asylum these roles were combined in one appointee, who was to 'perform all the duties of both offices', providing reports and acting as clerk to the quarterly meetings of the visitors. His overseeing of the day-to-day financial management of the asylum gave him considerable influence. A sound knowledge of book-keeping was required.

> He shall distinguish the building account from the maintenance account, and the accounts of the county from those of the unions and parishes; and shall lay an abstract of the accounts before the Visitors at the quarterly Meetings, showing the monies received and paid, and the unions and parishes in arrear.

The first clerk and steward, John Robinson, proved himself a diligent and able official.

General Management

Language

Rule No. 1 stipulated that 'All the Officers of this Institution whether Male or Female and whether Medical or otherwise are required to have a thorough Colloquial knowledge of the Welsh language.'[8] This public institution was probably unique for its time in promoting the use of the Welsh language, when many other forces of modernization were posing a linguistic threat. It was a fundamental tenet of the system of moral treatment that had so inspired the founders that words could only be therapeutic if uttered in the patient's native tongue. This had been one of the key arguments for rallying political and financial support, and representatives of the subscribers and justices at the first annual general meeting in January 1849 voted to award it primacy of place in the rule book.

Gender divisions

The second rule of government concerned the strict gendered division of the asylum, aimed first and foremost at protecting patients from any sexual abuse or impropriety, and staff from any unfounded accusations of such.

> The male and female patients shall be kept in separate wards; and no male attendant, servant, or patient shall be allowed to enter the female wards; nor any female to enter the male wards, except in cases where the resident Medical Officer shall deem it advisable to appoint nurses or female servants to attend for that purpose.[9]

This second rule was reinforced by various other clauses in the rule book. The visiting physician, for all his status, 'shall be attended by the Matron or a Female attendant' whenever entering the female ward.[10] Also, 'Upon every visit made by a male relation or friend, or by a parish officer to a female patient, the Matron or a female attendant shall accompany the visitor and remain in the room throughout the interview.'[11] These strict gendered divisions were observed in most public asylums and were one of the main principles of management.[12]

The strict segregation of the hospital extended beyond the patients, and the rules made clear that 'male and female attendants are not allowed to associate'.[13] Certain additional regulations were designed to maintain propriety among the male staff. The rule book laid down that they were only permitted to sleep in single beds, and not allowed to sleep in any dormitory containing less than three beds.

The role of the attendants

The rules prescribed the ratio of staff to patients, requiring not only that there should be at least one attendant for every ward, but that 'there shall be not less than one attendant for twenty patients who are tranquil or convalescent; and not less than one attendant for twelve patients who are dirty, violent, or refractory, or dangerous to themselves or others'. The attendants were to wash and dress those incapable of doing so for themselves, and to brush their hair each morning. Patients were to be provided with clean linen twice a week, and given a warm bath once a week. Each male patient was to have his hair cut regularly once a month, and to be shaved twice a week.

The working day was as arduous as it was long: 'The attendants are to commence their duties at six o'clock in the morning, and are to retire to bed at ten o'clock at night.' And during all that time they were expected 'to be occupied with the patients', and were not allowed to 'sit in their own rooms except at meal times, or when off duty', but must at all times be 'actively attending on their patients, or cleaning the rooms and galleries'. Furthermore, they were expected to be 'neat and clean in their dress, and respectful in manners'. They were not allowed to absent themselves from the asylum without the consent of the superintendent or matron.

Like nineteenth-century police officers and prison warders the male staff wore brass-buttoned tunics and peaked uniform caps. Together with the keys securely attached to their belts the uniforms conveyed the sense that the 'attendants' were keepers in a 'therapeutic' yet carceral institution, where the inmates were captives and not voluntary patients.

At the first annual general meeting in 1849 staff appointments were confirmed. There were four female attendants, Jemima Williams, Harriet Roberts, May Everett and Elizabeth Jones, and five male attendants, Edward Pierce, William Lloyd, David Jones, John Blewer and William Williams. When Blewer and Jones were detected climbing over the perimeter wall with the apparent intention of spending the evening in town the resident medical

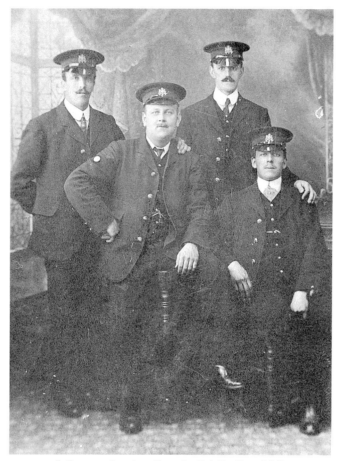

5. *Four attendants in uniform. Denbighshire Record Office*

officer summarily dismissed them. The house committee endorsed this action. By enforcing a strict disciplinary regime from the first, the resident medical officer swiftly established the norms and expectations of the asylum, and his own credibility as head of the institution.

A high standard of moral behaviour was expected of each and every attendant. They were to treat their patients 'kindly and indulgently, and never to strike or speak harshly to them'. It was their duty to act in accordance with this philosophy of care or risk dismissal, since any attendant 'found striking a Patient, or being intoxicated, shall be instantly dismissed'. Staff were also 'forbidden to use any angry or vindictive expressions towards the patients, or repeat out of the institution anything connected with it, or the names, history, or conduct of the patients under their charge'. Should a patient succeed in escaping 'through the negligence of an attendant' then the expenses of recapture were to be deducted from his or her salary. They were responsible for keeping any items, such as fire iron, or chamber pots, which might be used by patients to injure themselves or others, carefully under lock and key between use. Patients suspected of being suicidal were to be watched 'with the greatest vigilance', and their beds and clothing carefully examined every night, to 'guard against any possible accident'. Finally, attendants were forbidden from bringing any article of 'food, wine, beer or spirit' into the asylum for the use of either the patients or themselves; and 'upon penalty of instant dismissal' from accepting any fee or reward from any of the patients. Attendants played a 'pivotal role' in the day-to-day running of the asylum and the quality of staff was critical to successful management.[14] The supply of labour within the area was an important factor in recruitment. Over the years the Denbigh asylum managed to retain staff of high calibre and was in a position to dismiss staff who did not conform. This is one of the distinctive characteristics of this institution.

Ancillary staff

In addition to the nursing staff, or 'attendants' as they were called, a range of ancillary staff was essential to undertake domestic duties, to operate the heating systems, and generally maintain the institution. The first cook appointed was Eleanor Armour, and the kitchen maid was Margaret Williams. Anne Rogers was appointed as laundry maid, and Jemima Williams as under-laundry maid. Such staff were expected to conform to the house rules. At a meeting of the house committee in May 1850 Dr Jones reported that Anne Rogers, the laundress, 'still continued to stay out in the evening beyond the time allowed by the Rules of the house'. Since this was a second offence, it was resolved that she be discharged. Most staff lived in this total institution, so that the disciplinary regime of the hospital encompassed their entire lives.

Applying the Rules

The majority of both staff and patients spoke Welsh as their first language, and so most of the routine, daily communication in the asylum was through that medium. In order to make full use of the available beds and assist the finances, a number of non-Welsh 'out of counties' patients were accepted. Also, some of the first- and second-class patients were not Welsh-speaking.

Inspecting the asylum in February 1849, just three months after the opening, the Revd W. Hicks Owen, observed the beneficial effects upon patients of the everyday use of Welsh. He noted the 'soothing results of being spoken to in their own language, and the great comfort and happiness it seemed to afford them'. He affirmed the success of this Welsh institution, for he saw 'none of that fear and exasperation which was so distressing a symptom among the Welsh patients I have seen in the Asylums in England'.[15] Visiting the asylum some six weeks later he received further assurance that the laudable aims of the founders were being realized, when the patients ' "rejoiced" in having officers who could speak to them in their own language'.[16] By the end of that summer, many of the patients who had been noisy and truculent on first arrival had calmed down, so that the same visitor was able to remark upon the greater tranquillity and happiness which he observed, and upon 'The absence of that sullenness coupled with suspicion which is so marked a feature among the Welch patients in English Asylums'.[17]

The whole ambience of the asylum was Welsh, in both language and culture. Some of the patients were literate and a few were even creative writers, and the medical officers encouraged them to write. In 1855 William Edwards, who wrote under the bardic name of Gwilym Callestr (but was known simply as 'Wil Ysgeifiog'), died in the asylum, having been a patient there for about two years. He was a well-known character and stories about his exploits still circulated in his native village over a century later.[18] His writings, whilst humorous, reveal emotional sensitivity. In the asylum he wrote the winning *awdl* (ode) at the Abergavenny Eisteddfod of 1853, a tribute to 'Carnhuanawc'.[19] However difficult Wil must have found confinement in the asylum, there is little doubt that his love of writing was respected and acknowledged.

English remained the language of officialdom, and all records had to be maintained in English. Nevertheless Welsh remained the dominant language in the asylum's daily life throughout the nineteenth century and most of the twentieth. Neither the lay committee governing the asylum nor the medical or nursing staff sought to repress the Welsh language. With a regionally recruited staff, the Denbigh asylum, despite being part of an anglicized state system, was a uniquely organic Welsh institution.

Physical Environment and Provisioning

During the early years of operation the asylum was dependent solely upon candlelight. This deficiency had arisen because initially the issue of the gas supply, like that of the water supply, had not been resolved. For the patients during those first five years, life during the winter must have been dire as the staff were 'under the necessity of sending most of them to bed soon after dark'. Not surprisingly, patients found this to be 'a source of great dissatisfaction and annoyance, and causes many of them to be restless and noisy, to the injury and disturbance of others'.[20] The medical officers penned eloquent pleas in the annual reports calling attention to the seriousness of the situation, and contrasting their institution unfavourably with other asylums that had the benefit of modern lighting.[21]

A gasworks was erected in 1853 'thanks to the liberality and benevolence of Mr Townshend Mainwaring', MP for Denbighshire, who donated £200. The medical officers recorded their satisfaction: 'This is a boon which none can duly estimate, but those who have witnessed the former gloom of the Asylum during the long winter nights, and contrasted it with its present light and cheerful aspect.'[22]

In other ways, too, the officers were seeking to make the asylum more congenial and, by the end of 1853, attendants and patients had painted the galleries and most of the dormitories. Curtain hangings were placed over several of the windows in the galleries, giving them 'an air of greater comfort'.[23] To add to the visual comforts a measure of aural diversion was introduced – it was announced that 'A barrel organ has been purchased for the amusement of the patients during the winter evenings.'[24]

One of the major practical problems faced in running any large hospital and an important factor in selecting its site was obtaining a sufficient supply of water for drinking, sanitation and above all for the use of the laundry. Although a good source of pure water was claimed to be one of the benefits of the donated site, the adequacy and quality of the water was one of the most persistent problems that had to be confronted during the first fifty years of the asylum's history.[25]

Each day fifteen patients were employed in pumping water from the well. There was no covering or shelter and during the first two years they made strong objections to being forced to work outside in all weathers. Following these complaints, in January 1851 the house committee resolved that the Capstan pumps 'be roofed over with galvanised iron'. As the number of patients grew the demand for water was difficult to satisfy. In 1860 the house committee decided to build a brick tank to hold 10,000 gallons of water, collected from the asylum roofs, which helped, for the time being, to alleviate the problem.

The laundering was one aspect of the domestic arrangements which the architect had not adequately addressed. During the first year of operation the mangle was sited in an outbuilding 'originally intended for a straw-house'. (A supply of fresh, clean straw was needed for bedding.) In winter the unheated outhouse proved bitterly cold, and female patients chosen to operate the mangles complained of the physical hardship, and some even 'objected to go there'.[26] But the work of dealing with a continuous supply of soiled clothes and linen had to go on. New equipment was purchased which went some way to reducing the burden.

Provisions supplied to the hospital were not always of the best quality. One of the reasons for deciding to keep a herd of cows was to secure good quality milk and butter at a reasonable cost, and the visitors claimed that they 'have thus, in the important article of milk for their patients, placed themselves beyond the power of the contractor; an object of consideration, as such a contract admits of little competition, being necessarily confined to the immediate vicinity of the Asylum'.[27]

Traders sometimes tried to give short weights, or provide inferior quality goods, but the asylum was strict in checking deliveries and monitoring quality. In October 1853 a special meeting of the house committee was convened to consider the brewer's contract, the steward having reported that the barrels sent by him during the quarter were short in measure. The next contract was awarded to another supplier. Soon they decided to experiment with brewing their own beer, and baking their own bread. The contract to supply groceries or goods was a valuable one for local traders and, as the asylum grew in size, its purchasing power became an important factor in the local economy.

The commissioners in lunacy who visited in 1851 commended the asylum for its good management, and observed that 'The diet appears to be liberal and the provisions of good quality'. The steward, John Robinson, was strict in enforcing standards and, by setting these examples during the early years of the asylum, he sent a clear message to local traders that irresponsible dealings would not be tolerated.

In this public/private establishment, which included representatives of the subscribers on its management committee, the voluntary element played an important part. The asylum continued to benefit from gifts and bequests. Joseph Ablett's widow continued his support of the asylum and gave money to establish a special fund to deliver a form of 'after-care'. This was an enlightened project in terms of mid-nineteenth-century provision for the mentally ill. Clothes, tools or equipment were bought to enable discharged patients to earn a living. Prior to this the officers had found it necessary to discharge pauper patients 'without any pecuniary provision'. Many subscriptions were added to this fund over the years. In 1854 Mrs Ablett donated a very beautiful brass turret clock, which became a distinctive feature of the asylum.

The asylum was an important part of the region's social scene, and remained a focus of charitable endeavour. The committee of visitors recorded their gratitude to the Misses Luxmoore (sisters to the dean) and to the daughters of Dr Lloyd Williams and other ladies 'for their Christian consideration in attending the Patients Ball'. The Dowager Lady Willoughby de Broke gave £25 to the Reverend Hicks Owen to contribute to the Ablett Fund. Through many small donations the asylum built up separate subscription funds, providing a limited degree of financial autonomy, which enabled the management committee to initiate innovative changes, independent of statutory funding. Fee-paying patients similarly generated an additional private income, so that the management was not solely dependent upon gaining prior agreement from the five counties for improvements, a process that could be slow and cumbersome.

The majority of the beds were allocated to pauper patients and, although initially counties were slow to send lunatics to the asylum, the flow steadily increased and by 1855 additional space was urgently required. The committee of visitors decided to build a new chapel in the grounds and convert the existing chapel room in the main building to provide additional beds. An organ was presented by 'compassionate ladies of the five counties', its soothing tones to provide 'an unspeakable consolation to these afflicted ones'. This and other gifts served to underwrite the institution's voluntary dimension.[28]

Apportionment of Costs

The agreement to unite had required some system for apportioning the capital and running costs between the five counties. When Merioneth decided to join the alliance just as the asylum was reaching completion, it signed an agreement to contribute to the building costs. Merioneth magistrates then refused to pay, with the result that the asylum management had to take legal action, in the form of a mandamus, to recover the costs. The original formula for apportionment was based on the relative size of the population of the uniting counties, but over time industrialization and rural depopulation due to out-migration had a differential impact on each of these counties. The population of the eastern counties grew in proportion to that of the western ones. This led to recurrent demands to readjust the burden of costs.

In early September 1861 the visiting justices of Caernarfon and Anglesey expressed dissatisfaction with what they regarded as the unfair apportionment and agreed not to concur with any extension plans unless the costs were redistributed. They called for a new quota to be set on the number of patients from each county and for an adjustment in the charges so that any patients admitted in excess of a county's quota should be charged at a higher rate. They also demanded that, with the asylum full, any vacancies should be offered first to counties below their full quota. These demands reflected the clear sense of grievance that was felt by the western counties in supporting an asylum that they viewed as offering greater benefit to the more populous, wealthier shires of Denbigh and Flint. It was a tension that was to recur throughout the history of the asylum, on occasions being resolved, and then again at times giving rise to serious discord.

Anxious to proceed with an extension to the institution, the committee of visitors responded to these grievances. They resolved that, after the enlargement, patients sent from any county already beyond its quota should be charged as 'out-of-county' cases and the extra income credited to the asylum. It was also agreed that the quota would be recalculated to reflect changes recorded in the 1861 census. This established a precedent to be followed on future occasions.

In the mean time, the asylum was increasingly overcrowded, and a new extension not yet commenced, so that it was difficult to receive new patients. In October 1861 the committee of visitors asked the medical superintendent to identify all patients he considered suitable for removal to the workhouse and later directed him to negotiate their transfer to the workhouse. This temporarily relieved pressure on beds, a strategy resorted to time and again over the coming decades whenever the asylum reached full capacity.

In 1862 the counties finally approved an extension, completed in 1866, for 200 additional beds. The new wards allowed 'out-of-counties' patients to be accepted, thirty-nine from the city of Chester and fifteen from Abergavenny Asylum. This made immediate use of the extra beds and provided additional income to help cover the financial outlay.[29] Within only two years the enlarged asylum was again practically full to capacity and Abergavenny was asked to remove its patients. During the nineteenth century asylums frequently employed this tactic of leasing beds.[30]

The growing number of patients had not been matched by a commensurate increase in staff, and the lunacy commissioners complained about the adverse consequences of this staffing shortage. More patients were being kept in seclusion, and not enough were occupied in useful employment. The women's side of the hospital especially was understaffed, and Turner Jones complained of the difficulty of obtaining suitable nurses. He explained that one of the difficulties arose from the availability of work in other areas: 'The communication is now rendered so easy by railways that competent female servants seek for situations in the large English towns, thus securing to themselves higher wages and greater advantages.'[31] He recommended offering higher wages, and the following year succeeded in appointing three extra female attendants. The lunacy commissioners continued to complain of the insufficiency of staff, particularly on the female side, and drew attention to one ward where only two nurses had charge of about thirty 'very refractory' patients. After visiting no. 4 ward on the female side in 1872, they recommended that it would be better to avoid congregating 'so large a proportion of the worst cases' on one ward, and recommended 'less strict classification'.[32]

The visiting lunacy commissioners played an important role in inspection and monitoring. Each year they cast a critical eye across the fabric of the asylum, and alerted the committee of visitors to any deficiencies. They evaluated the performance of the asylum, in terms of rates of death and discharge, and advised on treatments and standards of care. Possessed of a good deal of authority they expected their recommendations to be implemented by the time of their following visit. Usually this occurred, and when it did not some explanation was required. During their inspection in May 1872 they recommended that a chief attendant be appointed on both the male and female sides of the asylum. That year the visiting committee took up this recommendation, this being but one example of many that suggests the commissioners' input over the years was formative.

In 1875, 'to the great grief of all', Dr Turner Jones died, leaving behind a strong personal stamp on the character of the institution. The asylum was overcrowded, and an ever-increasing number of patients were being sent for treatment. In the early days there had been some resistance to sending patients to the institution. That this hesitation was now partly overcome, his successor attributed to the wide respect earned by George Turner Jones. In the earlier years, he said,

> there was a prejudice against Asylums; but the kind and efficient manner in which my predecessor managed this Institution for a lengthened period, dispelled that feeling, and relations at the present time do not make the same efforts as formerly to keep their friends at their homes.[33]

✳

Inhabiting the Asylum

The asylum opened in October 1848 and during the following year 142 patients were admitted, many of them cases of long standing transferred from other asylums or workhouses, and some new cases sent by magistrates. This chapter will describe the daily routine and seasonal activities of the asylum and introduce some of the characters who inhabited this institution during its first quarter-century.

Management of Patients

On a patient's arrival the medical officer's first task was to ascertain that the committal papers were in order, since a patient could only be legally detained if properly certified insane. This required the signature of two magistrates and the medical opinion of an approved doctor, supported by sufficient and proper evidence of insanity. Information would be exchanged with either the police officer or relieving officer, or any relatives accompanying the patient. The asylum doctor needed to confirm the diagnosis of the patient's condition made by the certifying doctor. The attendants then gave the patient a bath and washed their hair and checked carefully for any signs of bruising or sores. The epileptic or suicidal were placed in wards where they could be kept under close scrutiny. Beyond this obvious precautionary division, the rules required further classification: 'The convalescent and quiet patients shall be, in general, separated from those who are refractory, noisy or dangerous; and that the clean shall be at all times separated from the dirty patients.' There were designated sick wards for the treatment of any with physical ailments. Once committed, patients were not allowed to go beyond the grounds of the asylum without the specific authority of the resident medical officer.

Near relatives and friends were permitted to visit, but no more than once a fortnight. If the medical officer felt that visits were likely to be detrimental to the patient, he had the right to withdraw the privilege, subject to appeal to the visitors, or to the lunacy commissioners. Parish officials too were encouraged to visit the patients belonging to their parish or union, at least once every three months, but more often if possible. They were expected to inquire about treatment, liaise with the hospital concerning the patient's fitness for discharge and make arrangements for placement or supervision following discharge. In the event of the death of a patient the clerk of the asylum was to notify the parish officers, and also one of the deceased's nearest relations. Should they request the body to be returned, it would be delivered forthwith; but if by the fourth day after death it had not been removed the body was to be buried under the directions of the superintendent.

Some asylums allowed interested visitors to enter the asylum or its grounds to view the patients. Such curiosity was not welcomed at the North Wales Asylum, and the rules stated that no 'stranger shall be admitted into any part of the Asylum occupied by patients', except by written authority.

Medical Treatments

The main emphasis in terms of treatment was on developing a 'therapeutic regime', providing a kindly, structured environment. However, Dr Jones also deployed a variety of medications in the treatment of his patients, such as iodine, quinine, hyoscene, digitalis. In January 1851 the house committee approved an order for four dozen bottles of port wine and a quarter cask of brandy. These were regarded as having medicinal properties, and were frequently prescribed by Dr Jones. He occasionally prescribed a mixtura of morphia, beef tea and wine. The medical officers also purchased various aids to employ in the care of patients. In August 1849 Dr Lloyd Williams was authorized to order articles for use in the refractory wards, including six gutta-percha chamber utensils, one night commode and three epileptic caps. The latter were protective skullcaps designed to prevent damage to the head during a violent fit. In October flocks were acquired for cushioning the walls of the padded cell. Although a system of non-restraint was operated at the asylum, patients were occasionally placed in seclusion if they became violent and unmanageable during periods of frenzied mania.

In May 1850 the steward 'paid £2:17s to Mr Abraham for a Galvanic Machine'. This suggests that Dr Jones was experimenting with the use of galvanic shocks as a treatment. In November 1852 a 'Water Mattress' was ordered from William Hooper of London. This was recommended for nursing patients who were bedridden, as it helped to prevent bedsores. A good deal of the everyday furniture, bed linen and clothing was actually made in the asylum, with the assistance of the patients.

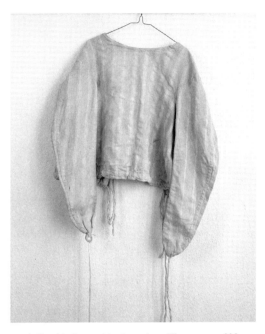

6. Straitjacket used in the asylum. The arms would be crossed over the front of the body and the sleeves securely tied at the back, thus preventing movement of the arms. Crown copyright: Royal Commission on the Ancient and Historical Monuments of Wales

In 1869 the medical superintendent announced that new Turkish baths had been in operation for about twelve months. Believed to have therapeutic benefits in the treatment of mental illness, these could also provide relief in the case of physical ailments, and so the facility was made available to others in the locality. George Turner Jones reported that the Turkish baths were being 'very freely used by the public and several who had been crippled for a length of time, after a few trials, were able to walk with comfort and resume their occupation. I can myself speak personally as to its efficacy in rheumatic attacks.' The popularity of the baths led the visitors in 1870 to authorize Dr Jones and Mr Robinson, the steward, to visit asylums in Cork and Limerick for the purpose of examining the construction of the Turkish baths. Dr Power at Limerick told them that he found the baths beneficial in almost all cases of insanity, but 'especially when combined with melancholia, scrofula, and rheumatism, and especially in the early stages of consumption', claiming that their use not only arrested but actually cured these diseases.[1] On their return they had additional baths built at Denbigh.

Moral Treatments

The value of purposeful employment, and of diversion and amusement, was a basic tenet of moral treatment as advocated by Tuke and Conolly. The visitors to the North Wales Lunatic Asylum explained their adherence to the principles of moral treatment:

> It is now happily notorious that through the truly humane abolition of all mechanical restraints and all bodily coercion the two great objects to be sought for in the moral treatment of the Insane are employment and recreation – that these are as much essentially necessary for the modern mode of treatment as medicine, or nourishing food, or warmer raiment.

Occupation was seen as a therapy, whilst the provision of amusements was regarded as just as important in the treatment of those 'brooding over their own delusions' as were medical appliances for the treatment of bodily disease.[2]

Female patients were employed in the kitchen, in the wash-house and in cleaning duties. Workroom facilities soon proved insufficient and during the first decade a new sewing room was provided. Spinning was described as 'a favourite occupation' with many of the women. The visiting lunacy commissioners clearly approved when they reported that 'we learn with pleasure that nearly all the stockings used in this asylum are knitted by the patients'.[3]

The male patients were employed in 'spade husbandry', gardening and other outdoor work, and when additional workrooms were equipped and skilled craftsmen appointed to the staff the patients began to assist in shoemaking, tailoring, painting and even worked with the engineer. As the farm developed, patients were encouraged to work with the cattle and horses as well as on the land.

Entertainments for the patients had not been planned during the founding stages of the asylum, but within the first year of operation the need to provide a variety of diversions became a priority. The medical officer reported that 'We are frequently at a loss to find suitable amusement for the patients, and we beg to propose to the Committee to have a portion of the ground allotted and levelled for a bowling-green.'[4] Over the following year a bowling green and quoiting and skittle grounds were laid out. This was accomplished at a 'trifling cost' through the use of patient labour. The report by the two medical officers also announced that money had been found from the subscription funds, and partly from increased fees for private patients, to finance the 'ornamental as distinguished from the profitable' laying out of the grounds.[5]

The summer months naturally afforded a greater variety of leisure possibilities. Besides the fact that more of the patients could be employed in daily outdoor labour, parties of patients and attendants made frequent excursions into the adjoining countryside. This proved to be 'a source of much gratification, as well as of utility in mitigating the tedium of confinement'.[6]

The Ball

In order to celebrate their first festive season in the asylum, the senior staff decided to organize a dance, which they cheerfully described in the first annual report:

> seventy of the patients, males and females, assembled, about six o'clock in the evening, in the corridor on the female side of the house, which was decorated for the season with evergreens, &c. A piano forte was procured, and dancing commenced with great spirit, and was kept up till nine o'clock. During the evening, the males were supplied with a moderate allowance of good ale, and the females with tea and a little negus.[7] It was truly gratifying and affecting to witness the decorum as well as the joyous delight of these poor people. The success of this our first experiment at an assemblage of the sexes was such as to induce us to hope that much good may result from an occasional repetition of a similar indulgence.[8]

This account conveys the sense of newness and experimentation that prevailed and nicely captures the benevolent concern of the medical staff. The emphasis upon the notion of an occasional indulgence, on the maintenance of decorum and on the sense of 'gratification' at seeing the 'delight of these poor people' supported the ethos of a benign and therapeutic establishment, wholly different from the workhouse. The sense of satisfaction with the institution at the end of this first year was further highlighted by the case of one 'poor young creature' who, prior to her admission, 'was tied down to her bed for many months'. Treated with 'kindness and freedom' she rapidly recovered, and after her discharge wrote to the matron requesting to be employed as an assistant in the wards. She was employed and soon became 'a general favourite with the patients'.[9]

The Annual Ball was to become the high point of the asylum calendar, where it was to feature for well over a century. In their fourth annual report the medical officers were pleased to claim that at Christmas 'the great event of the season, so long talked of, and anticipated with so much delight, the "Ball", as it is called, took place. We question whether any assembly in the Principality could boast of more happy faces.'[10]

Other progressive institutions introduced balls and dances, because they offered patients the opportunity to exercise self-control, and thereby played an important role in resocialization. Charlesworth and Gardiner Hill introduced them to the Lincoln Asylum, although Samuel Hitch claimed in 1841 that he had been the first to introduce them at Gloucester Asylum.[11] They became very fashionable and in 1848, the year in which the Denbigh asylum was opened, the 'Twelfth Night' celebrations at the Middlesex Asylum at Hanwell were featured in the *Illustrated London News*.[12]

Such was the success of this 'assemblage of the sexes' at Denbigh that the staff decided to institute a weekly dance. For some of the women patients especially, this provided a welcome relief from the monotony of institutional life. The resident medical officer took a close interest in the dance-room proceedings, seeing it as an opportunity to observe the conduct and interactions of the patients. Notes on behaviour patterns were entered in the medical records, with the doctor often remarking on the delight that patients took in dancing. Mary Ann Thomas from Caernarfon was admitted as a patient to the Denbigh asylum in 1858, aged twenty-two.[13] Although described as an idiot, it was said that once in the asylum she gradually became more amenable and helpful, and was sent to work in the kitchens. She was reported to be 'very happy if allowed plenty of dancing'. As the years passed she continued to work in the kitchens, where she was very industrious, and despite becoming 'immensely stout' remained fond of singing and dancing.

For the more energetic and gregarious patients the weekly dances provided an arena for a limited degree of exhibitionism, and for channelling their energies. Ellen Thomas, from Holyhead, was 'very noisy at times' but, according to the doctor, she was 'perfectly able to control herself'. She liked to assert her own individuality, and would stick 'bits of gaudy ribbon about herself'. Impulsive and dramatic, she once 'jumped out of a high window, and broke her leg'. She was in excellent health in the asylum, and described as 'very fond of attending the dances tho' she will not dance anything but the "clog dance"'. Another female patient was described as a 'zealous dancer'.

Private Patients

The need to provide accommodation in a Welsh asylum for patients of the private class was one of the rationales of the subscription account but the management committee was dismayed by the slowness of uptake of private beds. The fact that they had not 'reaped the benefit to any extent of the higher classes of patients' was cited as one of the causes of some initial financial difficulties.

Treatment of private patients raised delicate questions of etiquette for gentlemen versed in the niceties of Victorian class and religion. When the dean of St Asaph pursued his duties as visitor, it was his responsibility to meet each and every patient. In May 1849 he recorded his visit to Mrs Farrar, conducted at her request in the matron's room, where she expressed herself 'much pleased with her treatment'. The question of propriety troubled the dean. Should a woman of quality and high standing be subjected to the same inspection as pauper patients? He recorded his concerns in the visitors' book, and made a proposal:

> I would venture to suggest . . . that as a first class patient is now admitted some line should be drawn by the visitors in regard to their visits to such patients – that which is wholesome and deemed a matter of kindness and attention by pauper patients from their superiors might be deemed intrusive and impertinent by persons in a higher station. I would therefore suggest that the Visitors should avoid intruding themselves beyond what is absolutely necessary to feel assured that proper attention is paid to the patients.[14]

Dinah Farrar was the first of this class of patients to be admitted to the Denbigh asylum, and had her own personal maid. Aged sixty-two, her son was a high court judge, who when on circuit found it difficult to provide care. For months prior to admittance she had hardly slept and would pace up and down for nights on end. The doctor's case notes suggest that her illness had been attributed to a moral failing, for he wrote that she had 'been a person of great pride, which is supposed to be the Cause – constantly talking of the principality, aristocracy, and bringing forth quadrupeds'.

Difficulties frequently arose in obtaining the fees for private patients, a problem not usually experienced in regard to pauper patients, where the Poor Law union was liable. Collecting the fees proved a problem in the case of Mrs Farrar and by December 1860 a total of £124. 9s. 5d. remained owing on her account. In May 1862 the asylum solicitor was instructed to demand an immediate settlement, and to warn Judge Farrar that 'unless the accounts are paid punctually, half yearly, he will be required to remove Mrs Farrar'.[15]

This was not the only case of unpaid bills, and as the asylum became increasingly overcrowded the private patients were taking up valuable space which could more usefully be appropriated for pauper patients. Accordingly, in April 1862 the solicitor was instructed to 'press for the amount due for Mr O'Neil and at the same time to intimate to his friends the necessity of removing him forthwith'.[16]

Private patients who paid their bills regularly could be a lucrative source of income, but did require separate nursing and individualized care, and so involved higher costs. In 1860 the lunacy commissioners proposed a separation of functions, and suggested that the asylum cater solely for pauper patients. The management stood firm against the recommendation. The subscribers had played a vital role in establishing the asylum, and there was a good deal of loyalty to the idea of a dual function. This adherence to the voluntary or private function of the hospital endured until it was absorbed into the NHS in 1948.

In September 1860 a new first-class patient arrived. Robert, fourth earl of Kingston,[17] was sixty-two years of age and had earlier been committed to Chester Asylum. He was removed from there by his lawyer, who planned to escort the earl back to Ireland, the family estates being in Mitchelstown, County Cork. They got as far as Holyhead, 'when a scuffle ensued and the lawyer bolted'. The police were called after the earl attacked the waiters at the Castle Hotel. He was taken before the magistrates as not being under proper care and control, and committed to the Denbigh asylum. The medical superintendent noted that, although the earl's memory was reasonably good, he had a tendency 'to ramble'. During the interview the earl made the first of many accusations against other persons for alleged misdemeanours. He claimed that the landlady of the Royal Hotel, Chester, was 'keeping a House for the accommodation of Gentleman only'. This may or may not have been true, since 'moll houses' existed in several cities. Dr Jones was clearly doubtful and concluded that the earl had 'delusions about sodomy'. The earl accused the bishops of having arranged for him to be seized in front of the altar in Chester Cathedral, and taken before magistrates for the purpose of confining him in an asylum. This, he claimed, was 'in order to deprive him of his property', so that his brother might lay claim to his inheritance. According to the account given to Dr Jones, the earl had committed the indiscretion of entering Chester Cathedral with his hat on and, when he refused to take it off, was removed forcibly from the cathedral. The earl's state of mind was to become the subject of an inquisition carried out before one of the masters in lunacy in the hall of Clement's Inn, London, in April 1861.[18]

About a week after his admittance he made some mention of 'a John Jones wanting to take liberties with him and exposing his person'. The earl subsequently accused one of the attendants of 'entering his room after he had gone to his bedroom'. This indicates the potential difficulty of dealing with isolated patients and shows how the mixing of boundaries of class and sexuality rendered such a situation potent with danger. Power relations existing in the society outside the asylum were reversed inside, where the lower-class attendants were in control, and had authority even over the aristocrat. Accusations of sexual impropriety of male staff towards male patients were fairly rare. The word of the insane earl was pitted against the word of the servant. The earl claimed that 'he was sitting naked at his bedroom window looking at the glass and looking about his person', when the intrusion occurred, an encounter which the earl construed as an im-portunement. The attendant claimed that he had been instructed to enter the room to examine the patient's clothes, 'as he was supposed to have some of his faeces about his person, he having in the morning evacuated in the bath'. When the earl was admitted to the asylum Dr Jones had detected a very faecal smell upon the patient's breath and so the earl had been variously administered either figs or senna. The earl had repeatedly been observed to have traces of excrement on his clothes, but would stubbornly refuse to remove his shirt. After a few weeks the earl began to protest loudly about his detention, and spent much of his time hammering on his door. He requested an interview with the chairman of the visitors and, during a lengthy exchange, made what Dr Jones regarded as 'unfounded complaints of the Clerk and Steward and attendant'. Moreover, the earl was 'determined to give Dr Lloyd Williams at least two years in purgatory'.

The earl read the newspapers daily and wrote prolifically, regularly dispatching seven or more letters per day, although, as the doctor observed, he seldom received replies. The weekly charges for keeping him in the Denbigh asylum were set at 5 guineas. The earl was apparently a 'well known character for his eccentricity', and it was said that he came from an insane family. His father had reputedly died insane, and had also been regarded as an eccentric. During the years of the Irish famine his family were spending as much as half of the annual rental of their estates on the alleviation of distress in the district, and it was claimed that, 'but for the munificence of the Earl of Kingston', Mitchelstown district would surely have been another Skibereen.[19] At the inquisition heard in Chancery, the advice of Dr Seymour was that Lord Kingston was of unsound mind. His counsel withdrew from the case. It found Lord Kingston to be deranged so he lost control of his estates, and forfeited his seat in the Lords. Lord Wicklow announced the decision to the Upper House, noting with regret that it was unfortunate that the protection of the law had not been thrown over the unfortunate nobleman at an earlier period. For he had, he said, 'been insane twenty years, and had, during this time of unprotected insanity, dissipated a great fortune, and become, practically, a pauper'.[20] The earl was removed from the asylum by his lawyers in 1861.

Downward social mobility occurred for many of the patients labelled as insane. In the cases of a number of second-class patients their private means were soon exhausted if they became ill and spent time in a fee-paying institution. George Ellis, a thirty-four-year-old clergyman from Wrexham, was admitted to the Denbigh asylum for a second time in April 1861. Previously he had been a private patient, but he was 'now reduced to a pauper'. The doctor described Ellis's case as one of 'quite confirmed chronic mania'. The clergyman could not 'occupy himself in any way not even reading'. Without the ability to engage in intellectual endeavour the young clergyman would be unable to maintain a living.

The private patients were quickly outnumbered by a growing contingent of pauper patients. Who were these patients and how did they settle in to the routine and formal structure of the asylum that has been described here?

Pauper Patients

In 1862, when Edward Barker was appointed assistant medical officer, G. T. Jones, newly promoted to the post of medical superintendent, wrote him a brief summary of many of the patient case histories. These provide a lively synopsis of their idiosyncratic traits and characteristics.

Many of the patients had become long-term residents, and a few, such as Ann Owen of Beaumaris, had been there since the opening in 1848. There was little prospect of recovery for Ann, aged thirty-three, who was suffering from chronic mania and had previously been housed in an English asylum (case 4). Another of the first group of admissions was Jane Cooper from Hawarden, suffering from 'chronic mania with epilepsy', about whom Jones issued a warning: 'A very powerful woman. Is not at all ashamed of exposing herself before males' (case 13). Ellen Roberts, who like Jane had been transferred to the Denbigh asylum from Haydock Lodge in November 1848, was more docile. Jones explained to his new colleague that she was 'Very quiet and harmless as long as she has snuff'. This suggests that staff attempted to humour the patients. Mary Jarvis insisted that her name was Miss Hughes, and would be perfectly amiable so long as she was not addressed by her real name. Anne Jones, known as Mrs Arthur Jones (to distinguish her from the other Anne Jones in the asylum), had a 'great opinion of herself'. She had been in the asylum for over seventeen years when one day she became extremely excited, shouting and threatening, repeating every statement twice or more, and 'has not been this excited for more than five years'. It transpired that the attack was 'distinctly caused by an attendant refusing to allow her to smoke in the ward and insisting upon her going outside'. It appears that the females, as well as the male patients, were allowed small indulgences. Mary Roberts was described as a 'hard-working imbecile' who 'smokes and takes snuff'. Ellen Williams (62, 81), who was nicknamed 'queen', wore rings on her fingers and would sometimes lie in bed all day. She was 'constantly begging for Chloral' (a sedative) and if given an occasional draft she would afterwards become 'very amiable' and 'work well'.

Doubtless Dr Barker was given a guided tour of all the facilities and introduced to staff and patients. He would have met Catherine Ellis from Caernarfon, a patient in the asylum since 1854, who became 'cross if spoken to and fancies that the house belongs to her and nobody else has a right to be here' (case note November 1862), and Sarah Farrel from St Asaph, admitted in January 1858, suffering 'delusions upon religious (subjects) and very annoyed to the Roman Catholic priest. Has made an oath to do no more work.' The young medical officer evidently encountered similar problems when he came to manage these patients (and it was considered a problem when patients would not fit into the routine of the asylum), for he noted in

January 1863 that nothing would 'induce her to work not even the priest can alter her'. Sarah was still in the asylum in April 1877, when the medical officer at that time wrote that she 'makes sham banknotes which she gives away', and 'decorates her cap with all kinds of rubbish'.

Barker must soon have come to accept the authenticity of Jones's characterizations of his patients. Having been warned that twenty-four-year-old Ellen Hughes from Conway was the 'most destructive patient in the house', Barker wryly added his own case note: 'Is still very destructive, tearing her clothes, kicking patients, jumping through windows. Very strong and as elastic as an eel.' Not all patients submitted passively to their confinement.

Some were simply confused about where they were. Jane Hughes, transferred to Denbigh from Manchester two years previously, aged thirty-two, was incoherent and 'does not know where she comes from or where her home is'. Before Christmas she became very excited and wanted 'to go to her sister, but where her sister lives she cannot tell'. The medical officers believed that some of the patients became long-term chronic cases simply because it was very difficult to find any other place for them to go. Elizabeth Jones, aged thirty-three on admission, was 'quiet and harmless', but had been 'found wandering and could not give any account of herself'. She was diagnosed as suffering from dementia and in 1863 the doctor observed that none of her friends were willing to take charge of her or she 'might return home – but without being well looked after would soon be rambling about the country'. Fairly vigorous attempts were made to arrange for her to be cared for outside of the asylum, for in July the doctor wrote 'Does not alter in any way. Her brother has been written to several times but will not notice any letters.'

Domestic care was not always forthcoming, nor was it uniformly kind. Mary Evans of Trawsfynydd had been 'in restraint for many years' before her admission, and Mary Lloyd 'had the marks of cart ropes upon her body, where she had been tied to a bed'. For patients such as these the asylum may have offered more freedom, not less. It was not only women that had been restrained at home. Thomas Parry, a twenty-four-year-old, described as 'idiotic and epileptic' from Llanddona, had been fastened down in bed with ropes. It was said that he had been severely mistreated by a fellow manservant while at a farm near Beaumaris. His right femur was fractured and did not heal, so that he was quite crippled and so much 'in dread of the man who had beaten him that the very sight of him was sufficient to bring on a fit'. After arrival at the asylum he had several fits, and was very noisy, 'crying in as loud a tone as possible "Oh, mam bach" during the whole of the night'.[21]

The asylum was continually receiving new patients whose condition was of a chronic nature. Elizabeth Jones had been admitted only in May of the previous year, but she was aged forty-eight and suffering from chronic mania, and her case was 'of many years standing. Lately becoming very dangerous and rambling about without any clothes.' As families often declared their unwillingness to take care of wandering women, the asylum frequently took on a role of care and supervision. Another patient, Mary Roberts from Cilcen, aged fifty-four, similarly diagnosed as suffering from chronic mania, caused similar problems of management, since she (November 1862) 'Cannot be prevented rambling otherwise innocent enough'. In this case, too, attempts were made to return her to her family, but her 'friends do not seem to like removing her as they have been written to some months ago' (January 1863).

Some of the chronic patients were designated as 'Idiots' and had often been placed without success in the workhouse. Women like Jane Jones, an 'idiot and epileptic', had previously been discharged to the workhouse, but being 'very epileptic' was returned to the asylum. Patients such as these inevitably added to the growing number of semi-permanent residents. There was no cure, and they were only sent there when their health deteriorated or they became too difficult for their relatives to manage.

Some patients required very careful watching, such as women like Ellen Jones, from Ruabon, who had been admitted in 1855, aged thirty-nine. Still in the asylum seven years later, it was recorded that she was not 'to be trusted as she frequently attempts strangulation'. Her condition may well have become catatonic for the next case note, in January 1863, reported that she 'Never speaks but will remain in the same posture for hours'.

How would the scenes in the asylum wards strike this young doctor? He would have observed Elizabeth Bather, who was 'always trying to hide herself in a corner' and who had 'latterly become much thinner'. And poor Ann Chaloner, who was 'very cross at times and will not recognise any of her relations', and 'fancies that she had better never been born and has no hope'. There could have been few moments for silent reflection – not with patients like Sarah Rogers, aged sixty-five, who was 'Full of delusions and fancies herself robbed of her property. Her tongue never ceases.' Yet, as Barker noted in July 1863, she was 'the best worker in the house'. The noises of human disturbance must have reverberated through the asylum, a cacophony of sounds, day and night, caused by patients like Elizabeth Roberts from Llandegfan, on her second stay in the asylum, who was 'very noisy at night – breaks windows, etc.' Margaret Davies from Bala was 'very excited and violent at times and more especially at night [when] she will sing and scream for hours at a time'. Yet none, apparently, could rival Ann Blyddyn, referred to as 'The noisiest patient in the asylum'.

Many patients failed to respond to treatment. Eleanor Humphreys, aged fifty-three from Ellesmere, was admitted in 1859 suffering from melancholia. She was equally miserable in November 1862, 'always unhappy and crying. Fancies that she has every complaint imaginable. Appetite very good.' One can almost feel the doctor's dismay in the case note, written the following January: 'Continues in the same unhappy state and nothing gains her ease. Have tried every known preparation.' In July she was still 'in the same unhappy state of mind under witchcraft. Nothing gives her relief.' And over a year later, in January 1864: 'Is continually crying. A fresh mystery how she does not wear herself out.'

Among the patients there were networks of friendships and family ties. Maria Evans, for instance, would 'take to one of the other patients and nurse her' (71). There were always a number of patients who were related one to another. Some of these connections were pointed out to the young doctor in 1862, such as Jane Evans, removed from Prestwich Asylum in 1852, whose illness was described as 'Hereditary. Father also confined here.' Two sisters were admitted on the same day in April 1857. One was later discharged, but then readmitted on 23 December 1858. They were both diagnosed as suffering from chronic mania but, as Dr Jones observed, Elizabeth was 'as quiet if not crossed as her sister is excited'.

Words of caution were entered in some of the cases, to ensure that the doctor be on his guard against patients who were violent or potentially suicidal. Other aspects of behaviour were recorded which might compromise the young doctor should he not be careful in handling the patient. Hence the following comment in the case of Elizabeth Edwards, from Corwen, aged fifty-two in October 1862 and diagnosed a chronic maniac: 'Is very restless and fearful of being drowned. Charges attendants and other persons with improper conduct.'

On the male side too there were many chronic long-term cases, some of whom had been admitted when the asylum was opened in November 1848, often having already spent time in other asylums. John Jones was transferred to Denbigh from the Kingsland Asylum, and he would occasionally make his escape from Denbigh and walk for days before being apprehended. He suffered from very powerful delusions, and in 1863 the doctor's note recorded 'Has underground railways and aerial machines and travels the whole universe by day and night' (9).

A number of the male patients were described as 'idiot and epileptic', including David Jones, aged thirty-eight on admission, who was 'very strong and powerful and has the fits very severe' (82). John Jones, an 'idiot', was sent to the asylum 'for safety' for they could not keep charge of him at the St Asaph workhouse. He settled in well at the asylum, where he would 'work like a horse' although 'very idiotic'.

Some patients suffered terrifying delusions, such as William Daniel Jones who fancied that people were trying to steal portions of his intestines. Others had more agreeable delusions, such as William Jones who experienced 'the happy notion that he is to marry the Queen who frequently writes to him'. Two years later he was still contented, having 'daily communication with the Queen and Princess Alice'. Thomas Williams, of Caernarfon, was full of delusions about 'extracting gold from stones'. Prior to his admission suffering from 'chronic mania' he had scarcely ever been outside the door of his house. In the asylum he began to paint and, although continuing to have 'very strong' delusions, he became 'a great portrait painter'.

Various of the male patients were potentially dangerous and required close supervision. David Davies (98) would attack another patient without any cause 'if nobody is near and will charge attendants or other patients with having done it'. Moreover he was a potential threat to the safety of the institution, since he was 'very destructive more especially to gas pipes or anything else which is dangerous'. Edward Smith, an 'idiot' aged thirty-eight, had been sent from the Wrexham workhouse in 1861. He was described as 'a big unwieldy man', who was 'not to be trusted'. He had been an idiot from birth, and he died suddenly in 1863. A post-mortem was conducted, which showed 'no trace of disease' but indicated that he had an 'enlarged heart'. Many of the men had physical complaints, which may have given rise to violence, and the 'most dangerous patient in the house' was Richard Williams (116), aged forty-eight from Caernarfon, who was epileptic.

However, some of the patients were able to contribute to the work of the asylum, and fulfil a useful role in the institution. David Abraham (8) was 'very noisy at times' so that he could be 'heard from any distance', but nonetheless 'takes charge of the coal'. Richard Bullock (142), suffering from chronic mania and in a state of dementia following admission, within a year or so 'commenced working at his old trade of painter'. John Jones (9) would 'do a little at his trade of shoemaker when he feels well in himself'. Edward Owen (91), who had twice been confined in the Chester Asylum before being sent to Denbigh, had strong delusions about Roman Catholics, but he was still able to 'continue at his trade as a carpenter' and proved a useful craftsman in the asylum. Joseph Hughes (1), was the very first patient to be admitted to the Denbigh asylum, having been transferred from the Prestwich Asylum in 1848. He suffered from 'mental delusions', but at the Denbigh asylum he began running messages and was described in 1864 as 'Messenger and Porter', and 'one of the most useful in the house'.

Even the most difficult patients were placed in a useful occupation, so that the tradesmen in the asylum, such as the painter, the carpenter, the shoemaker, the tailor and the farm bailiff all required skills in handling the patients. They needed to be able to handle patients like Edward Griffiths (65) who would curse and scream, and was very threatening, especially towards the doctor. He was employed on the farm tending the cows, although he was 'not to be trusted'. Henry Williams (81), on the other hand, was 'very useful with the horses', but prior to being committed had attempted to set fire to a farm, and was 'addicted to drink and not to be trusted'.

When the medical officer felt that a patient, although not 'recovered', had the potential to cope outside of the asylum, negotiations took place to try and arrange a return home, negotiations which were not always entirely successful. William Evans (80), from Eglwysfach, had been discharged home once, but was returned to the asylum, as he had alarmed his neighbours, who were 'all afraid of him'. Once again resident in the asylum, and still suffering from 'religious delusions', he would nonetheless 'make his escape and return home for a day or so'. The asylum seems to have taken a surprisingly tolerant attitude to this habit, for a year later it was noted that he 'will now make his escape and return home for a day or two and return without any trouble and his friends not at all anxious to detain him'. Robert Robert Williams (84) (the middle name being used to distinguish him from all the other Roberts Williamses) was well educated and from a 'respectable family' in Abergele. He was 'fond of drink and tobacco' and suffered from epilepsy, and, although efforts were made to place him at home, his family were 'afraid of his being out of the asylum as he becomes excited and plagued by children'. So, to some extent, the fate of chronic patients depended on the level of tolerance in the locality as well as the willingness of family members to shoulder the burden of care.

Close liaison with both the relieving officer and the family was essential in securing the discharge of patients and in order to obtain background information on patients when admitted to the asylum In 1873 a newly admitted female patient committed suicide by self-strangulation. The verdict at the inquest was that 'no blame or neglect can be attached in the least to any of the officials of the Asylum'. One problem identified in this case was that insufficient information had accompanied the patient on arrival, which had it been provided might have alerted the staff to the danger of a suicide attempt. As a result the committee of visitors decided to take two steps. First, they insisted that all patients should be accompanied to the asylum by the relieving officer of the Poor Law district, and not, as was frequently occurring, solely by a police officer. The relieving officer was able to convey informal information about the background of the patient, for 'it is of great importance that the previous history of the Patient should be ascertained'.[22] Such information could make a material difference to the treatment and outcome of the case. The committee of visitors, after careful consideration, decided that all of the facts and particulars of the case of each and every patient should be entered by the medical officer into a book, 'for the information and guidance of the Matron and Head Male Attendant'. The lunacy commissioners were consulted, and approval was given for a new form for 'setting forth such particulars'.

The new case books came into operation in 1875, and thereafter record detailed background information concerning each patient provided on their admission to the asylum. The richness of contextual detail in these subsequent case books provides a treasury of social as well as medical documentation.

By 1875 the asylum had admitted 2,711 patients. Between a third and a half of the patients had recovered, one-third had died, and between 10 and 15 per cent of the cases had left the asylum 'not improved'. The patients who remained accumulated year on year, so that by 1875 there were 394 patients in residence (32 private and 362 pauper patients), some newly admitted, but a large proportion, probably about two-thirds were by now chronic long-stay patients. Some years the recovery rates were better, as high as 50 per cent of admissions in 1866 and 1867, but as the asylum filled up with cases unlikely to improve, and only the most urgent cases were admitted, the opportunity for recovery lessened and only 30 per cent of those admitted in 1875 were discharged recovered. This was the pattern which was to dominate over the coming years, putting increasing pressure on the management of this, along with so many other asylums, to build, build, build![23]

CHAPTER SEVEN

1874–1914

In 1874 William Williams, an assistant medical officer of the Middlesex Lunatic Asylum at Hanwell and with recent experience at the Bethlem Royal, was elected as the new medical superintendent to replace George Turner Jones. Evan Powell, who had been acting medical officer in charge during Jones's final illness, then resigned and his successor Mr Lloyd Ellis stayed only six months before leaving for private practice. In the absence of a Welsh-speaking candidate, George Miles was provisionally appointed as assistant medical officer while the committee considered waiving the Welsh-language rule. Miles performed his duties well, and the post was confirmed. He remained there for five years, and was replaced in 1880 by Llewelyn R. Jones, who was a Welsh-speaker. The appointment of Llewelyn Jones was welcomed for he was 'possessed of great musical ability' and arranged several 'musical and dramatic entertainments', and when he began to accompany the Sunday services the house committee appointed him to the additional position of 'Asylum Organist'.[1]

By 1875 the asylum was operating at near full capacity, and only the most serious cases could be admitted, including a high proportion of elderly patients. In addition a number of chronic and imbecile patients were transferred to the asylum from the workhouses. Dr Powell attributed this to the advent in 1874 of a central government subsidy, granted 'for the maintenance of pauper lunatics in the Asylum'.[2] As a result it proved cheaper for Poor Law unions to accommodate lunatics in the asylum than in the workhouse. Given the pressure on beds, it made more sense to discharge chronic patients to the workhouse to create room for more acute cases. On the women's side of the asylum the average number in residence was only five short of the total number of beds.[3] Dr Powell recommended the removal of the chronic and harmless patients to the workhouses. However, new statutory requirements had been placed upon workhouses to provide special accommodation, and few of the workhouses in north Wales were able to comply. Hence the asylum doctors experienced more resistance than usual to their proposal. Despite negotiating some transfers, by 1876 the asylum had exceeded its capacity of 400 beds and the chairman of the visitors announced that either the asylum would have to be enlarged or another built. In the mean time he urged all boards of guardians to consider accommodating their 'many harmless and incurable Patients' in the workhouse.[4] Twenty-eight unrecovered patients were discharged that year to either the workhouse or the care of their friends. Discussions over the best way to cater for patients with long-term chronic conditions were taking place in many regions. Some counties were considering the establishment of branch asylums or other types of establishment to provide long-term care for the chronic insane, to enable existing institutions to treat recoverable cases.

Besides chronic cases, the Denbigh asylum continued to receive patients who were in the terminal stages of illness. In 1875 three patients died within one week of admission, and the commissioners in lunacy directed the clerk of the asylum to forward the medical officer's report on each of these patients to the relevant board of guardians, with a warning against sending dying patients.[5] Once again in 1878 Dr Williams was obliged to complain that many of his patients arrived in a very feeble state of health, and that two from the same union 'who were admitted in a moribund condition, died within 20 hours after arrival'.[6] The committee of visitors sent an immediate letter of protest to the union concerned. By increasing the death rate this practice reflected badly upon the asylum's performance, but more seriously it caused unnecessary suffering to the patient.

By 1878 the medical superintendent was warning that the strategy of removing harmless and incurable cases was exhausted, 'as there are no such patients now remaining in the Asylum'.[7] Only the most urgent cases could be admitted, and these were of an 'increasingly unpromising nature'. Dr Williams announced that there were only twenty patients for whom 'any reasonable expectation of cure can be entertained'. He expressed grave concern regarding the prospects for practising therapeutic care in the institution, and delivered a gloomy prognostication for the future. 'I fear that the Asylum will become less a hospital for the cure of insanity, than of a receptacle for the care and custody of the incurable.'[8]

The asylum was only able to continue accepting patients by putting up beds wherever room could be found. The option of placing patients at other asylums was resisted, partly because it would have proved twice as costly, but, more importantly, because the patients 'would have had to reside in an Institution in which their native language would probably be unintelligible'.[9]

There was little alternative but to approve another extension to the asylum and so in 1878 it was agreed to build a new wing for male patients, to provide 130 additional beds. Until that work was completed, however, the situation steadily worsened and in 1880 the visiting commissioners condemned the overcrowding, pointing out that 'Many beds are now made up in the corridors, all the dormitories are too crowded, and some of the patients have to sleep on the floor'.[10] By the time the new wing was completed it was already necessary to contemplate a further extension.

The likelihood of a patient's becoming a long-term inmate continued to depend upon family circumstances. The new medical superintendent acknowledged the willingness of relatives to take responsibility for patients, and the affection they showed towards them. He remarked upon a 'striking instance' of 'a miserable looking Epileptic, who had been in only two months before his friends urgently requested his discharge'. Although it seemed a 'most unpromising case' the committee agreed, and the patient returned to live with his father.[11] Many patients settled down fairly well in the asylum as their health improved. The critical factor in whether or not they then remained was the willingness of family to reclaim them.

The asylum continued to observe the principle of moral restraint. Physical restraint was occasionally employed, sometimes for surgical purposes. Seclusion was also used, but only where 'the condition of the patient urgently demanded it'.[12] However, over the following decade, as the hospital became more crowded, and the ratio of staff to patients worsened, there was increasing reliance on seclusion as a tactic in the management of difficult patients. The padded cell seems to have been used mainly for violent epileptic patients. There appears to have been rather more reliance on this method of restraint on the female side of the hospital where the nurses would separate and seclude patients who became frenzied.

Despite the insufficiency of staff, the visiting commissioner drew attention to the ambience of goodwill that existed in the asylum, and in 1880 remarked upon high proportion of long-serving staff.

> The attendants seemed to us to be kind to the patients, and evidently much good feeling exists between them, and we have much pleasure in recording that out of the 30 attendants on the male side, not one has seen less than 2 years' service, and 24 out of the 30 have been here for more than 5 years.[13]

Over the years the lunacy commissioners made recommendations for extending the range of employment opportunities for patients. In 1879 out of 190 male and 198 female pauper patients, 139 men and 110 women were 'usefully employed'. For example, fifty of the men worked in the garden and forty-two were ward cleaners, and on the women's side sixteen women worked in the laundry and fifty-four were occupied with sewing. There were very few men engaged in trades, and this was attributed to the lack of workshop space, and the general shortage of staff.[14]

The visiting commissioners repeatedly expressed worries about the inadequate arrangements for night attendance. In 1880 there was still only one nurse on duty in the whole of the female building by night. The commissioners deplored this situation, declaring: 'It is obvious that she cannot bestow that care and attention upon 14 epileptic and 16 actively suicidal patients, which their condition requires.' On the male side they found that a male pauper patient was newly appointed to assist the night attendant.[15] The commissioners were to become increasingly critical of this practice, which most asylums had abandoned long since.

Shortage of staff and insufficiency of water were two problems that beleaguered the asylum. Following the dry summer of 1874 a new solution was found to the perennial problem of the water supply. At one point during that summer, reserves of water had fallen to only one day's consumption. The committee of visitors made use of the Ablett Fund to purchase some nearby land upon which there was a good source of spring water – yielding about 5,000 gallons in twenty-four hours. The fresh supply was said to be pure and had a beneficial impact upon the health of the asylum, and over the following two summers there was a notable absence of diarrhoea amongst the patients. Before long, with ever-growing demands as the number of patients increased, a further attempt was made to secure an additional supply. A reservoir was constructed to conserve the water and, because of its proximity to the asylum, a 10-foot fence had to be erected around its perimeter to deter suicidal patients. In 1877 fire hydrants were connected to the town's water supply in order to secure the higher pressure required.[16]

Each year the visiting commissioners monitored the food being served to the patients and made enquiries about the diet. In 1876 they tasted the dinner of beef, pease pudding and potatoes, and found it to be of good quality. They observed that the allowance was 'very liberal', and recorded that the meat allowance was 7 ounces weight for the men and 6 ounces for the females on three days of the week. Twice a week the patients were served rice and meat pie, containing 3 ounces per person of Australian meat. Pea soup was served on another day, and once a week patients were given suet pudding.[17] This was probably a better diet than many of them received at home. Sometimes, however, the commissioners were to find the food less palatable, and complained of the thin, poor soup, or the insufficiency of vegetables.

Ever since the opening of the asylum, the male pauper patients had been given an allowance of beer, but in 1879 Dr Williams sought permission from the visitors to discontinue the practice. Beer had already been withdrawn from general use and was only given to male patients who were fully employed. This allowance was now stopped, although beer continued to be provided during harvest and other seasonal operations. Besides saving money this curtailment apparently had the added advantage that it 'prevented jealously amongst the inmates'.[18]

With patients obliged to wear hospital clothing, the commissioners regularly reported upon the standards of dress of the patients. Most of the men had only ever been issued with one set of clothes. In 1876 fifty 'Sunday Uniforms' were provided for them, and these gave 'such satisfaction that fifty additional ones were immediately ordered'.[19]

The commissioners were required to offer all patients the opportunity of speaking to them during their visit, and putting forward any complaints or matters of concern. It was also the commissioners' responsibility to ensure that they had physically seen every patient in order to ensure that there were no hidden cases of abuse or physical restraint. Checking over 400 patients at the Denbigh asylum was not without its problems, as the commissioners explained in their report for 1881: 'In this Asylum so many patients have the same surnames, and not a few the same surnames and Christian names, that the task of identification is not easy, but we satisfied ourselves we saw all of them.'[20] Quite how they managed to converse with the patients is not clear, since the majority of the patients were 'not familiar with the English language' and the commissioners spoke no Welsh.[21] Presumably they relied on staff members to translate for them.

Many of the patients regularly attended the chapel but, although designed for 200 worshippers, it was only possible to seat 130 and so in 1880 an extension was approved to provide seating for 400. Religious worship and hymn singing provided an opportunity for communal activity. Another collective activity was provided by the long country walks in which about a third of the patients participated. In 1879 about 130 patients of both sexes were taken out beyond the grounds.[22] They would be seen filing past local farms, walking in a long column two by two. Many of the walks took two hours or more and the exercise was deemed beneficial for both physical and mental health.

The asylum had by this time become one of the 'sights' for tourists to the area to see, and was identified as an attraction in *The Gossiping Guide to Wales*. From the grounds of Denbigh Castle there was a fine view of the asylum and, according to the *Guide*, one local lady conducting a family of tourists through the grounds was heard to say 'My goodness! – I forgot to bring my glass, or you could have seen the lunatics walking beautifully in the grounds of the asylum!'[23] Beatrix Potter used to visit her aunt in Denbigh and heard many stories about the locality.[24] Her aunt considered the old ladies in the asylum quite amusing, and told the story of how one had 'appeared and stopped for tea in the servants hall'. Beatrix heard that there was a reward of 5*s.* for capturing 'a strayed one' but remarked that in her opinion it was not worth the risk. She had heard that one patient, 'described as very dangerous and prepared to kill anybody, got into Miss Foster's garden, and being after dark could not be found, so a watch was set in the house, and the following morning he was found sitting among the potatoes, very damp'.[25]

These were the perceptions of a few of the local inhabitants of Denbigh. What more do we know about the patients incarcerated in this asylum? The new case books adopted in 1875 provide a much fuller picture and, in order to obtain a better understanding of the social profile of the inmates, a 10 per cent sample of all patients admitted between 1875 and 1914 was analysed.

Out of the total of 578 patients comprising the sample, 272 died in the asylum and 306 were discharged, 208 of whom were discharged in less than one year. This outcome corresponds closely to the pattern found in studies of other asylums, where about a third of patients were discharged within a year and a smaller proportion released over the ensuing year.[26] A significant proportion of the patients who were sent to the asylum responded positively to the care and treatment provided and were considered well enough to go home. However, once a patient had been in the asylum for more than two years, the chances of discharge fell dramatically. The average length of stay of those discharged was 482 days, and the average length of stay of those who died in care was 2,114 days. The latter average conceals an enormous degree of variation, since forty-eight patients died within three months of admittance, many of whom were suffering from terminal illness prior to admittance. Other patients remained for varying amounts of time, and thirty-five patients in the sample stayed for fifteen years or more in the asylum. Of these, twenty were male and fifteen female. Nine patients in the 10 per cent sample spent over thirty years in the asylum, and one, a former coalminer, was an inmate for over forty years. Amongst these very long-stay patients there were three quarrymen, three colliers, a seaman, a shoemaker, a Baptist minister and a 'gasfitter and bellhanger'.

A comparison of the occupational background of patients admitted to the Denbigh asylum in 1891 with the occupational census for that year showed a surprisingly close correspondence, suggesting that, despite the label 'pauper lunatic', patients were drawn from a cross-section of occupational backgrounds. Few people had the resources to withstand long periods of ill health and mental illness could very quickly result in diminished resources so that a person qualified as a 'pauper lunatic'. Anyone for whom the state made a partial financial contribution was labelled a 'pauper lunatic' under the terms of the 1890 Lunacy Act.

A majority of the very long-stay patients were diagnosed as suffering from mania (twenty-one of the thirty-five) and six of them had epilepsy alongside either mania or dementia, while five suffered from melancholia. The figures for length of stay show that there were essentially two classes of patients – those who were discharged within two years, averaging just over a third of the admissions; and those who stayed for more than two years and were likely to become chronic, long-stay patients.

Many elderly patients were admitted and these were more likely to be chronic cases with no chance of recovery. Of the 578 patients over eighty-seven were aged over sixty years of age on admittance. Twenty-seven patients were over seventy years of age on admittance (thirteen females and fourteen males), and only three of these were subsequently discharged; the other twenty-four all remained in the hospital until they died. The female patients over seventy lived longer on average (777 days) than the men (574 days).

The gender balance of admissions was fairly even, with 3,241 males and 3,208 females having been admitted to the asylum by 1914 since its opening in 1848. There were slight variations from year to year, but over the period there was a close correspondence between male and female admissions. The gender imbalance in asylum populations noted by many feminist writers did not apply in north Wales.

A careful analysis of the certification of pauper lunatics highlighted the diversity of circumstances that led to patients being certified insane. Out of the sample of 578 patients, no less than 174 were described as being 'violent' prior to committal. The level of violence could vary. Often patients were committed to the asylum following outbursts of domestic violence. The wife of William Jones, a thirty-four-year-old labourer from Tremadoc, informed the doctor that her husband had attacked her and the children with a poker, inflicting severe wounds on their heads, and that he also attempted to destroy himself with the same implement. He had always been a sober, hard-working man, on the best of terms with his wife and neighbours. Since his father had died the previous year friends noticed that he had been 'a little peculiar'. Subsequently, he injured his hand severely in the quarry and in consequence had to give up work. This caused him great anxiety and was thought to be the cause of his aggressive behaviour towards his family. There were many cases of extreme violence and patients who had committed serious assaults were more likely to remain in the asylum. James Williams, who had been beating his mother and sisters, was detained in the asylum until his death twenty years later. The wife of John E. of Hawarden told the magistrates that she lived in fear of her husband and had to have a man with him always. He 'talks queer and to people who are not present and if she tells him so he flies into great passion and attempts to strike her'. His blindness and dropping, staggering gait indicated that he was suffering from general paralysis of the insane, a terminal stage of syphilis. This was not sufficiently understood at the time and the example of cases such as this would have added to the dread which ordinary people had of mental illness.

The anxieties which patients suffered often reflected the social and political upheavals of the day. The slate-quarrying industry of Caernarfon-shire was fraught with industrial conflict. The work was extremely hazard-ous and the industry was in the hands of a small number of employers who determined the rates of remuneration. The workmen struggled to gain better pay and improved working conditions. Whole communities were dependent upon the slate quarries for existence, so when industrial conflict broke out everybody was affected. There were many long and bitter disputes, and anyone accused of black-legging found it difficult to survive the social disapprobation of their work-fellows and their neighbours. The repercussions of standing apart from the other workmen could have profound psychological consequences.

Thomas M., a forty-six-year-old quarryman admitted to the asylum in 1875, was one of the few men who kept working when the Penrhyn quarrymen were on strike, and being 'greatly annoyed by them it preyed on his mind' and produced attacks of insanity. On admission to the asylum he said that his mind had given way and that everybody, as he thought, was conspiring against him and that he was now being punished for his sins. His neighbours had found him beside the lake, crying bitterly and preparing to commit suicide. In the asylum his condition improved and he was discharged recovered.

The industrial region of north-east Wales was particularly susceptible to fluctuations in trade and the economic hardships would affect the families of employed men. In March 1875 a thirty-seven-year-old mother, Ann Owens, from Llanasa was admitted to the asylum. Her husband was a labourer in the coal works and his income was insufficient for the needs of the growing family. Ann had been suffering for many months from what was described as melancholia. She had felt suicidal and left the house with a razor with the intention of killing herself. She later told the asylum doctor that she had succeeded in overcoming the temptation. In the asylum she was tormented by illusions which were constantly before her, often of her children eating one another on account of hunger. She had five children, and the youngest was a baby only a month old. She had very little breast milk and could not satisfy his hunger. In a ward filled with many other restless patients, and with mice scuttling under the beds, she imagined that she was being righteously visited by a plague of rats, and that she was being punished for her sins. She died five months later from phthisis, the term then used for pulmonary tuberculosis.

Elizabeth Evans from Ruabon was mother to six children. Her husband had been on strike and they had not lived very well in consequence. The 'exciting cause' of her insanity was said to be 'debility from poor feeding and having a child suckling'. Jane, aged thirty-one, was the wife of a leadwasher earning 16*s.* a week, and had recently given birth to her seventh child, after which she had become 'suddenly maniacal'. She was admitted to the work-house but refused food and all attempts to make her comfortable. She was said to be very poor and her husband in debt.

About a fifth of the patients admitted to the asylum were transferred from the workhouse, and about a fifth (119 of the 578 patients in the sample) of all patients admitted were described as being suicidal. Fear that a patient would commit suicide proved a strong incentive for relatives to seek certification for they were afraid of the consequences of not taking action to prevent a suicide.[27] There were strong social taboos in Wales concerning suicide. The gender balance of suicidal patients was roughly equal, unlike the pattern of suicides recorded by coroner's inquests, where men tended to predominate in the successful completion of suicide acts.

The case notes provide vivid accounts of the anxieties of the age, which often drove patients to attempt suicide. Fears about sexuality and ideas about contamination abound. In the parish of Llanymawddwy, Merioneth, in 1879, Owen Parry, a thirty-two-year-old son of a farmer, was tormented by the conviction that he was suffering from syphilis and that he had infected his father, brother and sister, the sheep, the cattle and the domestic animals such as dogs, fowls and so on. He said that he could no longer stay at home because he had tainted everybody and everything with this loathsome disease, that the meat, butter and milk alike were infected. Life, he said, had become unbearable and he wanted to die. He had run away from home on several occasions, and once been found hiding in an old mine. His family had been searching the river for him. The local doctor's certificate stated that he was perfectly free from any such disease. The case papers stated that some time ago he had slept with a man in Leicester, and on being told that his 'bed-fellow' was suffering from venereal disease, had become convinced that he too had become infected and had gone on to imagine, and believe, all the ensuing disasters. He and his family were Wesleyan Methodists. In his notes on the patient's mental state on examination the asylum doctor entered the additional information which he acquired from the relieving officer who brought him in to the asylum. It appeared that 'His paternal grandfather, a paternal uncle, a paternal aunt; also two maternal uncles and two maternal aunts all adults died of pulmonary consumption'. Contemporary medical opinion was drawing a link based on observation of kinship patterns, between insanity and 'consumption', a term commonly used for tuberculosis.

Within a week of his admittance to the asylum Owen again attempted to commit suicide. He was found by an attendant between 5.30 and 6 o'clock in the morning, having inflicted two small wounds on his scalp with the key of the bath tap. He was lying with his head on the floor and his feet on the bed. However, he seemed none the worst, and managed to eat his breakfast well. He was a full year in the asylum before he began to show improvement, but then he began to 'improve very much, became cheerful, active, assisted daily in the wards, gained flesh'. His dirty blotched and pimpled complexion was replaced by a clear appearance of skin and he was soon discharged recovered. Cases such as these illustrate how the asylum could have a therapeutic effect and assist patients on the road to recovery.

Changes of Staff

In 1882 William Williams resigned and Llewelyn Cox was appointed as his successor. A member of the Griffiths family of Taltreuddyn Fawr in

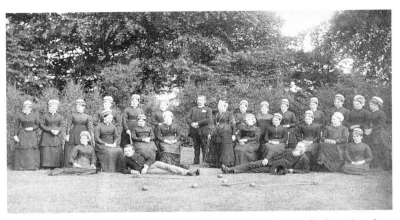

7. Officers and staff, 1884. Standing in the centre is Dr Llewelyn Cox, medical superintendent, and Miss Pugh, matron. Seated nearest to Dr Cox is Mrs Hannah Jones, the head nurse from 1861 to 1898. Lying on the ground on the left are Dr William Whittington Herbert, assistant medical officer, and on the right Mr John Robinson, clerk and steward from 1848 to 1888.
Denbighshire Record Office

Llanbedr, Merioneth, his brother practised in Caernarfon and later opened a sanatorium for tubercular patients in Hueres in the south of France.[28] Prior to his appointment to Denbigh Llewelyn Cox had been assistant medical superintendent at the Wiltshire Asylum. The following year the assistant medical officer, Llewelyn Jones, left to join a general practice in Abergele and Rhyl, and Dr William Whittington Herbert took his place. Brought up in Briton Ferry, Glamorgan, Dr Herbert had experience of working as a ship's doctor. Dr Herbert was placed in charge of the women's side of the hospital, although both he and Dr Cox had to cover both sides of the asylum as necessary. Dr Herbert often wrote warmly and sympathetically of his patients, occasionally writing comments such as 'this is a very nice little woman'. Occasionally he would reveal his attitudes towards his northern brethren, as when he wrote of one patient from Llanerchymedd, 'this woman is lacking in intelligence even by the standards of the Anglesey peasantry'. He published an article in the *British Medical Journal* describing the technique that he developed at Denbigh for the treatment of patients who refused food. He would force-feed the patient by means of a rubber tube inserted through the nose and down into the stomach. He asked the blacksmith at the asylum to make a metal collar to fit over the neck of an old sweet jar, which he suspended from a metal bracket attached to the ceiling in order to dispense the liquid mixture, usually either beef tea or milk and brandy. Such were the innovations devised by staff at the Denbigh asylum. About 5 per cent of patients had been refusing food prior to admission and surprisingly many of them recovered following this treatment.

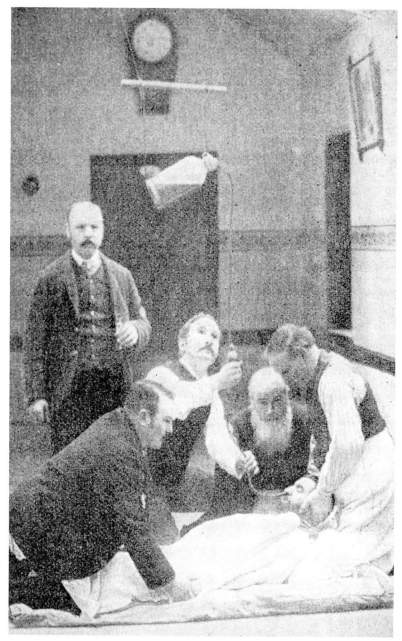

8. Dr William Whittington Herbert force-feeding a patient. British Medical Journal, *3 March 1894. Reproduced by kind permission of the Wellcome Institute Library, London*

In 1888 John Robinson, clerk and steward since 1848, died in service. He was succeeded by his assistant, William Barker, who was to serve for an even longer period, thereby ensuring an extraordinary degree of continuity in the management of this asylum.

When Llewelyn Cox took up post he spent his first summer holidays visiting nine different asylums, mainly in south Wales and the border counties.[29] He observed that the North Wales Asylum did not compare favourably with its counterparts in south Wales so far as employment opportunities for patients was concerned. He concluded that the main explanation was the deficiency of accommodation for various trades and the lack of sufficient numbers of male attendants to provide indoor occupation for those patients not suited to farm work. His sole innovation to address this deficiency at the time appears to have been to depute an attendant to supervise those patients not suited for outdoor work, in hair and flock cleaning, and the general repair of bedding.[30]

The asylum was again overcrowded, especially on the women's side, and in 1885 the visiting commissioners called attention to the seriousness of this, suggesting it 'probably accounts, to some extent, for the many black eyes which we saw in the wards'.[31] Once again attempts had been made to discharge as many patients as possible. Some elderly patients, who had been in the asylum almost from the beginning, were sent to workhouse wards. Mary Davies, for instance, who had been admitted in 1851, was transferred to Holywell workhouse in 1883, at the age of seventy-four. A letter was sent from the Local Government Board in Whitehall, instructing the clerk to the board of guardians that she was to be cared for either in the workhouse infirmary with a paid nurse, or in an ordinary workhouse ward. Also, that she was to be provided with the special dietary for the 'aged and infirm'.[32] Such transfers required official sanction and could only marginally improve the situation in the asylum.

By the late 1880s it became clear that a major decision had to be taken regarding the future of institutional provision for the insane in north Wales. The constant pressure of admissions, and the accumulation of around half to two-thirds of these each year as candidates for long-term care, drove the asylum towards expansion. County magistrates began to baulk at the expense. The whole of north Wales was suffering economic decline, as the agricultural depression hit the livestock industry during the late 1880s, and a slump in world trade affected manufactures. The committee of visitors knew that they would soon have to seek overspill accommodation in other asylums. Yet, they 'preferred the risk of this rather than recommend a large outlay in additional buildings, in these depressed times, and, with a possible change in the government, and arrangement of Asylums, in prospect, under a County Government Bill'.[33] This anticipated change arrived in 1889. Up until then the county magistrates held responsibility for the funding and

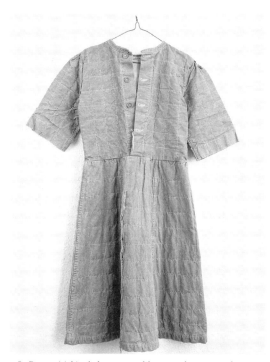

9. Strong 'ticking' dress secured by screw buttons at the rear.
For use with patients prone to tear their clothing, the material
was virtually indestructible, and the screw buttons at the back
prevented the patient from removing the dress. Crown
copyright: Royal Commission on the Ancient and Historical
Monuments of Wales

administration of public asylums. This responsibility was transferred to the new local authorities, and so elected county councillors assumed the duty of nominating representatives to the committee of visitors of the asylum. The 1890 Lunacy Act strengthened the legal dimensions of certification, further emphasizing the custodial aspect of asylum care.

The pressure on space led the commissioners in lunacy to become increasingly critical of standards of care at the Denbigh asylum. They complained about the gross overcrowding in the female wards, which led to 'many quarrels'. The beds were packed tightly into the wards and in the dining room tables were so close that 'discomfort arises'. An unduly large number of the women were in strong dresses. These were made of ticking and secured at the back with screw buttons to prevent the patients from pulling them off or tearing them. Special boots with locked buckles were made in the asylum to fit patients who kicked off their shoes. Evidently

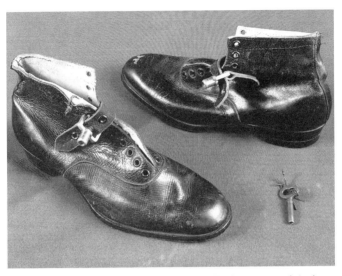

10. *Leather boots with locked buckles and key. The boots were made in the cobbler's workshop in the asylum. They were put on patients who habitually kicked off their shoes, since they could only be removed when the key was used to unlock the fastening. Crown copyright: Royal Commission on the Ancient and Historical Monuments of Wales*

there was increasing resort to seclusion as a method of control, and the commissioners recorded their disapproval:

Fifteen males have been secluded on various occasions for a total of 1,853 hours, two of them accounting for 1,400 of the total hours. Fourteen women have been secluded 16 times for 76 hours. One woman has been restrained twice for surgical reasons, and another woman has worn gloves to prevent her from scratching her face. Two males have also been restrained by jackets and sleeves on account of suicidal propensities, and for surgical reasons; and another man by sleeves only, also for surgical reasons, but in no case is the duration of the restraint recorded as it should have been.[34]

A Second Asylum?

The commissioners recommended that the committee of visitors give serious consideration to the option of erecting a second, branch asylum. There was a lot to be said for having a second asylum in the western part of north Wales to provide a service for Anglesey, Caernarfonshire and

Merioneth. This would have the advantage of cutting two hours off the journey for patients from these areas, and would enable relatives to maintain better contact with patients, improving their prospects of rehabilitation and discharge. The disadvantages to this proposal were that suitable land would have to be acquired, and it would be considerably more expensive to build a new asylum, including all of the core amenities, than it would be to extend the existing one. Delay was anticipated, since 'the usual battle of the sites would have to be fought out' and there was already strong political pressure to choose Caernarfon.[35] A site with an adequate supply of pure water would have to be located, be approved by the lunacy commissioners and then there would have to be unanimous agreement between the counties. Investing money in a second asylum would leave the Denbigh asylum with its existing deficiencies. Having appraised the situation carefully the visitors voted to enlarge the existing asylum. In fact, two committee members representing the western counties of Caernarfon and Anglesey proposed the motion. Draft plans were prepared early in 1891.

However, the commissioners were unhappy with this outcome, since they favoured the option of building in Caernarfon. There seems, at this stage, to have developed a good deal of ill feeling between the lunacy commissioners and the committee of visitors. The commissioners ruled that the enlargement of the Denbigh asylum be subject to two provisos. First, the purchase of additional land and, second, confirmation of a sufficient supply of good quality water. The purchase of the adjacent Kings Mill property appeared to answer these provisos as it offered an additional supply of water as well as power for generating. However, the sufficiency and suitability of this water soon became a point at issue. Despite having received two favourable reports, the lunacy commissioners insisted on sending down their own analyst to take samples. His report suggested that the water was open to pollution, and that the sources of water used in the asylum were of an unreliable character. The committee of visitors then called in another expert, Mr Chas. E. de Rance, 'a very high authority on underground waters', to examine the geological strata in the vicinity of the asylum.[36] His report too was very unfavourable. The only way to circumvent the danger of pollution in the water supply was to take waters from higher up the hill, above the line of human habitation. Accordingly they employed a water engineer to investigate and estimate the cost of bringing water to the asylum from a distance. The management argued that, since the water supply would have to be improved anyway, it would not seriously affect the price of the extension to the asylum building. Therefore, in cost terms, they believed the advantage still lay with the enlargement.

After visiting and seeking advice from asylums in north-west England, the visitors submitted plans to the lunacy commissioners for approval.[37] However, Caernarfonshire was by now determined to have a second asylum, preferably in Caernarfon town. County councillors in Anglesey and Merioneth came out in favour of an extension to the existing asylum. The county of Caernarfon then voted to withdraw from the alliance and build for itself. It asked for compensation for its share of the capital costs of the Denbigh asylum, and demanded that the money should be transferred to them as retiring partners. During this dispute W. A. Darbishire and J. Issard Davies, representatives of Caernarfonshire County Council, were in direct contact with the lunacy commissioners, and making detrimental statements about the North Wales Counties Lunatic Asylum.[38] The constitutional situation regarding the alliance of the counties was very complex, and the commissioners in lunacy decided to submit the case for legal opinion to Sir Horace Davey, QC. His interpretation of the law was that it was not possible for one party to withdraw from the alliance, without a complete dissolution of the agreement. It would not be possible to reconstitute the alliance minus Caernarfonshire, because the legislation no longer allowed for an alliance between local authorities and subscribers. Therefore it would be necessary to devise an entirely new scheme. In his opinion, however, it was not possible for the county of Caernarfon to retire, without a majority vote by the committee of visitors, which included representatives of all counties and the subscribers, in favour of dissolution.[39] At the annual meeting of the committee of visitors held on 17 January 1893, Mr W. A. Darbishire proposed a motion that the existing agreement to unite be dissolved. The motion was rejected by ten votes to three. The matter was further debated at the meeting on 24 March and again at a special meeting held on 23 June, when the committee decided to proceed 'without further delay with the enlargement at Denbigh'.[40] In August 1894 a special conference of delegates was held at Conway, Caernarfonshire, where a resolution was passed stating that it was 'in the true economic interests of the five Counties in Union' that the union be maintained, and that additional accommodation be provided 'by the extension of the present Asylum at Denbigh'. It was unanimously adopted, although the visitors and delegates from Caernarfonshire abstained. Finally the case was referred to the Secretary of State, who recommended the enlargement.

This had been a lengthy, bitter dispute and the outcome determined well into the future the provision of hospital care for the insane in north Wales. Concentrating resources on one site did facilitate the development of a modern hospital with a wide range of resources. However, by opting to develop one centralized institution for north Wales, the question of the distance and remoteness of some areas from the service was to remain a contentious one.

While these deliberations were taking place, the asylum became ever more overcrowded. Discharges and asylum transfer strategies were implemented. In 1887 twenty-five female patients were transferred to the Abergavenny

Asylum, and by 1893 the management had boarded out a similar number in asylums at Derby, Shrewsbury and Bristol. This proved costly, and was isolating for the patients if they lost contact with relatives who might have visited. To reduce pressure on the hospital, alternative accommodation in the vicinity was sought. In 1894 a five-year lease was taken on Glan y Wern Hall near Llandyrnog, and the mansion was converted to accommodate eighty female convalescent patients.[41] The opening of a branch asylum necessitated the appointment in October 1894 of Mr Corbet William Owen. An additional medical officer had long been required, and this finally enabled the medical superintendent to concentrate more on his management role.

An ambitious scheme was approved for the expansion of the asylum, including a new isolation hospital for infectious cases, a large 'chronic' block for females, a new laundry, wash-houses, boiler and engine house. New kitchens and a new dining hall also formed part of the scheme. There was to be a large investment in new sewerage and sanitation for the asylum complex, and all of the old barrel drains were to be replaced by earthenware pipes. A new system of steam heating came into operation in 1898 and was welcomed as providing a more constant, reliable and easily controlled temperature. The new boiler rooms necessitated the construction of an enormous new chimney-stack, which became a distinctive landmark. A good deal was done to improve the ventilation throughout the asylum. A large investment was made in the new reservoir at Llyn Brân, piping the water a distance of eight miles to the asylum. Llyn Brân was connected in April 1900, and the use of water from the Ystrad River was discontinued. An Act of Parliament had been required to obtain the water rights for this reservoir project. Since the present gasworks were already inadequate to supply the needs of the asylum, a decision was taken to install a system of electric lighting. In 1901 the estate was consolidated when the committee purchased Parc y Twll farm, which provided additional land suitable for cultivation, conveniently situated adjacent to the boundaries of the existing asylum.

A large building scheme was bound to be disruptive and, since it involved alteration of some of the existing accommodation, it necessitated relocating patients while work was in progress. Therefore the initial impact was to worsen the situation as far as patient accommodation was concerned. Visiting the asylum in October 1898, the commissioners 'were struck by the dull and cheerless aspect' of many of the wards, and when they reached female no. 3 block they were clearly shocked. They declared that 'there were too many box beds and straw beds on floors of single rooms' and protested that the rooms were unsuitable for occupation.[42] The pressure of numbers was having a deleterious effect on patient health, and in February 1899 Dr Llewelyn Cox reported on the prevalence of pulmonary tuberculosis, which accounted for 26 per cent of total deaths during the previous year. The high incidence of the disease amongst patients was the result of 'a combination of insanitary elements, due to overcrowding, defective ventilation and drainage, with an impure and unreliable water supply'.[43] An improvement in the standard of accommodation at the hospital was long overdue.

Unfortunately, the building programme was facing serious problems. The architects to the Lunacy Commission had suggested various amendments to the original plans. These changes had not been included in the specifications provided by the architects, which had provided the basis for the competitive tenders. The building contractor, Warburtons, complained bitterly that the work had been under-costed and that it was impossible to meet the modified specifications for the amount quoted. In addition, problems were experienced in sinking the foundations for the new female blocks, leading to delays and additional costs. The architects were not closely supervising the work, and there were complaints that the quality was substandard. In October 1899, the committee voted to dismiss Ellison and Co., and to appoint instead the company of Messrs Lockwood and Sons of Chester. There were delays in handing over the plans, and charges and countercharges flew between the architects and the asylum committee. The differences became the subject of litigation, and led to the work being halted for several months.[44] The builders then refused to recommence without an adjustment of the pricing and after work had been at a standstill for an entire year the committee of visitors terminated the builders' contract. Messrs Jones and Sons of Liverpool, a firm with a high reputation, then completed the abandoned work. The same firm was retained for the remaining work on phases two and three. The female chronic and quiet and the female epileptic blocks were erected, followed by the new dining hall, kitchen, female attendants' block and female recent and acute block.[45] In 1902 an arrangement was made with the town council of Denbigh to connect the asylum main drainage to the town sewers.[46]

In May 1903 the tenancy for Glan y Wern, which had been held for nine years, terminated, and the seventy-three patients in residence there were moved into one of the newly completed blocks at the hospital. Patients boarded out at Derby and Middlesbrough were also returned, so that all of the patients were once again resident on the main site. This meant that a lack of accommodation remained a major and still unresolved problem. The buildings constructed so far had increased the accommodation for patients from 500 to 760, and had provided bedrooms for sixty-four of the staff. However, the number of patients in the asylum was by now 795, with some patients still accommodated in a temporary building.

When the Secretary of State had given approval for the extension, he had agreed that the ambitious plans be embarked upon in two stages. The first of these now being completed, it was time to move forward to the second stage. In the original proposal this had included two further residential blocks for pauper patients, and a separate annexe for private patients. The visitors decided to press ahead immediately with the two additional blocks to accommodate another 152 patients, and to leave in abeyance the plans for the annexe for private patients. These buildings were completed in 1907, concluding this long phase of expansion. At the annual general meeting the chairman expressed the feelings of relief at the imminent completion of this extended project:

> Thus will be brought to an end a matter which has occupied a great portion of the time for the Visitors from the first establishment of the County Councils in 1889 until the present time. Practically, during these 18 years there has been established what is nearly equivalent to a new asylum.[47]

Once again, however, the question of future enlargement reared its head, and on 4 September 1905 a special conference was held between representatives of the asylum committee and representatives of Caernarfonshire County Council. Delegates resolved that consideration should be given forthwith to the needs for additional accommodation. It was further resolved that 'the Conference is of opinion that no further extension should be made to the buildings at Denbigh, but that the proper course to pursue would be to erect a new and separate Asylum on some suitable spot in the western portion of the five Counties'.[48] The question of a second asylum was back on the agenda!

During all these years of uncertainty and disruption the medical work of the asylum had to continue. There were practically no changes in the diagnoses given to patients, and there was little change in the treatment either. With only three medical staff and no pathology laboratory the scope for variation was limited. Much depended on the expertise and willingness of the nursing staff, and on basic care and provision of food, warmth, raiment and shelter. Amongst the patients there were always some spontaneous recoveries. There were also many patients who suffered from long-term chronic complaints where the hopes of discharge were small. The overcrowding caused serious problems in regard to patient care and staff morale. In June 1901 a female patient complained to the visitors that she had been ill-treated by the attendants. They saw her breasts 'which were very black apparently caused by blows', but the attendants denied having struck the patient.[49] Within such a large and overcrowded institution the standards of patient care were apt to decline, and the loneliness and isolation of patients increased as the space for individuality shrank. Women particularly found themselves lost and excluded in the crowded wards and long corridors of this custodial institution.

In 1902, after seven years as assistant medical officer, Dr Corbett Owen resigned and was replaced by Dr Frank G. Jones, who became another long-serving officer of the institution, commencing work alongside Dr Cox and Dr Herbert and learning from their experience. Dr Frank, as he was soon called, made an immediate impression in the asylum, being a talented musician and keen footballer. He arranged 'a variety of excellent indoor musical entertainments throughout the year' and formed a cup-winning football team.[50]

Over the years many patients had been admitted to the asylum following florid expressions of religious beliefs. Before certification Mary Roberts had been 'preaching and praying all the last two nights'. Owen Pritchard had been incessantly talking about religious affairs and singing hymns[51] and David Williams claimed that he had the Devil inside him and that he was 'a little Jesus one week old'.[52] Sin and guilt were prevalent in a society dominated by religion. Catherine Lloyd of Lon y Popty, Bangor, told her doctor: 'My conscience accuses me of disobedience and want of faith and forces me to pray.' She had a disagreeable smell in her nostrils that she associated with brimstone and images of hell. All night long she would wander about the house impelled by her 'guilty conscience'. Another patient in Bangor was 'always accusing herself of having committed sin in reading novels, titbits being contrary to her religious training'. She was shouting prayers at all hours over the house and had become terribly agitated.

It is difficult to underestimate the centrality of religion to many people's lives in late nineteenth-century Wales, but by the early twentieth century new secular trends were beginning to undermine its position. Then in 1904–5 a remarkable wave of religious enthusiasm swept across Wales. The chapels filled with worshippers and revivalist hymn singers toured the country. Preachers appealed to the hearts and sentiments of congregations, there were many new conversions and chapel members took the lead in an upsurge of spontaneous prayer. The movement gained dizzy heights, only to collapse as quickly as it had erupted. In 1905 Dr Cox reported that 'early in the year an exceptional number of patients were admitted suffering from "religious mania" attributed to religious fervour due to the Revivalist movements'.[53] About 11 per cent of male and 4 per cent of female admissions were said to be attributable to religious mania. Edward H., a milk purveyor from Corwen, had been rushing about the yard with a wheelbarrow 'shaking and shouting about his soul and body'. Cadwaladr L., a farmer from Llanegryn, had become violent, was refusing food, and praying, shouting, singing and constantly talking about religious matters. A weaver from Talybont became very emotional, praying and singing religious verses and so excitable at night that he would not go to his bed. His sister, a farmer's wife, had been attending religious revival meetings and suddenly without warning became insane. She was certified as 'manical, constantly praying, singing hymns, thinks herself lost to God, says she saw Christ' and referred to the medical attendant as 'God's deputy'. She remained in the asylum until her death in 1942. A sixteen-year-old butcher's boy from Barmouth ran around the town shouting through people's windows, 'telling them to take care of their souls, singing hymns and praying constantly'. In the asylum he made a rapid recovery and told the medical superintendent that before admittance he went to prayer meetings for five successive nights and was there until 2.00 a.m., and that boys of ten and twelve years were also there until that hour. The Revival of 1904–5 was followed by a popular reaction against enthusiastic religion and sentimentality and the asylum case notes of the twentieth century are no longer so saturated in religious images and delusions. Following a careful investigation, Dr Cox concluded that in the majority of cases there was distinct evidence of 'hereditary predisposition' to insanity.

In 1910 Dr Llewelyn Cox retired due to failing health after twenty-nine years in office. In his place the committee elected Dr W. Stanley Hughes, a senior assistant medical officer on the male side of the Claybury Asylum. Other Welsh staff had already been recruited from Claybury. The medical superintendent there was Robert Jones (later Sir Robert Armstrong-Jones) who came from Portmadoc in Caernarfonshire.[54] He took a keen interest in the organization of psychiatry in Europe and believed strongly in the hereditary nature of mental diseases, also perceiving a close link between tuberculosis and mental disease.[55] His influence on the thinking of practitioners in the Denbigh asylum is clear. His approach to the treatment of mental illness was progressive, and he advocated early treatment and the development of after-care work. Helen Boyle, who went on to pioneer the development of early treatment for women patients, referred to Claybury as a 'first-rate mental hospital . . . under the inspiring superintendency of Sir Robert Armstrong-Jones'.[56] Dr Stanley Hughes came direct from Claybury, bringing with him many progressive ideas about the treatment of 'incipient insanity', and the importance of after-care of the insane and these were fed into the plans for future developments at Denbigh. A new reception hospital for incipient cases of insanity was proposed along with a comprehensive system of outpatient clinics to extend care into the community.

✸

CHAPTER EIGHT

The First World War and its Aftermath

Poised to begin a building extension and develop outpatient clinics, the hospital staff anticipated another phase of modernization, only for it to be abandoned when events in Europe culminated in armed conflict. The war declared in August 1914 was to have profound repercussions on Wales, accelerating economic, social and cultural change. For the most part, people supported the war although there was an active protest movement whose most articulate spokesman was the Christian pacifist, George M. Ll. Davies. The influence of such conscientious objectors was small in a world caught up in war. Nonetheless, according to poet and academic W. J. Gruffydd, the existence of a Welsh monthly pacifist publication *Y Deyrnas*, which spoke for the conscience of Wales, was one of the main reasons 'na chollodd Cymru ei henaid yn hollol yn nydd y gwallgofrwydd mawr'.[1]

As the government took war measures it immediately sought to secure emergency accommodation for expected casualties. Hospitals were ordered to make beds vacant and some were converted entirely to military use. The Denbigh asylum was full to capacity, with numbers rising to a new peak of 1,040 during 1915. When ordered to make emergency provision, the visiting committee took steps to secure alternative accommodation. They arranged to take a tenancy on Plas Caermeddyg, Llanbedr, Merioneth (the home of former medical superintendent, Llewelyn Cox, where he and his sisters had begun running a private asylum) and the Heath Convalescent House, Llanfairfechan, 'the Trustees of which have met them in the most accom-modating and patriotic spirit'.[2] In the event they did not need these provisional arrangements. The Lancashire asylums which were seeking overspill accommodation in north Wales in order to release their beds for war victims secured placements within their own area. Hence the Denbigh hospital continued throughout the war to function as a mental hospital serving the five counties of north Wales.

Impact of the War on Insanity

Initially the conflict had no marked impact upon the level of admissions, although thirty of the cases admitted during 1915 reported suffering from war-related anxiety. A phenomenon of enduring interest to social scientists, as well as to medical professionals, is the fact that the rate of insanity and of suicide amongst the general population diminishes during times of war. Or at least the level of admissions to mental hospitals and the numbers of recorded suicides usually diminish.[3] Whether this is due to a real decline in the experience of insanity, and in the numbers committing suicide, or whether it is rather a reflection of the increased reluctance to commit people to mental hospital, or lack of evidence to substantiate suicide, is a matter of some contention.[4] Such a trend was experienced in north Wales during the First World War. 'Throughout the country', remarked Frank Jones in 1916,

> there has been a marked decrease in the number of admissions into Asylums. This is attributed to higher wages and the abundance of occupation and employment. This decrease would have been more marked had not the war itself been the actual cause of some cases of Insanity both among the military and civilians.[5]

He and his medical colleagues considered the war to have been the principal or contributory cause of insanity in the case of forty-seven of the civilian patients in 1916.[6]

Amongst staff belief in the hereditary causes of insanity remained paramount during this period. In 1914 Dr Jones reported that 'an hereditary taint has been traced to 30 per cent. of the admissions'.[7] The medical superintendent had begun to forward a special enquiry card to families following each admission. This asked close relatives to answer a number of questions about the health of relatives, etc. and signified a new sense of scientific enquiry. The cards may have been similar to those used by Frederick Mott, the pathologist at the Claybury Asylum in Essex, who was carrying out an extensive investigation of family trees using a card system.[8] There was regular professional contact between Frank Jones and Robert Jones at Claybury Asylum, who like Mott was a firm adherent to the view that mental illness had an organic basis, and was unsympathetic to a psychodynamic approach.[9] Mott believed 'shell shock' to be the result of organic lesions to the brain. Medical staff at the Denbigh asylum remained equally committed to a hereditary/organic disease model as an explanation for mental illness.

During the period of the war ninety-eight military patients were admitted to the Denbigh asylum, thirty-three of whom were discharged. Nine died, leaving fifty-six remaining at the end of the war. There is no evidence to suggest that these patients were treated in a different way from the civilian patients in terms of clinical or therapeutic approach, although as their numbers increased they were put in separate wards. The records of the Denbigh asylum reflect none of the contemporary interest in psychotherapy, such as that employed in the treatment of military patients at the Craig-lockhart Asylum by W. H. R. Rivers and his team.[10] There was little alteration in the practices of the Denbigh asylum as a result of war, and any changes had more to do with the adoption of basic public health measures than with alternative psychiatric practices.

Scientific enquiry was becoming the accepted path to a fuller under-standing of mental illness, and small laboratories were attached to the leading hospitals. Medical staff at Denbigh felt hindered by the lack of such a facility, especially regarding pathological investigations. During the war there was growing concern about the increase in venereal disease. The connection between syphilis and general paralysis was more widely recognized, but in Denbigh, wrote Frank Jones, 'as we have no Laboratory and no Pathologist we are unable to carry out the blood test necessary for its detection'. And yet, for an 'annual expenditure of about £20 all these blood tests could be made'.[11] Annual reports were a good way of drawing attention to deficiencies in resources, and by the following year his public statements had borne fruit. He was able to report that Wasserman's blood test 'is now being carried out by Dr Distaso, of Cardiff, in all suspected cases, and is a great aid to diagnosis and treatment'.[12] The practice of sending specimens to laboratories in Cardiff for analysis was to continue until the appointment of a pathologist in 1928. The blood of forty-four patients was tested for syphilis by the Wasser-man reaction in 1916, and of these twenty gave positive results.

Dr Distaso identified many cases of dysentery and suggested a new treatment, which was adopted with satisfactory results.[13] Measures were taken in an attempt to curtail the spread of disease from one patient to another, and a new disinfecting tank was constructed for the sterilization of all soiled and infected clothing. This attention to cleanliness highlighted the deficiency of washing facilities. In 1918 the commissioner urged that every effort should be made to use the lavatory basins attached to each ward, particularly after using the WCs. He recommended that basins should be placed in the kitchens and elsewhere, for the use of all officers and patients engaged in the handling of food.[14] The following year the commissioners noted with approval that these recommendations were being carried out, and reported on further ingenious attempts to stem the spread of dysentery:

> The manufacture of a very useful pattern of loose drawers is being hurried on (some 80 pairs being now available for the worst cases), an open-air tank with steam disinfection fittings has been placed near the laundry, and portable iron receptacles are now in use for the transport of foul-linen from

the dormitories to this tank. The willingness to fall in with the Board's wishes in these directions is gratifying.[15]

Dysentery and chronic nephritis had been the cause of nine and seventeen deaths respectively during the year 1918–19.[16] Further action was required to check the spread of dysentery, colitis and enteric fever. In 1919 there were thirty-four cases of colitis, twenty-nine cases of diarrhoea, five cases of enteric fever and one of erysipelas. In response to the situation, 'Spraying with germicide sprays is being carried out systematically, and Sulphome fumigation of even the largest Wards and Dormitories is done at intervals.'[17]

Experimentation with New Therapies

Despite the lack of interest in psychotherapy, a new atmosphere of experimentation was discernible in other areas of patient treatment. Dietary provision was one aspect of patient care that was receiving renewed attention. General health was closely observed, and in 1914 'an excellent weighing machine' was purchased, so that 'all the inmates are systematically and regularly weighed'.[18] Diet attracted special scrutiny in regard to a number of disorders, particularly that of epilepsy. In 1917 Frank Jones reported that a number of epileptic patients had been given an entirely vegetarian diet for the last ten months, and that a 'decided decrease in the number of seizures has taken place in most cases'; although in a few cases they had increased.[19]

Wartime shortages had some impact on diet generally in the asylum, as flour, meat and sugar became subject to rationing. However, there is no evidence that patients suffered disproportionately as a result of wartime privation. Early in the war, food shortages caused problems and there were cutbacks in the amount of food available. When the visiting commissioner made his usual inspection of the fare during his visit in September 1917, he recorded that: 'I saw dinner being served to some 340 patients of both sexes in the dining hall. It consisted of a stew made from meat, carrots, turnips, and onions, with curried rice and potatoes, and appeared to be enjoyed by the patients.'[20] He discussed the impact of rationing with the medical superintendent, and was clearly interested in his response.

> Dr Jones told me that when first the patients' rations were diminished, he at first noticed a marked falling off in their bodily weight, but that since porridge has been issued daily for breakfast, and oatmeal scones have been given to the workers for lunch, they have again put on weight, and are gradually getting back to their normal condition.[21]

The evidence from the Denbigh asylum does not therefore support the contention that mental hospital patients were systematically deprived of food during the First World War. Cranmer has suggested that there was a deliberate policy of semi-starvation in the Buckinghamshire Pauper Lunatic Asylum during these years.[22] Russell Davies concluded that patients in the Carmarthen Asylum were treated contemptuously and starved of food. Neither the official reports nor the patient case records would uphold such an interpretation in the case of the Denbigh asylum. There were privations, and it may be that a relative deterioration in the diet made patients more susceptible to disease, but similar trends occurred amongst the general population too, and there is disagreement as to the relative contribution of poor diet to the rise in tuberculosis death rates.[23]

It was increasingly recognized that an overactive thyroid could make a patient appear manic, so the quality of drinking water also received close attention at this time. The asylum began to boil all drinking water, with a view 'to diminishing the prevalence of Goitre' (an enlarged thyroid), and subsequently staff noticed an improvement, particularly amongst the younger patients, and even found that 'a very large Goitre in a boy has entirely disappeared'.[24] In 1910 David Marine and others had shown that goitre was caused by iodine deficiency in the water, and could be treated by the use of iodine.[25] It is not clear whether the medical staff were administering iodine as well as boiling the water, but it is the case that they were monitoring the relationship. One of the first books to be purchased for the medical library, established in the asylum in 1914, was *The Causation and Treatment of Goitre*, by Dr McGarrison.[26] Also, an additional question was inserted on the printed forms used in the medical case books of patients, regarding the presence of goitre.

Epilepsy continued to be a significant physical cause of insanity. In 1914 about 10 per cent of cases admitted to the Denbigh asylum were attributed to it, which was somewhat higher than average, but at least 6 per cent of the admissions were recorded as epileptic in each of the First World War years. No further mention was made of the dietary trials, but in 1919 a much more drastic treatment was attempted, when Dr Thelwell Thomas performed an operation on a patient's brain for the relief of epilepsy. The operation itself was successfully carried out, but 'the result on the mental condition of the patient' was disappointing.[27] This seems to have been one of the first experiments in brain surgery carried out in the asylum, other than surgical attention to fractured skulls.

In 1918 the hospital purchased an electrical apparatus, with the intention of treating several forms of mental disease by cerebral galvanism. It was used on five cases the following year, but the results did not appear promising. However, staff discovered a hidden bonus, for the galvano-set proved 'very useful in treating local disease by ionization'.[28] These experiments might be seen as early precursors of more ambitious applications of psycho-surgery and electrical shock treatments which emerged in the Denbigh hospital during the Second World War. There is no suggestion of any further improvisation with such techniques at this earlier time.

The spirit of experimentation extended to methods of nursing, as exemplified in the innovative treatment of patients suffering from tuberculosis. Since the development of sanatoria in the late nineteenth century, specialists in the treatment of tuberculosis had argued the need for special provision being made for open-air treatment and isolation of infective cases. Plas Llangwyfan, an estate near Denbigh, had been purchased by the Welsh National Memorial Association in 1913 to provide a sanatorium for the treatment of tuberculosis in Wales.[29] Outdoor provision with plenty of fresh air and daylight was advocated. This method of nursing tubercular patients was first introduced on the male side of the Denbigh hospital, and statistics soon supported its merits.

Tests were also made to establish the cause of tuberculosis, which was by now accounting for roughly 20 per cent of the deaths in the asylum. Deaths

Deaths from tuberculosis during the First World War

Year	No. of deaths
1914	18
1915	22
1916	27
1917	31
1918	36

from tuberculosis in the asylum rose steadily during the war, as the table illustrates. Tests by the inoculation method were carried out on dairy cows at the asylum farm. All of the samples proved negative, indicating that 'milk supply was not infective'.[30] The conclusion was therefore drawn that 'the cause is in the buildings, just as is that of dysentery'.[31] A series of recommendations followed from this deduction, and a new regimen was imposed. Increased ventilation was considered necessary although there was need to be cautious about offering too many opportunities for patients to escape or to commit suicide; enlarging the openings on the upper floors was not compatible with other safety considerations. The obvious course was to locate all of the tubercular patients on the ground floor, but this too went against the grain of established practice, for 'it is not desirable to congregate all forms of Insanity in one Ward'.[32]

In 1914 there were fifteen deaths from tubercular disease on the female side, while on the male side, where this new provision was introduced, there were only three deaths. Verandahs were constructed outside both the male and female infirmary wards, and this enabled the patients 'to be bedded out of doors in favourable weather'.[33] The next step was to experiment with special outdoor huts for the isolation and fresh air treatment of consumptive patients. Two outside shelter huts were erected in an airing court on the female side and each became the temporary home of a female phthisical patient. It was necessary to make provision for the nurse in charge of these patients also to be located outside.

The medical superintendent was enthusiastic about the new fresh air therapy, and decided to recommend the purchase of a number of tents 'so as to enable all meals to be partaken out of doors'. This would ensure that for seven months of the year patients could remain outside all day. By 1918 there were eight open-air huts for phthisical patients on the female side, these beds being occupied day and night, and on the male side the new open-air verandah was being used chiefly for the same purpose. At the end of the war the male isolation hospital, erected in the grounds in 1902, was reopened for the purpose of isolating and treating tubercular cases. During the year 1919 phthisis was the cause of death of fourteen patients in the asylum. In 1915 Nurse Jane Jones had died after several months of treatment in a sanatorium, and in 1919 Dr Manifold, who had replaced Dr Herbert, suffered a complete breakdown of health. He was admitted to the Matlock Sanatorium, and died in 1921.

The problem of tuberculosis was by now being taken increasingly seriously. When Commissioner Hubert Bond visited the hospital in December 1921, eighteen months after the last official visit, he noted that in the mean time there had been twenty-nine deaths from the disease. At the time of his visit there were twenty cases under observation. This led him to conclude that it was 'unsafe to regard the existing ten cases as representing the true number of patients who are suffering from it in an active and communicable form'. He suggested that, in addition to the regular monitoring of weights 'which is now practiced', he would like to see a 'much more frequent use of cod liver oil in cases that show loss of weight'. He also recommended that each patient should receive a full physical examination every six months, 'for it is only by being constantly on the look out for, and promptly dealing with the first signs of this disease, that its incidence is likely to be sensibly diminished'.[34] He advised the fitting up of a small laboratory that need not be a costly matter but would facilitate the examination of sputa of suspected tubercular cases. It would also be advantageous for many other clinical purposes, such as the control of dysentery and diarrhoea, cases of which were now being 'adequately segregated', but which nonetheless needed closer monitoring.

It is clear from this discussion that the overwhelming focus of both staff and official visitors was on the material fabric of the asylum and the physical health of its patients. The Board of Control officials consistently directed their inspection reports towards the condition of the buildings, water-supply, bedding and furnishings, standard of clothing of the patients and the general health of the asylum as expressed by death rates and outbreaks of infectious diseases. The attention paid to the methods of treatment of mental illness was remarkably slight. Hubert Bond expressed surprise at the small number of patients taking medicines, and at the fact that so few patients were ill in bed, and he 'could not help thinking that a few of these patients manifesting active and acute excitement might benefit by a period of rest in bed, and perhaps by some medicinal treatment'.[35] A modified form of Weir Mitchell's rest cure was in use at this time in the Bethlem Hospital, but does not seem to have been used in Denbigh, where the emphasis was always on useful activity.[36] Apart from the brief and unsuccessful experiment with the new galvanic machine, there was virtually no innovation in the treatment of mental afflictions within this asylum. The 'management' of the insane continued in much the same way, with all of the emphasis being on basic nursing and care and on the provision of occupation and amusement for those who were well enough to take part. The most significant new additions to the technologies of therapy seem to have been the purchase in 1914 of two gramophones and a cinematograph. These proved immensely popular. During the winter of 1915 16 nineteen cinema shows took place, and were welcomed by the medical superintendent as an important therapeutic innovation: 'No other form of entertainment has created such an interest among the inmates, and this form of recreation will become a powerful factor in recovery.'[37] Of psychotherapy there was never a mention.

Staffing

The mobilization of men for the war created serious staffing problems in the asylum. By April 1915 a total of nineteen men, over 20 per cent of the male staff, had volunteered, including twelve male attendants. Following the precedent set during the South African War the committee of visitors voted to award staff formal leave, and to count military service towards service in the asylum. Furthermore, they agreed to augment army allowances from asylum funds so that married men would continue to receive full pay and value of emoluments, and single men full pay without emoluments. Compensating for the pay difference continued throughout the war. This act of generosity was important in securing the loyalty of staff, and contributed generally to the ethos of institutional allegiance and identity. It also encouraged men to return to their posts on the cessation of war. A similar policy was adopted at the Northampton Asylum.[38]

Meanwhile, several of the vacancies were filled by the recall of retired nursing staff, and by the temporary appointment of artisans. No permanent appointments were made, protecting the posts of the men in military service. The departure of experienced staff resulted in a considerable burden of overwork for those remaining. The visiting committee recorded their appreciation of the 'willing and loyal co-operation' of staff in helping to overcome the difficulties created by this sudden exodus of key staff.[39]

Alternative employment prospects further influenced the staffing situation, since the war created many new opportunities for women.[40] During 1915 seventeen nurses resigned. Already, the pay of staff had been 'adjusted' during the first year of the war, in order to establish 'a satisfactory basis and rate of remuneration'. Dr Frank Jones requested permission to classify the nurses and attendants 'according to merit', and with some relief noted that this was 'so far with satisfactory result'.[41] This 'classification' exercise had enabled him to give monetary recognition to skills and qualifications.

By the following year the institutional dislocation and personal strain caused by staff departures were presenting acute problems. One of the pensioners who had returned to work, Stephen Batten, a former charge attendant, died while on duty in the asylum. Conscription was now coming into force and, in light of serious staff depletion, discussions were held with the Board of Control. An agreement was secured to exempt four of the attendants likely to be called up, and a temporary exemption for three months was allowed for a further four attendants. By April 1916 thirty-three of the staff had been on active military service.

When commissioner Fraser Macleod inspected the asylum in December 1916, he noted that Dr Jones had within the past two weeks placed male ward no. 2 under the care of female nurses. There were seventy-two male patients under the care of four nurses, an arrangement which, Macleod observed, was not uncommon in other institutions, and which 'so far as one can judge . . . promises to work admirably'.[42]

The difficulties faced by the medical superintendent were exacerbated by the sudden departure of one of his medical officers. The appointment of Dr Benson Evans had been a successful one. He ran training sessions for the male staff, fifteen of whom passed the St John's Ambulance examination in 1915, and he lectured both attendants and nurses in preparation for the examination of the Medico-Psychological Society. What was more, he became fully involved in the life of the asylum; as an excellent musician, he organized theatrical entertainments, and played the piano for church services. In May 1915 he joined the RAMC. Eventually a locum tenens was appointed, Dr Eustace Hutton, who was to remain on the staff of the asylum for the next thirty-one years. Dr Jones reported that 'He very quickly gained a knowledge of his patients', and was soon doing 'very good work for the institution'. This was certainly a relief, for by this time his first assistant medical officer, Dr Manifold, was suffering ill health. In his place, Dr Jones managed to secure the assistance of Dr Corbett Owen. These two new appointments enabled Dr Jones to maintain standards of medical care during an extremely difficult period. On his visit to the asylum on 12 September 1918, Commissioner A. Rotherham congratulated the three doctors 'on the excellent condition in which I found the Asylum to-day'.[43]

By the end of the war, nursing attendant W. M. Williams and T. A. Davies, a painter, had been killed in action. A third, W. J. Pritchard, was reported 'missing, presumed killed in action'. A number of the retired staff who responded to the call to return to duty at the asylum died in service, including night charge attendant Thomas Jones, charge attendant Edward Williams, attendant John Jones and the carter, Robert Roberts.

By March 1919 the number of staff employed at the asylum had reached forty-one male attendants and forty-six nurses. The commissioner observed that a 'very large proportion of the Attendants have seen Military Service'. Consequently, some of these men had seen at first hand the horrors of the First World War, an experience which was to shape their respectful and sympathetic attitude towards the cohort of ex-service patients who were to become long-stay patients at the asylum.

For staff who survived the war unscathed, life began to return to normal. An extremely successful staff football XI, comprised mainly of ex-servicemen, was formed, and in 1920 they won the Rhyl and District Challenge Cup, to the enormous gratification of their medical super-intendent. The gate money on their matches was donated to the patients' recreation fund and was used to purchase new gramophone records and music, and to provide the summer sports. In this and other ways, good relations between the staff, patients and management were forged again, allowing strict rules of discipline to be maintained during the inter-war years.

Further improvement began to occur in the hours and conditions of work of the asylum staff after discussions took place between the National Council of Visiting Committees and the National Asylum Workers' Union in 1919. The management of the Denbigh asylum had a direct involvement in these negotiations, since Thomas Williams, chairman of the visiting committee, was elected to the executive committee of the national council. Over the years the Denbigh asylum was well represented on many such national bodies.

The goodwill shown towards the staff in trying to meet the increased cost of living, and accord them better conditions of service, along with the generous treatment of servicemen, pensioners and widows during the war, benefited the management of the asylum. When prices fell, and the cost of living decreased, the scale of wages was decreased accordingly, as negotiated by the conciliation committee. The working hours of nursing and artisan staff were simultaneously increased, and yet the chairman of the visitors was able to report that these new arrangements 'have been carried out with good will and without friction'.[44]

The Patient Experience

Forty thousand Welsh servicemen lost their lives, and thousands of others were maimed and injured in the 1914–18 war.[45] The extraordinary conditions created by trench warfare and modern weaponry led to an unprecedented incidence of mental illness amongst soldiers. Men became paralysed and mute and yet showed no signs of physical injury. Psychiatrists recognized in them a form of hysteria, usually only associated with women.[46] To make the condition sound more acceptable it was given a new name – 'Shell-shock'.[47] Some members of the medical profession engaged in mental hospitals remained hostile to the notion that cases of paralysis could have a purely psychological basis, and still argued that organic lesions must be at the basis of these physical manifestations. However, the War Office was prepared to take the suggestion seriously and to employ psychiatrists at its military hospitals to undertake psychoanalysis and employ a psychodynamic approach. Treated expeditiously, 'shell-shocked' soldiers could be given effective help enabling them to return to the battlefield. The pressure to get men back into action was enormous, and acted as a forcing house for psychotherapy. At the same time, the conditions of war created casualties even amongst those who were not in front-line service, as the records of Denbigh show.

The political and social upheavals of war brought patients from other countries and regions to the Denbigh asylum. During 1915 a number of alien soldiers were admitted, four of whom were transferred from the prisoner of war camp at Queensferry. Amongst them was Arno Bohnert, a forty-year-old clerk who had become violent and attempted to 'throw a Harmonium about'. He was a tall, healthy-looking man of middle age, who spoke English fairly well, although 'not disposed to do so'. Dr Benson Evans noted tremors on all parts of this patient's body, and that 'he declares that hypnosis is working through his system and that he cannot prevent these tremors'. He was constantly, recorded Dr Evans, 'writing short notes on the edges of newspapers and then wrapping them up in several pieces of paper, he also cut out a piece of newspaper with £1,000 printed on it and gave it to me as a cheque'. In March 1916 he claimed that he was 'in the state of mesmerism, and that it is a tradition in his family that all of them should be mesmerised, he cannot say by whom but thought that Professor Klaus of Berlin should know all about it'. In November 1916 a Wasserman test (for syphilis) was carried out, but this proved negative. In January 1917 he still claimed to be under the influence of mesmerism. His mental condition did not improve. In March 1919 he was still suffering from 'delusional insanity' and claiming that he was in 'telepathic communication with certain Professors in Berlin'. There was no further change in his condition, but he was 'well behaved' and had by now made himself very 'useful'. Finally, in September 1920, he was discharged to Colney Hatch Asylum, in Middlesex, ready for repatriation to Germany.

Another group of men brought to Wales during the war were the interned Irish rebels. After the 1916 Easter Rising over two and a half thousand of them had been transported to the mainland and dispersed for imprisonment. In June most were sent to Frongoch, in a sparsely populated moorland area of Merioneth. Here a former distillery had been converted into an internment camp to hold German prisoners. They were transferred to Queensferry and some of the leading political thinkers and military strategists of the Irish republican movement were interned at Frongoch, including Michael Collins, and so the camp became known as a 'University of Revolution'.[48] The health of a number of prisoners broke down and three were transferred to the North Wales Counties Lunatic Asylum. William Halpin of Dublin had attempted suicide in August 1916, by cutting his throat. According to fellow detainees Halpin suffered from an obsession that he had 'funked' in the Rising and that for a small sum of money he had betrayed his comrades. He believed that the other men accused him of being an Orange man and intended to shoot him. He kept muttering to himself 'my God what is going to happen to me'.[49] On admittance to the asylum he was depressed, crying, and in 'poor physical condition'. He was still in the asylum the following January, and although he 'seldom speaks' he could answer questions when addressed. In May 1917 he was transferred to the Grangegorman Asylum in Dublin, where he died the same year.[50]

The war saw an extremely vigorous public health campaign aimed at warning people of the dangers of venereal disease.[51] Its alarmist and censorial tone must have added considerably to the anxiety already experienced by anyone who was unfortunate enough to contract some form of sexually transmitted disease. In May 1915 a Swansea soldier was transferred from the Bangor Military Hospital to the Denbigh asylum after trying to cut his throat. An army doctor had already confirmed that he had previously contracted syphilis. While on the train from Rhyl to Denbigh he 'would make sudden dashes to get away' and while in the station he tried to jump on the line. Due to these suicidal attempts he was immediately put on a 'caution card' at the asylum. He was 'dull, self absorbed and depressed' and said that he wished he was dead. A month later he was still depressed, and was convinced that, due to the Army typhoid injection, he had 'been thoroughly spoilt by inoculation'. He was kept on a caution card, but by August was improving and talking rationally. In October 1915 he was discharged recovered. Whether or not he then fought in the war, the asylum records offer no indication.

By 1916 war casualties were mounting and many families were receiving news of the loss of loved ones. Janet W., the mother of three young children, was thirty-five when she received a telegram informing her that her husband was reported 'missing in action'. She then received a second, telling her that he was reported dead. He had in fact survived, but the shock of the telegrams left her distraught. She was committed to the Denbigh hospital after being examined by the Poor Law doctor. She claimed that someone had attempted 'to poison her last week with fluid to burn her throat and that the room was full of poison gas, which prevented her sitting down'.[52] Her husband obtained special leave to visit his wife. He found that she had been taken to the Denbigh asylum and his sister-in-law, Mrs M., was left in charge of the children. He was finally discharged from the army in 1919. When he returned to north Wales he found his wife still detained in the asylum, and his sister-in-law returned to Liverpool, taking the children with her. He followed them to Liverpool, where he settled. His wife lived out the rest of her days in Denbigh. For years Mr W. used to receive a monthly report on his wife's condition from Dr Jones, and this always said the same thing, 'Bodily well but mentally just the same'. The children visited her once a year until her death in 1957. In later life her sister, who had reared the children, joined her as a patient at Denbigh.

The new technologies of war created horrific wounds and unimaginable ways of death.[53] Some of the victims did not enter the mental hospital until after the war, with a history of medical examinations. S.T.H., Private 25804 of the East Surrey Regiment had his foot amputated in March 1918. The stump healed and a surgical boot was supplied, with which he could walk aided by a stick. He suffered from recurrent attacks of mania and was seen by military doctors at Woolwich, Wrexham, Cardiff, and again at Wrexham on numerous occasions between 1919 and 1923. The calf muscles of his leg were wasting, and the attacks of mania kept recurring. He and at least 158 other service patients were admitted to the Denbigh hospital in the years during and after the war. The majority of them were classified as suffering from mania, or delusional insanity, but a surprising number were diagnosed as 'feeble-minded'. A very few had been labelled as suffering from neurasthenia.

One man believed to be suffering from neurasthenia was a private in the Labour Corps. He was examined and diagnosed at Oswestry by the military doctor, who found him 'hard to understand (because he is Welsh)', and he was registered as 30 per cent disabled by his condition. He was examined in Bangor in 1918, 1919 and 1920, and then in July 1920 given an extended consultation at the National Assistance Board in Wrexham. It was recorded that he 'Complains of sleeplessness at night, gets very excited in noise and traffic. Noises in head. Awakens suddenly from sleep and sees shadows which he cannot describe . . . also complains of weakness in legs.' Following numerous other medical examinations he was examined again at a special board at Wrexham in October 1922, where he was described as a 'hypo-chondriac'. In 1923 he appeared before another special board at Wrexham; this time a neurological examination took place, and recorded his condition in these terms: 'disturbed sleep, nervous, giddiness, apprehensive'. The repeated examinations were associated with the deliberations of the Ministry of Pensions concerning the appropriate apportionment of pension allowance. In 1926 he was being treated at a Poor Law infirmary and in May was transferred to the Saltash Hospital in Cornwall. Here a doctor decided that he had the 'physical stigmata of degeneracy' and described him as a 'mental deficient with psychotic symptoms'. He was disorientated as to time and place, and was suffering from auditory hallucinations. Later that month he was finally designated as 100 per cent disabled and certified to Netherne Hospital in Coulsdon, Surrey. He was now described as 'Acutely hallucin-ated and deluded, has noisy outbursts also persecutory ideas fixed on various people – Is a very inferior type with high falsetto voice, speech almost unintelligible. Ideation is limited and childish. Quite incapable of ordinary life.' He was transferred to the Denbigh hospital in 1927 where he was to remain a long-term chronic patient. For men such as these their war-time experiences did not end in 1918. The method of screening meant that they had to be subjected to these demeaning examinations time after time.

As already indicated, servicemen sent to Denbigh had suffered a variety of physical injuries as well as problems of mental health. William L. was hospitalized suffering from melancholia and 'mild trench feet' in 1915. Thomas H. had extensive scarring on the spine due to burns, and had been invalided twice suffering from nervous debility and once from loss of memory. J.G.L. and Sidney T. had suffered the effects of gas poisoning, and the latter had multiple wounds to the arm and head and was treated for bronchitis which was present in both lungs. R.A. had shell wounds in the region of his left hip, his thigh and his calf muscles were wasting, and his movement at the knee and ankle was limited. He had wounds to the scalp, which although healed had left irregularity of cranium. R.A. believed that he had been infected by syphilis at a medical board. A number of the men had fears about sexually transmitted diseases, which they believed were exacerbating their condition. E.T. from Llanuwchllyn was found to be in a delusional state in 1917 after he had gone missing in action. When taken to the military hospital he feared that he would be killed, and said that someone had stood over him at night with a knife. He also stated that he had gonorrhoea (which was untrue according to the medical report) and so kept his penis tied up in brown paper. He would occasionally wet the bed. Cases such as these create a powerful sense of the fracturing of masculinities which some writers have claimed was engendered by the First World War.[54] There are many examples amongst the service patients' record cards of men demobilized only to find themselves unable to settle into the ways and rhythms of their former existence. Some sent to the asylum were still having battle dreams a decade and more after the events. Men who returned to a life that seemed strange and unfamiliar would stand in the dark on street corners, or wander abroad at night. The tribulations of the composer and poet Ivor Gurney, who would go on long tramps, are echoed in the stories of some of these men.[55] Like him, they were labelled as suffering from delusional insanity. Whether they would have become mentally ill if the war had not intervened to shatter their lives is a question that can never be answered. But it is clear from the stories contained in hospital files that, in the words of historian Gwyn Alf Williams, 'the war was an unhinging shock of the first order' – not only to a nation but to the individuals caught up in that grotesque and momentous affair.[56]

Epidemics and 'War Worry'

As the First World War drew to close a frightening bacteriological infection swept across the globe.[57] The influenza epidemic arrived in Europe in March 1918, and a second wave followed in the autumn. Two hundred thousand people died in Britain alone, and worldwide it may have caused thirty million deaths.[58] When the commissioners arrived at the Denbigh asylum during the epidemic's second wave in October 1918, they found the medical superintendent Frank Jones infected, as were several staff and at least thirty patients.[59] Altogether that autumn eighty-eight patients and thirty-six members of staff were attacked by influenza.[60] There were a number of deaths from pneumonia, some of which were associated with the 'flu outbreak.

After this, the asylum death rate which had increased during the First World War soon began to fall, from 15.1 per cent in 1918 to 11.1 per cent in 1919, so that during the 1920s it again averaged under 10 per cent. Whether this easement was due to less overcrowding or partly attributable to the more ample supply of food is difficult to say. Certainly by 1921 the hospital diet had considerably improved, so that 'the scale is now liberal, as well as largely freed from monotony'.[61] An additional meal was provided in the form of a supper of 'bread and cheese with coffee', a welcome improvement as it broke up the 'long interval between tea and breakfast'.

The mental burden of war was mirrored in many of the patient case histories, with 19 per cent of the admissions for 1918 being attributed to 'war worry'. This was the first time that a social causation had replaced 'heredity' as the principal causative factor in admissions.[62] Catherine J., a spinster housekeeper admitted in November 1919, had kept house for her brother, who had become a war casualty and since then she had become 'troubled and fretted much'.[63] When visited by her doctor she told him that he was 'the Angel of Mons'. A doctor and two magistrates certified her insane. Once in the asylum she was found to be in poor health and very deluded. She talked of seeing visions and flashes of light and claimed that she was 'full of spiritualism'. In 1920 the doctors diagnosed her as suffering from 'mania', in 1921 from 'delusional insanity' and by 1925 she was simply said to be 'deluded, simple and childish' but usefully employed and in fairly good health. She was discharged in June 1926.

Richard A., a thirty-five-year-old farm labourer, was an army veteran and the 'principal aetiological factor' in his case was recorded as 'war stress'. He had a discharging sinus on his left arm, the result of a shell wound, and had 'requested a razor to cut his throat'. He claimed that the powders sent to him by his medical men were poisonous, and refused to take them. Admitted to the asylum in March 1919 he showed little progress and was described as solitary and depressed, although his physical health improved. In 1921 he was suffering from melancholia, and continuing to experience aural hallucinations. In September 1934, having been 'quiet and well behaved' for a period, he was allowed out on trial. The placement was successful and he was fully discharged in December 1934.

There is no knowing how many men experienced similar feelings of depression and disenchantment, or were suspicious and morose, but lived their lives outside any asylum. A Caernarfonshire quarryman, who joined the Royal Welsh Fusiliers and was wounded in the attack on Delville Wood in 1916, kept a diary of his war experiences. He was said to have returned home deeply traumatized, and for the remainder of his life he suffered from a 'deep and unremitting melancholia'.[64] He died shortly before the outbreak of the Second World War, without appearing amongst the statistics of the 'mentally ill' in north Wales.

✳

CHAPTER NINE

The Inter-War Years

The First World War has been seen as a watershed in the treatment of mental illness. It is argued that the psychological impact of that war on soldiers who came from a variety of social backgrounds led to a paradigm shift in the theoretical and practical approaches to mental illness.[1] In 1927 a Harley Street doctor held that the 'Great War, with its crops of "shell-shocks" and nervous troubles, has entirely changed the outlook of the modern physician'.[2] Those outside asylum practice are said to have become more aware of 'functional nervous disorders', and the general public became more accepting of mental disturbance. Health policy analysts have contended that, whereas previously the public asylums only dealt with a 'narrow band of "riff raff"', namely the 'pauper lunatics', after the First World War they catered for a wider spectrum of the population.[3] The notion that insanity had a somatic basis, and was a condition which was invariably inherited, was replaced, it is argued, by the view that mental illness was primarily a psychological manifestation of the pressures of daily life. It could therefore affect anyone who incurred severe social stress or underwent traumatic experiences. A new cohort of patients is said to have entered the hospital arena seeking treatment voluntarily. They came increasingly from the middle and lower middle classes and altered the social profile of the patient population. To what extent is such a change evident in north Wales? Can we detect such a sharp dichotomy between the pre-1914 and post-1918 period in the psychiatric practices and patient population of the North Wales Counties Asylum?

First, on the theoretical front there is no evidence that the hereditary model was overturned. Throughout the inter-war period, hereditary tendencies continued to head the list of ascribed causations of insanity amongst patients admitted. The range of illnesses diagnosed was much the same as before. No new nosologies were introduced and the diagnoses remained in a very traditional mould, with 'mania' at the head of the list, followed closely by 'melancholia'. This is the pattern of illnesses amongst patients admitted in 1930:

Mania	29.5%
Melancholia	22.7%
General Paralysis	5.1%
Epilepsy	5.6%
Delusional Insanity	7.3%
Dementia Praecox	5.6%
Senile Dementia	11.2%[4]

By 1939 there was only one new addition to this list – 'confusional insanity' representing 5.7 per cent of admissions.[5]

Secondly, it has already been argued in this account of the Denbigh hospital that, even during the nineteenth century, the patient population had a much wider social basis than might be supposed from the attachment of the label 'pauper lunatics'. An analysis of the occupational profile of 'pauper' patients admitted between 1914 and 1939 suggests that the social pattern of admissions did not change dramatically. Whilst numbers increased steadily, the range of occupational and social backgrounds continued to parallel roughly the range of social categories and the employment patterns of the general population. If anything there is a slightly higher proportion of labourers in the inter-war period.

In some regions outpatient departments were developed. In Oxfordshire, for instance, the Littlemore Hospital operated an extensive outreach service in conjunction with the Radcliffe Hospital, and its origins lay in the treatment of soldiers during the First World War.[6] However, the outpatient services planned in north Wales in 1913 were long delayed due to the intervention of war. Very few patients were admitted on a voluntary basis and the work of the clinics was still in its infancy by the time of the Second World War. Such delays also contributed to the persistence of the existing patient profile so that by far the majority of patients occupying beds at any one time were chronic, long-term cases. New treatments and practices made little impact until the end of the 1930s.

Dealing with 'Mental Deficiency'

The institution might have modernized more quickly had it not been for the large number of 'mental deficiency' cases more or less permanently housed there. When the Mental Deficiency Act of 1913 recommended the establishment of special colonies for the housing and training of 'mental defectives', there had been some anticipation that this situation might change. The committee of visitors took the initiative to call a meeting of the five counties to discuss the new obligations placed upon them by the 1913 Act.[7] They favoured the establishment of a parallel institution to provide for mental deficiency cases and felt a joint venture would make financial and logistical sense. Discussions took place with representatives of Montgomeryshire County Council with a view to forming an alliance between six counties, mirroring the original attempts to secure such a union for the formation of the lunatic asylum itself. However, the idea never gained support and the hospital had to continue receiving a group of 'mentally deficient' patients, for which it was ill equipped to provide. In 1921 a group of male imbecile boys were separated off from the main male patient population, and placed in a part of the old isolation hospital, with the aim of providing more appropriate care.[8]

The majority of the mentally deficient in north Wales remained either at home or boarded out with relatives. Those requiring institutional care were mainly housed in workhouses. In Merioneth in 1924 there were twenty-three male and twenty-seven female adults classed as 'defectives' residing in the old Ffestiniog union workhouse in Minffordd. In Flintshire there were twelve adults of each sex, located in the old workhouse at St Asaph; and in Denbighshire twelve of each sex resided in the Ruthin union workhouse. In Caernarfonshire fifteen males and fifteen females were placed in Bodavon, and in Anglesey ten adult females who were classed as mentally defective were placed in the Holyhead union workhouse in Valley. There is no mention of any institutional provision for male 'mental deficients' in Anglesey.[9]

Following the Mental Deficiency Act, 1913, the Denbigh asylum continued to receive on average about fourteen patients of this class per year. By 1925 there were 150 'Mental Deficients' resident, representing almost 15 per cent of the total patient population. As hope of securing alternative provision faded, the medical superintendent urged the 'removal of suitable cases to the Workhouse'.[10] The expectation of the counties and of certifying magistrates that the hospital would continue to take responsibility for cases of mental deficiency ran counter to the expectations of central government that mental institutions would become more like hospitals, developing a more curative regime. As Dr Frank Jones wrote in obvious exasperation, 'The question of hospitalising this Institution cannot possibly be taken in hand seriously until the removal of most of the Mental Deficients can be carried out.' Recently two little boys aged seven and six respectively had been certified by magistrates and sent to the asylum. 'Owing to arrested development with paralysed limbs and no speech they are practically babies and are treated on the Female side.'[11] There was no prospect of successful treatment for sad cases such as these, ill-advisedly certified insane. But the power of certification did not lie with the asylum doctors. A decade later there was still no significant change in the situation, and the Board of Control singled out north Wales as the one region which had done the least to address the issue of care for the mentally deficient.[12]

The Board of Control recognized that 'in many parts of Wales the sparsity of the population makes the problem peculiarly difficult'. They also acknowledged that the weak position of agriculture 'on which they mainly depend' was the main reason why county council resources were insufficient to develop institutional care for the mentally deficient.[13] It was not until after the Second World War that these patients were finally removed.

Year by year, additional accommodation was becoming increasingly urgent. In 1922 there were 140 patients in male ward no. 5, situated in the old recreation hall. One hundred and sixty patients were obliged to take their meals in this same ward.[14] A hard-pressed institution was urged to modernize in line with new expectations in relation to the quality of care, but without the underpinning resources becoming available.

Reforming the System

In the years following the First World War a major re-evaluation took place of the role of mental hospitals in England and Wales. As with many changes in social policy this was partly precipitated by the eruption of a 'scandal'. In 1921 Dr Montague Lomax published his *Experiences of an Asylum Doctor*.[15] His exposé of seemingly intolerable conditions caused a public outcry and righteous indignation on the part of asylum superintendents. The majority of Lomax's allegations related to the Prestwich Asylum in Manchester, though the thrust of his argument was that the nature of the entire asylum system required questioning. He alleged that patients were housed in 'gloomy and often dilapidated barrack asylums' where they were systematically abused, confined under restraint, sedated and administered purgatives. During the First World War dishonest staff misappropriated patients' food rations. Many of the patients became chronic long-term cases simply by virtue of the lack of any therapeutic regime. Obliged to respond, in 1922 the government established a departmental committee to investigate the administration of public mental hospitals. After examining the evidence, the committee dismissed Lomax's 'sweeping allegations' and 'gross exaggerations' and concluded that the 'treatment of the insane is humane and efficient'. Nonetheless, it made a series of recommendations, amongst which were that the size of an institution should not exceed accommodation for 1,000 patients and that reception wards and convalescent wards should be in separate buildings.[16] The North Wales Counties Asylum already exceeded this threshold, with the result that the guideline was to be employed as an argument against building additional facilities, including the new reception ward, at the hospital.

Lloyd George's war-time coalition government had already considered reforming social policy in relation to the lunacy system. In 1916 the

Reconstruction Committee consulted the Board of Control, which suggested provision for early treatment, investment in psychiatric research, and a change in the admission requirements to enable patients to seek help on a voluntary basis.[17] Such sweeping changes did not sit comfortably within the existing framework, still based upon the legislation of the 1890 Act. The proposals went far beyond reformism effectively to promulgate a new philosophy of care. A Royal Commission on Lunacy and Mental Disorder was appointed in 1924 under the chairmanship of the Rt. Hon. H. P. Macmillan to consider the legislative implications. Its recommendations, published in 1926, formed the basis of a parliamentary bill introduced to replace the Lunacy Act of 1890. The Mental Treatment Act became law in 1930. Its primary aim was to extend the facilities for early treatment by means of greater provision for the reception of voluntary patients, introducing a new code for the admission of temporary patients, extending the Urgency Order procedure to rate-aided patients, and encouraging the development of outpatient treatment. The Act was radically to alter the whole basis of patient referral, admission and detention. However, the extent to which it brought about material change varied considerably. Whereas some mental hospitals moved rapidly to a system of voluntary admissions, others, including the North Wales Counties Mental Hospital (NWCMH), as it was now to be called, did not. Even shortly after the implementation of the Act a wide divergence between regions was evident. By 1932 not a single voluntary patient had been admitted to any public mental hospital in the area covered by the Lancashire Mental Hospitals Board. In other areas, where the Act had been energetically embraced, as many as 45 per cent of admissions in 1931 were either voluntary or temporary patients.[18]

In 1930 the NWCMH Chairman Aneurin Evans welcomed the new legislation and the 'broadening of public opinion on this question' as heartening to those with lengthy experience of administration in mental institutions. But a meeting of the house and building committee early in 1931 to consider the implications of the Act resolved that 'the applicants for voluntary treatment are not deemed suitable for treatment here'.[19] Effectively, the door was shut on voluntary patients, for the time being at least. Instead, a special subcommittee was formed 'to consider and co-ordinate with Public Authorities and General Hospitals in the formation of clinics and out-patients' departments'.[20] In this way a clear division was envisaged between the traditional work of the NWCMH in receiving certified patients, and the new type of work with non-traditional patients who would henceforth be referred to out-patient clinics.

The 1930 Mental Treatment Act had far-reaching implications for the whole structure of the mental health services in England and Wales. It implied a widening of provision, and the opening out of psychiatry to meet the needs of anyone seeking medical help for their distress. The Denbigh hospital had been established at a time when the only entry routes were either as a wealthy private patient, or as a pauper patient through the judicial system, with the subsequent loss of liberty and status. With the reform of the Poor Law and the transfer of health and welfare responsibilities to local government in 1929, the old designation of 'pauper lunatic' disappeared forever. The 1930 Act signified a repudiation of the legalism of its 1890 predecessor. Henceforth, certification was intended only as a measure of last resort. Yet in many regions the institutional provision remained very much the same, and the evidence for north Wales certainly suggests that changes were not brought into being simply by legislation. A much wider cultural shift had to take place, encompassing the attitudes of the general public, a commitment to reform at local level and the willingness of general practitioners to alter their procedures and strategies for patient care. In order to bring into being the spirit of the Act a new outreach system had to be created. In the absence of wider change, the new certification procedures might represent no more than a modification of the old forms of paper documentation.

Building Again

Within the hospital there was a great deal of sympathy towards the notion of providing modern care, but with only three medical officers responsible for well over a thousand patients resources were fully stretched. In 1922 a special subcommittee had been appointed to consider the proposal to provide a reception ward and separate convalescent wards, but 'under the pressure put on all Public Bodies to economise in their expenditure' they had not been able to progress. However, in 1923 there arose an opportunity to consolidate the land around the asylum and acquire the substantial Gwynfryn House for £5,100. The asylum's own funds were used, so avoiding recourse to seeking the financial support of the county councils.[21] This was a shrewd decision, allowing development of modern facilities on a site which appeared detached from the main hospital, yet sufficiently close to share all main amenities. The management proceeded to convert the mansion to house a group of twenty female convalescent patients.

There was ample scope for more ambitious schemes, and in 1928 the visiting committee appointed Messrs Lockwood, Abercrombie and Saxon of Chester, a prestigious practice closely associated with the garden city movement, as their architects. In consultation with the Board of Control it was decided to implement ambitious plans for a modern hospital complex, allowing the adoption of the 'most up-to-date methods of treatment'. It was envisaged that the development would include a reception ward for new admissions on the Gwynfryn site, and facilitate the treatment of cases of incipient or transient mental illness, 'with discharge on recovery, without

contact with the parent institution in any shape or form'. A new convalescent home would rehouse the female patients already placed in
Gwynfryn. An equivalent male convalescent home would be provided at
Trefeirian, a house on the outskirts of the estate. Six new patient villas
would be built and a new hostel to accommodate eighty nurses. In view of
the high costs of the project it was decided the following year to implement
it in stages. The county councils agreed to proceed with the first phase of
the scheme at an estimated cost of £80,000, and work commenced.

The adaptation of Trefeirian was completed by spring 1930, but in the
mean time the structural alterations being made to the main building were
creating a severe shortage of space. Admissions were still rising, and so
another property, namely Pool Park, a large mansion on the outskirts of
Ruthin suitable for eighty or more patients, was purchased for a sum of
£2,000.[22] Although the building required some modification, in the short
term it was considerably cheaper than the option of proceeding with the new
villa accommodation. Pool Park was officially opened in 1937, and was soon
to became home to about one hundred of the more 'easily manageable'
patients. A senior nurse, Richard Blythyn, was put in charge of this new
annexe, and medical staff visited regularly.

The nurses' hostel and the reception ward were formally opened in May
1934 and, along with the convalescent home and the male villa, 'proved
admirably suited for the purposes for which they were designed'.[23] When
the commissioners visited they were 'much struck by the beauty of the
surroundings of the new buildings, and of the new Villas'.[24] The new model
hospital was ready to move forward in the treatment by modern methods of
incipient and early cases of insanity. All that was now needed was the new
model patient.

At this stage there were few clinics available to the public that would
facilitate voluntary referral. In 1935 outpatient clinics were established in
three regional general hospitals, but they were only offered once a month.
By 1939 the psychiatrists from Denbigh were holding a monthly clinic in
five centres: Wrexham, Colwyn Bay, Mold, Bangor and Dolgellau. The
grand total of patients dealt with in all of these clinics catering for the whole
of north Wales during that year was forty-four, hardly a great expansion.
The number of voluntary and temporary patients admitted to the NWCMH
remained extremely low. When commissioners visited the hospital in
October 1936 there were 1,384 patients in residence. Of these only eleven
men and nine women were on a voluntary basis and five men and six women
were temporary patients.[25] This was in sharp contrast to the situation in
south Wales where nearly three-quarters of the patients admitted to the
mental hospitals in Cardiff and Swansea were voluntary admissions.[26] In
1938 the Board of Control produced a table ranking the different mental
hospitals according to the proportion of voluntary patients to total direct

admissions. Denbigh came near the bottom of the list, in the band 15–24 per cent, although Lancaster fell below, with only 10–14 per cent, and Prestwich worst of all, with only 5–9 per cent of admissions in the voluntary category.[27]

In terms of outpatient services and adoption of the provisions of the 1930 Act there seems to have been little progress during the inter-war years, but this does not necessarily mean that no changes or improvements were taking place within the hospital. In some areas, as will be seen, there was evidence of good practice.

Modernizing the Asylum

The committee of visitors made the key decisions in the management of the hospital and it was fortunate that it included members of high calibre, keen to be abreast of the latest innovations in treatment, and conversant with current official policy. Mr Branthwaite of the Board of Control met the committee for the first time in 1925. He was interested to note that 'some five or six of its members are medical men, and that the recently appointed lady member is a medical woman, who is anxious to make a specialty of matters relating to the comfort and welfare of female patients'. Dr Katherine Drinkwater was the first woman member of the committee of visitors, and gave many years of valuable service. In 1928 a delegation of members attended the National Health Congress in London and took the opportunity to visit three London County Council mental hospitals of the most modern design, where they were 'afforded valuable information and advice on the latest developments in the treatment of mental disorders'. In this way the committee kept informed of the best of contemporary practices.

In 1931, the hospital's committee chairmen attended a conference of the Mental Hospital Association in London where they agreed to 'fall in with' the resolution for reducing the number of working hours of indoor staff to fifty-four hours per week. The committee of visitors accordingly agreed that all cuts previously made in the pay of officers and staff of the NWCMH be restored, backdated to 1 July of that year.[28] This also followed the active opposition of the Asylum Workers' Union to the cuts in salary and altera-tions to conditions of service.

These wage cuts had been the result of the deteriorating economic situation nationwide that had left the county councils strapped for cash. As indicated earlier, a problem of the system of funding which prevailed up until the Second World War was that, while central government set standards and could recommend improvements, investment decisions were delegated to local government. Now local authorities were being forced into financial retrench-ment with the committee of visitors trapped in the middle. They could listen to advice from the Board of Control, observe good practice and make recommendations, but as representatives these delegates had to obtain the backing of their full county council for major capital expenditure decisions.

Within its allocated budget the house committee gave considerable thought to the purchases of technical equipment. In 1934 the committee of visitors decided to investigate the purchase of new X-ray equipment. They deputed Dr J. H. O. Roberts, the assistant medical officer, to attend an international exhibition at Zurich, 'with a view to securing information as to the most recent and up-to-date appliances'.

Some basic equipment installed early in the century also required upgrading. The internal telephone system was replaced in 1931 by a new and superior one. Telephones were becoming more available generally in north Wales, but were still restricted in terms of private use. The North Wales Counties Mental Hospital was known to many simply by its telephone number. It is said that if any member of a local family behaved strangely the usual response was to exclaim 'Oh dear, it looks as if we'll have to phone Denbigh 7'.

New Treatments

The classification of diseases and the treatments may have been slow to change, but a number of new therapies did emerge to displace some longer established approaches. One of the first diseases to be treated by a new and novel method was general paralysis of the insane (GPI). During the second half of the nineteenth century experts on the disease began to identify evidence of the link between syphilis and general paresis. Research by Krafft-Ebing in 1897, and more by Nissl and Alzheimer, published in 1904, brought about a general recognition of its syphilitic origin. In 1913 Noguchi and Moore demonstrated the direct link between syphilis and paresis when they identified the syphilitic spirochete in the brains of paretics.[29] In 1916 Wasserman introduced a serum test to show up active and latent lesions produced by syphilis. The link between syphilis and GPI was thereby firmly established.

Long before this, practitioners had observed that, when patients suffered a high fever, the development of general paralysis was often checked. In 1917 Wagner-Jauregg began infecting patients who were suffering from GPI with malaria, and saw significant improvements. By 1921 he reported that a quarter of the first 200 subjects so treated had improved sufficiently to be able to return to work.[30] The treatment was rapidly adopted outside Austria, and was first introduced in Britain at the Whittingham Mental Hospital in Lancashire in 1922.[31]

There were wide regional variations in the recorded incidence of general paralysis of the insane. At Whittingham Hospital GPI was a significant problem, accounting in 1924 for 26.5 per cent of the male deaths at the hospital. In north Wales there were never more than a few cases, although inevitably the results were fatal. In the years following the First World War the NWCMH, like other hospitals, witnessed a rise in the number of admissions of GPI patients as a result of men having contracted syphilis during military service (see table). Screening of all patients was first carried out in 1929, confirming that the percentage of patients testing positive for GPI was very low for a mental hospital. The reason, according to the newly appointed pathologist, was that north Wales was 'mainly an agricultural district, with few large towns and without a floating population'.[32] The proportion was usually much higher in cities, especially in large ports.

	Incidence of general paralysis of the insane at Denbigh, 1924–30
	Cases admitted
1924	3
1925	3
1926	6
1927	8
1928	12
1929	7
1930	8

Malarial treatment of GPI commenced at the NWCMH in January 1924, when a patient was transferred to Upton Mental Hospital in Chester, which offered the required facilities. After receiving inoculations of malaria the patient was discharged to his home, having in the opinion of the medical staff 'recovered'. Dr Frank Jones was very positive about the benefits, stating that in his opinion 'in early and suitable cases of G.P.I. the disease can be arrested by this Malarial treatment'.[33] The claim was not that it would be cured, but that it could be kept in abeyance if treatment was available soon after the onset of the paralytic stage.

Inoculating with malaria could be dangerous, and not only to the patient, since malaria could be transmitted to others by a bite from an infected mosquito. Therefore, elaborate isolation precautions had to be taken. Before the process of infecting patients could be commenced at Denbigh it was necessary that a facility be 'lined with wire gauze and the exit and entrance door doubled and lined with wire gauze to prevent the exit of any mosquitos from the ward'.[34] By 1930 eight patients had visited Upton Mental Hospital for treatment, and three of them had recovered.[35]

Finding any treatment for GPI was a major breakthrough because it rendered a disease hitherto regarded as both incurable and fatal susceptible to medical intervention.[36] If this dreaded disease could be challenged, what other treatment might not emerge to release other patients from their imprisonment within differing forms of insanity? For the nursing staff this one breakthrough had a significant impact on their outlook and approach to their own role in the hospital. They began to identify themselves more closely with the mainstream nursing profession as it increased their general faith in scientifically grounded progress towards conquering mental illnesses. Therefore, although the numbers of patients affected by this new therapeutic innovation were very small in terms of the total patient population, the implications were broader.

In 1930 medical staff at the NWCMH decided to experiment with the sulphur injection method as an alternative to malarial treatment. This proved equally successful in producing high temperatures, and similarly resulted in 'improvement in some cases'.[37] The treatment of GPI created the opportunity for experimentation with a growing array of pharmacological preparations, so that the room just sealed with protective wire was no longer required. Only one case was treated with induced malaria during 1936–7, and that case failed to show any improvement.[38] When seven cases of GPI were admitted in 1937–8, four of them were treated with TAB or pyrifer injections followed by tryparsamide and bismuth injections. Of these, three showed a clinical improvement.[39]

In an interview a retired member of staff, charge nurse Kearns, recalled the malarial treatments for what he described as the 'cruel and crippling disease' of GPI. By the end patients could do nothing for themselves. Their knees would be contorted right up to the chin and nurses fed them with a spoon. 'If they had been an animal they would have been shot', he said. Sufferers of GPI invariably had 'delusions of grandeur', and some had 'the most fantastic ideas'. One man claimed to own a fleet of silver submarines patrolling the coast off Rhyl. Often men believed themselves to be king of England, and at one point in time they had two patients claiming the throne, each one angrily maintaining that the other was an impostor. To survive nursing on a ward where there was so little hope of recovery, a sense of humour was helpful. Some men developing GPI in the 1930s after earlier contracting syphilis during war service were by then in their mid-thirties, with wives who had no knowledge of this past episode in their husbands' lives. The staff found it very difficult to explain to a wife the nature of her husband's disease, and the morbid prospect before her – that she would be left a widow, perhaps with young children to raise alone, even that she herself may have contracted the disease. Nursing attendants were taught that only about 4 per cent of all cases of syphilis resulted in GPI.[40] They knew that the patient's destiny was simply 'the luck of the draw'.

Dementia Praecox

It was in the inter-war years that psychiatrists in Europe and America devoted themselves to the search for an effective treatment for schizophrenia, which was now recognized to be the cause of much long-term chronic illness. Research work was focusing primarily upon biological treatments. At Denbigh, in 1931 Dr Sidney Davies treated five cases of dementia praecox with colloidal sulphur, but the results were unpromising, and the experiment discontinued.[41]

Neither the annual reports for the NWCMH nor the patient case notes make use of the term 'schizophrenia' during these years, although it was by this time in general use. It is evident, nonetheless, that staff were conversant with the latest treatments for this condition, so it is unclear why they retained the older term of 'dementia praecox'. They were well aware that this was the one condition that produced a majority of their long-stay patients. As Dr Frank Jones explained: 'Although responsible for only about 15% of admissions into a mental hospital, the fact that dementia praecox was rarely recoverable and occurred in young people likely to live many years, resulted in these patients forming well over half the chronic mental hospital population.'[42]

Jacob Klasi of Zurich first introduced prolonged sleep therapy in 1920, employing the drug somnifen, already adopted for its calming effect in cases of delirium tremens and tetanus. Klasi thought that it might help in 'breaking the vicious cycle between psychic excitation, psychomotor activity and the increase in psychic excitation' so typical of agitated schizophrenics.[43] First used at NWCMH in 1937, five cases of agitated melancholia and mania were treated with somnifane injections to induce prolonged narcosis. The outcome was disappointing. As only one case recovered and the others showed but a short, temporary improvement.[44]

The discovery of insulin in 1921 by two Canadian researchers, Frederick Banting and Charles Best, turned attention to the role of the pancreas in maintaining the equilibrium of glucose in the body. A lack of insulin causes diabetes, whereas an excess of insulin causes hypoglycaemia, inducing the body to go into a coma or convulsions through lack of glucose reaching the brain cells. In 1927 a young Polish neuroscientist, Manfred Sakel, was experimenting with insulin when he accidentally caused convulsions in a patient by administering an overdose.[45] The patient experienced a remarkable recovery in her mental condition. In 1936 a representative of the British Board of Control, Dr Isobel Wilson, visited the clinic in Vienna where Sakel had later pioneered the technique of insulin shock therapy. She recommended that one hospital in the UK should trial the approach. It was taken up by Dr Pullar Strecker at the Royal Edinburgh Hospital for Mental Disorders, and was later adopted by other mental hospitals in England and Wales.[46]

Meanwhile, in Budapest, Ladislaus von Meduna had been experimenting with another form of shock therapy. Noting what appeared to be a biological antagonism between epilepsy and schizophrenia he reasoned that artificially induced epileptic convulsions might potentially offer a cure for schizophrenia and proceeded to develop a compound (subsequently marketed by a German company under the trade name of cardiazol). The results published by von Meduna claimed an 80 to 90 per cent remission in cases of under six months duration. However, where the illness was of over one year's duration the chance of success would sink rapidly. After his findings were communicated to the international psychiatric community in 1937, two representatives of the Board of Control were deputed to visit Budapest to evaluate the technique. The treatment was then taken up swiftly at mental hospitals in the United Kingdom, initially at Bexley, West Park, Goodmayes and Arlesley.[47]

Medical staff at Denbigh began to conduct their own tentative experiments with the new therapies becoming available. During 1938 fifty cases at the NWCMH were treated with cardiazol, and following the treatment half of these were discharged, eighteen of them as having recovered and eight as 'relieved'. Of the patients who still remained in the hospital an improvement had been detected in eight and according to Dr Jones this meant that they had become 'more useful and happy members of our community'. These outcomes appeared very favourable, and suggestive of a significant breakthrough in the treatment of dementia praecox. Cardiazol had to be administered intravenously, and an alternative, triazol, which could be administered intramuscularly was also introduced. This was beneficial in some cases.

Dr Jones had by this time learned that insulin shock treatment was considered superior to cardiazol, and that it was likely to give better results. Presumably he had either read or been informed of a recent evaluation report by two commissioners of the Board of Control,[48] or perhaps he had spoken to colleagues elsewhere.[49] A special unit was set up and six male patients began to receive insulin shock treatment in March 1939. If cardiazol required careful monitoring of the patient's condition, insulin shock treatment required even more. It was very exacting in terms of nursing, as staff who worked at the hospital during these years recall it as potentially dangerous.[50]

Less radical therapies also played an important part in conveying to the public the idea that the hospital provided a modern curative regime. Patients were carefully screened on admission, and those with the best prospects for early recovery were nursed in the new reception unit in Gwynfryn and offered what might be seen as more benign therapies. In 1935 the visiting commissioners reported that 'Plombiere lavage and continuous baths are now available'.[51] This therapy had been in use for some time in Cardiff and other hospitals.[52] Patients would usually be placed in the bath at 7 o'clock in the morning and would remain there until 5 in the afternoon. They would be served breakfast, lunch and tea in the bath. It was considered especially efficacious in the case of very agitated patients.

The new facilities at Gwynfryn were also equipped to provide infra-red and ultra-violet rays.[53] Some patients were said to respond well to this therapy, particularly those suffering from melancholia. Some psychiatrists believed that it worked to best effect on those patients who were open to suggestion, and that its success was mainly the result of psychological influence rather than any physiological benefit. Whereas relaxation and water therapy were considered suitable for some patients, exertion and activity were considered beneficial for others. At both the reception ward and the main building, attendant Kearns led suitable male patients in physical drill in the open air.[54] This was thought bracing, a good way of channelling energy and was based on the assumption that a healthy body is the foundation for a healthy mind.

Dental Hygiene

There was an increasing emphasis on all-round health and hygiene, and on the unity between bodily and psychological health. Attention to teeth was all part of the new philosophy of care. In 1921 the Board of Control inspector noted with approval that at last 'Tooth brushes are now available for all patients desiring one', adding cryptically that he hoped it would be possible 'to persuade a still greater number to use them'.[55] The appointment of a dental surgeon to attend to the patients was also proposed at this time. In 1924 the visiting committee appointed Charles Hubbard to the post of visiting dentist, one he occupied for the next thirty years. During his first year he attended to 846 patients, and extracted a total of 1,862 teeth with local anaesthetic. He treated only 230 female patients, compared with 616 males, which he attributed to the fact that females 'are as a rule, more nervous than the males'. Several cases of gingivitis, stomatitis and pyorrhoea were notified, and one patient was found to be suffering from a tumour in the mandible.[56]

Research work being carried out at the University of Birmingham was suggesting a startling link between focal sepsis and insanity.[57] Adherents to this notion believed that bacterial poisoning caused by rotting teeth could trigger mental disorders; thus dental treatment could be a key to preventing mental illness. A dental service was completely lacking in most parts of Wales, and people would often resort to having their teeth pulled at fairs. Most patients arriving in the 1920s and before would never have visited a dentist prior to admission. In 1928 it was reported that one patient in the NWCMH had recovered as soon as the dentist had removed his very septic teeth.[58] There is little doubt that improved dental hygiene worked to the benefit of the patient's health and well-being, but there is no evidence to suggest that in Denbigh it led to any increase in the rate of recovery from mental illness.

Occupational Therapy

Ever since the establishment of the asylum in 1848, employment had been regarded as a primary tool in the therapeutic regime of the institution. As has been shown, patient labour played a vital role in much of the routine work of the asylum. The laundry and the kitchen, even the wards, operated with a large input from patients. Male patients contributed much of the outdoor labour in the large kitchen garden and fields of vegetables. Their work was integral to the domestic economy of the asylum.

The newly emerging discipline of occupational therapy (OT) involved a rather different emphasis. The normal routine of the hospital was for the working patients to go to their posts immediately after breakfast. It was customary for the remaining patients, other than those on the sick ward, to be turned out into the airing courts, where they would be left to wander around until lunchtime. After lunch they would once more be put outside. Rainy days were the occasion of some difficulty, and awnings and corrugated iron coverings were erected over the airing courts. There was a strong emphasis on outdoor exercise, but it was often rather purposeless. It was for these patients that occupational therapy was urged as much as for those already considered 'useful'. Patients with little interest or ability were to be encouraged to do simple tasks and, with repetition, to acquire skills that would help them, if not to recover, at least to gain basic competencies. Advanced ideas on OT were developed by Dr Hermann Simon at the mental hospital at Gutersloh in Germany, and were adopted by the Dutch. Between 1928 and 1931 members of the Board of Control went to Germany and Holland and were so impressed with the atmosphere of harmony and high recovery rates they found in the continental establishments that they returned determined to promote occupational therapy in the UK.[59]

In 1934 committee members of the NWCMH paid a visit to Upton Mental Hospital, Chester, where Dr Hamilton Grills's enthusiastic adoption of the new practices had earned the praise of the commissioners. The introduction of modern occupational therapy required trained staff and it also required suitable accommodation, not easy to provide in an overcrowded hospital with resources fully stretched. Once again a step-by-step approach was adopted at Denbigh. Mrs Howe Thomas of Mold was appointed to attend the hospital two mornings a week, instructing a group of male patients on one morning, and female patients on the other.[60] Additionally, in

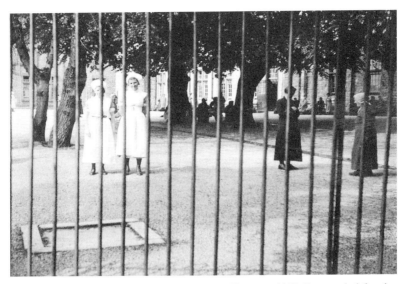

11. Nurses and patients in the airing courts, 1939. The nurses, Nellie Jones on the left and Betty Davies on the right, both became ward sisters. The airing courts were an original feature of the asylum and patients who were unable to work were put in the airing courts and allowed to wander around for most of the day. High iron railings surrounded them to prevent patients escaping. Denbighshire Record Office

1937 charge attendant Jones was selected to pay weekly visits to the Upton Mental Hospital, and 'through the kindness of Dr Hamilton Grills' he was given free instruction in handicrafts.[61]

A temporary room was made available by partitioning off part of a corridor and new brush-making equipment was installed. The bulk of the articles produced were used within the institution, but some would be put on sale to visitors. An informant recounted how he never knew of his father's stay at the asylum until the day he casually inquired about a stool in the living room, and to his surprise was told that it had been made by his father when he was a patient at the Denbigh asylum. The period of mental illness had never before been spoken of, but the plaited leather and wooden stool remained as proof of his father's brief incarceration. Not hidden away, it had become a familiar piece of household furniture.

The output of the new occupational therapy workshops in 1938–9 included seventy-three floor rugs, twelve willow hampers, thirty-five shopping baskets, sixty-six scrubbing brushes, thirty-one stools, and 430 dish cloths and pieces of furniture, embroidery, knitted goods and raffia work.

However, the number of patients involved in OT remained proportionally very small, particularly on the women's side of the hospital. Commissioners inspecting the asylum in October 1938 urged the committee of visitors to appoint without delay a full-time occupation officer who would train the nurses, in order that they could cooperate 'whole-heartedly in training the patients'. The commissioners also administered a sharp rebuke: 'The depressing sight of hundreds of patients walking the ward gardens for hours every day should exist no longer.'[62]

Nonetheless, the overall impression gained by the visiting inspectors during the inter-war years was of a hospital where close attention was given to the basic needs and care of the patients. Two commissioners, one of whom had inspected the institution in 1933, visited in July 1939 and were favourably impressed with the changes that had taken place, and the 'rapidity of modernization in all directions'.[63] They admired the abundance of flowers and pot plants, the 'gradual improvement of female under-clothing', the new medicine cupboards and the well-equipped operating theatre. 'In the wards the patients are given the benefit of the most up-to-date forms of treatment including cardiazol, triazol and insulin in dementia praecox and epanutin in epilepsy. All of these drugs have given results sufficiently encouraging for their continued use.'[64] From providing pot plants to cardiazol treatment the hospital was at least seen to be making an effort on behalf of its patients.

✳

CHAPTER TEN

Patients and Staff in the Inter-War Years

While medical and policy changes were taking place in the wider world, life within the asylum maintained its own even momentum. The institution was still organized according to the old hierarchical structure, although with a tiny, if stable, medical staff it was the nursing and artisan staff who did most to sustain the continuity of care. On the nursing front there was a distinct pattern, whereby a solid core of extremely long-serving male and unmarried female staff persisted alongside a fairly rapid turnover of newer recruits. Despite the economic depression it proved difficult to retain female nursing staff at Denbigh. The work demanded long hours and an enormous amount of patience and stamina.

Medical Staff

The appointment of Welsh-speaking staff continued to be a priority since the majority of patients used Welsh. Dr Frank Jones welcomed the appointment of Dr Sidney Davies as junior assistant medical officer in 1921 and considered that his knowledge of Welsh would be 'a valuable asset in carrying out his duties'.[1] Davies remained on the staff until 1933 when he moved to take up the position of medical superintendent at the Carmarthen Asylum.[2] He was succeeded by another Welsh-speaking psychiatrist, Dr J. H. O. Roberts, who eventually became medical superintendent in 1940. This ensured a continued succession of staff familiar with the unique linguistic and cultural facets of the hospital.

The asylum was overcrowded to the extent of about 20 per cent and a medical staff of three was quite inadequate for over a thousand patients. There was pressing need for additional medical staff. The visiting commissioners were insistent that the hospital should have its own laboratory and appoint a pathologist. Although discussed in 1922 the matter was deferred owing to lack of financial resources.

In 1926, with another severe outbreak of asylum dysentery, swab cultures had to be sent for analysis by the Chester Royal Infirmary Laboratory. Dr

Frank Jones sought advice from Rainhill Asylum, where they 'claim to be stamping out the disease'. Usually, their pathologist told him, the disease could be traced to a carrier and strict isolation of cases was necessary.[3]

Recurrent outbreaks of dysentery and colitis increased the pressure on management to make a pathology appointment. Finally in 1928 this was agreed and Dr Jones sought candidates who could combine the role with that of relief doctor. He asked the Welsh School of Medicine, Cardiff, if it could recommend someone who was Welsh-speaking.[4] Dr Ceinwen Evans's name was proposed. She had 'extensive experience of pathological work', gained in the laboratories of the university and the Welsh National Memorial Association, the voluntary body established to tackle the problem of tuberculosis in Wales.[5]

Laboratory Work

On arrival at Denbigh, Dr Evans was surprised to discover no equipped laboratory.[6] However, she was offered the services of a carpenter to construct one and within nine months she fitted a laboratory with enough scientific equipment to commence regular work. As a medical officer, Dr Evans was on duty on the evening and weekend rotas and sometimes deputized on the wards. Primarily, however, she considered herself a pathologist, and there was ample work to keep her busy.

Her first objective was to identify the dysentery carriers; she analysed over 500 specimens of faeces. She also performed twenty-nine postmortems and at the end of 1929 began systematic tests on all the male patients for general paralysis, using both Wasserman and flocculation techniques. In all she conducted 772 Wasserman and 765 flocculation tests and 660 bacteriological examinations, as well as routine analysis of blood, urine, and throat and nasal swabs.

In 1932 the commissioners spoke approvingly of the useful work being undertaken in the bacteriological laboratory, where more than a thousand excretal samples had been examined for dysentery.[7] The incidence of dysentery at Denbigh now compared unfavourably with that of other mental hospitals. The Board of Control drew attention to this, pointing out that an 'outstanding feature of the health statistics of this hospital is the high incidence of dysentery. Whereas the mean rate of new notifications of dysentery in all Mental hospitals of England and Wales in 1931 was 3.5 per thousand of population, in Denbigh the rate was 38.'[8] The problem was stubborn and recurrent, and Dr Evans's systematic work of identifying carriers and isolating infective patients was carried out over a period of years.

After repeated attempts to bring the situation under control, in January and March 1938 the hospital experienced yet another outbreak of dysentery, this time involving 129 patients. Dr Evans's analysis identified an organism that had the same morphological and biochemical characteristics as one found in 1935, designated 'atypical B. dysenteriae'. She sent specimen cultures away to Dr W. M. Scott of the Ministry of Health. He identified the organism as B.dynsenteriae Schmitz., previously unknown in the United Kingdom, and believed to have been the cause of the recurrent dysentery outbreaks in Denbigh. From her analysis of the evidence Dr Evans concluded that the Schmitz bacillus was a pathogen.[9] Her findings were published in *The Lancet.*

This success reflected Dr Evans's continuing interest in research and involvement with a wider academic community, particularly with her former colleagues in Cardiff. Together they carried out joint investigations into tuberculosis, which similarly presented a problem of considerable proportion for the Denbigh asylum. In 1931 she began to follow a line of inquiry initiated by Professor Cummins of the Welsh School of Medicine. She inoculated 304 patients intradermally with old tuberculin in varying strength, and then performed sedimentation tests on blood from fifty patients who had the highest positive reaction and fifty who had the lowest.[10] Results indicated that there was a marked variation in reactivity amongst patients who were free from active tuberculosis, leading to the conclusion that probably many of the 'healthy' patients had encountered minute doses of tubercle bacillary infection, but had developed a resistance. She also detected a marked difference in the pattern between males and females. These points of scientific interest were published in the *British Medical Journal* in a paper co-authored with Professor Lyle Cummins.[11]

Pathology might have seemed an unusual choice for a woman, but a minor physical handicap partly contributed to Dr Evans's decision to follow this career path. A childhood ailment caused mild deafness, but the condition was forecast to become progressively worse. It presented a problem when it came to detecting a heartbeat. Her professors in Cardiff advised that it would be better for her to concentrate on dealing with people who no longer had a heartbeat, so she became a pathologist! It was not uncommon for women to be directed into this occupation, and also into mental hospitals, which had low status relative to general hospitals, as another pathologist, at the Royal Edinburgh Asylum, Isobel Hutton, recalled in her memoirs.[12]

Dr Ceinwen Evans remained at Denbigh for the rest of her career. She was an exceptional woman, yet one who also represents the situation and dilemmas of other professional medical women of her time. She was sensitive to the social difficulties of female patients. However, as pathologist she was also convinced that many patients were in fact suffering from physiological diseases, such as cancers, heart conditions or diabetes, which went undiagnosed by psychiatrists. 'They were too busy looking for the neuroses', she said.[13]

Another New Appointment

Due to increasing patient numbers and the demands of providing a more modern hospital service, the insufficiency of staff again became a pressing problem. Dr Evans's ward duties interfered with the smooth running of the laboratory and, in the absence of either Dr Davies or Dr Hutton, the medical superintendent had to cover the male or female wings. His own administrative duties were becoming more onerous, and he was increasingly involved with outpatient clinics, a time-consuming task in a vast rural area. In 1936 it was officially put on record that the hospital was understaffed medically, and the following year the committee of visitors decided to approve the appointment of an additional doctor. The scientific orientation of the establishment was reinforced by the arrival in November 1937 of a young doctor with an interest in the application of new treatments, Dr Ernst Schwarz.[14] He was a German refugee who had come to the UK in 1934. He requalified and took a psychiatric qualification in Scotland. 'Very method-ical' was the phrase most used in staff recollections of this new appointee. According to Dr Evans, he was 'taken aback' by the number of long-term chronic cases in the hospital, and quickly tried to distance himself from dealing with them. He must also have experienced a 'culture shock' on his arrival at Denbigh, where the language was predominantly Welsh, and the customary practices little changed from the previous century. Within a short time of his taking up post the house committee accepted a motion to the effect that in future the special linguistic needs of the hospital should be taken into account when appointing new staff. This was the first of a series of objections to the appointment of non–Welsh-speakers.

Multiplication of the Unfit?

Although long since retired, Dr W. W. Herbert continued to take an interest in matters of public health and patient welfare. His election as chairman of the Denbighshire County Council 'Committee for the Care of Mental Defectives', gave him a platform from which to advance eugenicist views. In this way one of the controversial politico-medical debates of the day obliquely touched the NWCMH. In 1930 Dr Herbert proposed to his county council that the 'multiplication of the unfit' should be limited.[15] He advocated instructing all married women in birth control, justifying this proposition from his certain knowledge that 'Vast numbers of wives suffered insanity due to pregnancy.'[16] He also began to petition the management committees of the NWCMH with a resolution in favour of sterilization of the mentally defective.[17] His proposal was treated with the utmost caution. When first presented in April 1930 it was considered by the finance committee, which deferred discussion in order to allow time to receive a report from the medical superintendent.[18] A further resolution was received from Denbighshire County Council in July and was tabled together with the report from Dr Frank Jones. This time consideration was postponed 'until after receipt of a report by the Mental Hospitals' Association of the result of their deliberations thereon'.[19] Clearly the hospital management, alert to the political nature of the issue, was anxious not to act precipitately. In August 1930 members received a letter and pamphlet from the Eugenics Society.[20] The rationale used by the Eugenics Society for advocating sterilization was that, whereas the higher social classes had taken advantage of contraceptive information, 'the class from which defectives tend to spring cannot practise the abstinence recommended by the Churches, and it lacks the self-control and intelligence necessary to use existing contraceptive methods'.[21] The pamphlet in question outlined a draft for a parliamentary bill. This would consist of clauses designed to facilitate the voluntary sterilization of 'three classes of person: (1) mental defectives (2) the recovered insane and (3) persons suffering from grave transmissable diseases and defects other than insanity and mental defectiveness, or those desiring to avoid procreation on eugenic grounds'. Since there were ongoing professional discussions of the issue at national level, the finance committee of the NWCMH deputed Dr Frank Jones to attend the National Health Congress and report back. Eventually a printed report of the congress was received, and there followed no further debate on the question of sterilization. Whilst Dr Herbert's own position indicates an adherence to eugenic views, it also displays a genuine concern for the women in question. He advocated setting up Women Welfare Clinics to which sufferers from tuberculosis or heart or kidney diseases, for whom pregnancy would be especially dangerous, could be referred. He envisaged clinics providing advice 'and subsequent supervision' for 'women on discharge from mental hospitals', adding that 'The propagation of their kind by these unfortunates account for the steady increase in number and size of our Mental Hospitals with corresponding cost.'[22] Although the committee of the NWCMH never adopted Dr Herbert's views, birth control clinics were established by Denbighshire County Council to pioneer the provision of birth control advice in north Wales.[23]

Nursing Staff

During the inter-war years there was a gradual change in the status of the nursing staff. Mr Tom Hughes, Bangor, joined in 1918 at the age of twenty-one.[24] He mainly learnt his nursing craft from older colleagues, although he received some formal instruction. During the 1920s Dr Eustace Hutton gave lectures in 'Mental Nursing' to apprentice nurses, although this only amounted to one hour per week.[25] Candidates had to learn the content of what was referred to as 'the Red Book', the colloquial name given to the *Handbook for Mental Nurses,* a text authorized by the Royal Medico-Psychological Association.[26] This textbook provided basic instruction on general nursing, dealing with anatomy and physiology, first aid, hygiene, bodily diseases and the principles of nursing the sick. The second half was devoted to psychiatry, introducing the notion of the 'healthy mind', outlining the causes of nervous and mental disease, cataloguing signs and symptoms of mental disturbance and explaining the special nursing requirements of certain mental disorders. The course introduced the students to hereditary, physiogenic and psychogenic explanations of mental illness. Candidates might sit the examination of the Royal Medico-Psychological Society, although there was no requirement to obtain this qualification. Indeed very few succeeded in passing, although it was explained that 'the small number of nurses who hold the Medico-Psychological Certificate is due to the fact that many of them understood English insufficiently well to do credit to themselves in an examination held entirely in that language'.[27] By 1934 thirty-one of the men and nineteen of the female staff were certificated or registered as mental nurses, and twenty-six men and twenty-three women had passed the preliminary examination.[28] With the opening of the new nurses' home and the appointment of a sister-tutor, greater emphasis was placed upon staff training.

The promotion of nursing staff took place in strict accordance with length of service.[29] This meant that advancement was based on age and experience, but helped to ensure a career structure for all, giving continuity of long-serving staff.[30] The committee of visitors always warmly acknowledged the contribution of senior staff on their retirement. Mr Collins, the head attendant on the male side, retired in 1934 after thirty-six years service and deputy head attendant, John Evans, after forty-four years service. They retired to what was in the period of economic depression a relatively generous pension, compared with their contemporaries who had not had the opportunity to work steadily in superannuated employment.

This workforce stability not withstanding, there was a considerable turnover, particularly on the female side. Some of the trainees did not take to the work, while others stayed and became very proficient, only to have to resign upon their 'impending marriage'. The marriage bar resulted in a considerable drain on experienced female staff.

Daytime shifts began at 7.00 a.m. and finished at 8.00 p.m. There was some variation in hours during the inter-war years, as the trade unions won and lost concessions, but, even when there was a reduction, staff still worked a split shift in order to provide cover for the same length of working day. General nursing standards were maintained during the inter-war period and, as far as their physical welfare was concerned, the patients seem to have been well cared for. Tom Hughes recalled that everything was kept spotlessly clean, with careful attention to standards on the sick wards. The commissioner wrote in his report for 1929: 'I gladly record the freedom from bedsores in all the 111 deaths. This speaks well for the care given by the nursing staff.'[31] He also noted that the medical needs of the patients were well supplied, and that sedatives were used sparingly. Patients continued to assist in cleaning the wards, and carried out various tasks under the direction of the staff.

Unmarried staff had to live in, and if a member of the male staff wished to marry and live outside he had to ask the permission of the medical superintendent at least six months in advance. Although this was never refused, it was a strict requirement, and highly symbolic of the patriarchal structure of the asylum. The strict marriage bar for women was enforced throughout the inter-war period.[32] Fraternization between male and female staff was still strictly forbidden, and a male member of staff was never allowed to talk to a female member in the corridors, even if it was his own sister.[33] In the case of any breach of discipline or detection of improper behaviour staff were called upon to resign. The large collection of personal records of members of staff employed at the hospital revealed a surprising number of examples of female nurses brought before the medical super-intendent and 'asked to resign'. Occasionally breaches of discipline on the male side led to summary dismissal.

Prior to the opening of the nurses' home, staff quarters were situated in cramped conditions in the main hospital building, and a shortage of night staff often meant that off-duty staff would be called upon to help out in emergencies. Nurses' lives were dominated by the institution, but for all the hard work and discipline it was an interesting place to be employed and offered a variety of social experiences. A grand ball was held over the Christmas season. This was the great event of the year, the staff counterpart to the patients' Christmas Ball. The dining hall decorations were a work of art. Many members of staff recalled Dudley, a patient who spent much of his life making the decorations. Once all the lights, tinsels and paper chains were taken down at the end of the dance, he would begin preparing for the following year, working diligently to create a wonderful atmosphere for the next Christmas. His dedicated activity filled the entire twelve months, but for most inhabitants of the asylum the annual festivities were but a brief highlight of the entertainment calendar. The summer picnics and sports day and harvest thanksgivings were similarly welcomed as diversions from the weekly routine.

Such festive rituals fulfilled a role in marking out time in this long-term institution, and for people confined within its walls they imposed a rhythm. They were important not only for the patients but for the staff, symbolically signifying that the institution constituted an organic whole, of which everyone was a part. Functionally, then, they served to bind the staff together and to underpin a very necessary sense of shared identity and common purpose. This observation is not intended to convey the impression that harmonious relationships characterized every aspect of the institution's life. Power struggles, conflict and accommodation are also detectable, although it is possible to argue that, given the long-stay nature and the less differentiated professional structure of this type of hospital at this time, a sense of 'community' prevailed.

Artisan Staff

The craftsmen and artisans as well as the nursing staff were valued for their skills. In 1937 the chairman of the committee of visitors expressed his regret at the loss sustained

> in the death of their Waterman, William Williams, who had been in their service for 35 years and who, with his native shrewdness and expert knowledge of conditions in the hills round about the source of our water supply, has been of considerable value to the Institution.[34]

The inadequacy of the water supply had for so long been a problem at this institution that the skilful conservation of this resource was vital. Williams was responsible for the reservoir at Llyn Brân, which drew water from the peaty moors above Denbigh.

The bailiff at the asylum farm was an experienced stockman who bred pedigree pigs. In 1932 over one hundred home-fed bullocks were slaughtered for food, while the pigs slaughtered that year were worth £1,560. The value of the beef, veal, mutton and lamb was £3,574 and the fresh daily milk worth £1,237.[35]

When new staff came to the hospital they were introduced to a work culture where long-serving members of staff had well-established reputations, contributing positively to the general ethos of the hospital. The permanency of some staff may have inhibited change during certain periods, but it did perpetuate a strong sense of occupational security. Many families in the surrounding area had relatives who had worked in the asylum for generations. Of course, more cynical observers have sometimes claimed that the asylum was run for the employees' benefit rather than for that of the patients.

The hospital did employ some female staff with married names, but usually they were women who had been widowed. When Mrs May Jones, the head laundress, retired in 1923 after thirty years' service, the committee awarded her a period of four years' additional service, in order that she could qualify for a full two-thirds pension.[36] It was gestures of this kind which members of staff valued so much. Dr Ceinwen Evans singled out the super-annuation scheme as being one of the main reasons why the hospital succeeded in retaining such loyal staff. Few other employers in the area offered a generous pension, giving the hospital staff an advantage that counted for a great deal in pre-war Wales.

Recreational Life

A high priority was still given to the provision of entertainment. The commissioners frequently recorded their approval of the activities. In 1922, for instance, they reported that 'A good deal is done at this institution to amuse and occupy the patients', and remarked upon the excellent bowling green, the weekly cinema entertainment and the 'ample opportunity for dancing'.

Football continued to be of importance in the asylum's recreational life. Both staff and patients took great pride in the hospital's team. The male patients, in addition to playing, were also admitted to away league matches free of charge. Cricket featured during the summer months and there was still croquet on the lawn. Selected patients could even go for a round of golf at the local club. During the 1920s tennis became 'exceedingly popular' with the staff, so that it was found necessary to lay out new tennis courts on the recreation ground 'in order to meet the great demand for the game'.[37] There was an annual sports day, in which many patients competed, and others watched. They also had summer fêtes, picnics by the hospital reservoir and days on the beach at Rhyl and Pensarn.

Indoor amusements included twice-weekly cinema showings.[38] Some whist drives and dances were open to guests from outside. The proceeds of these events were used to improve the facilities and purchase a new 'talkie' projector. In 1933, before this equipment was purchased, a special programme for patients was provided at the cinema in Denbigh on Friday afternoons.[39] To the great delight of patients and staff the new sound projector was installed in the large reception hall in 1934.[40] Unfortunately the Board of Control inspectors criticized the fire safety measures, and its use had to be curtailed. Amateur dramatics companies from the surrounding counties continued to visit, and musical concerts were performed before the patients. Since such activities involved many outsiders this rendered them an important means of integrating the hospital with communities throughout north Wales.

Standards of Care

The emphasis on occupation and entertainment that helped to promote healthy interaction between staff and patients is what many members of the staff have remembered. The reminiscences of ex-patients are less readily available, but the rapport between staff and patients was observed by the commissioners, who could be censorious enough if they observed deficiencies in the system. When they inspected the asylum in 1924 they remarked upon 'the good feeling existing between patients and medical and nursing staff', and saw this is as the basis for the 'general tone of contentment', and the minimum of excitement amongst the patients.[41]

The commissioners would scrutinize the standards of cleanliness and the quality of food. They approved a 'good dinner of boiled bacon and potatoes, with rice pudding to follow' and deplored the amount of tinned milk being used. They disapproved of the use of corned beef. Many patients required assistance in cutting it up, and it was not a popular dish.[42] The commissioners were legally responsible for monitoring the dietary standards and after the accusations of Montagu Lomax there followed a thorough review of diets in all mental hospitals. On the whole the committee of inquiry found that the dinners provided in most mental hospitals were of good quality and sufficient in quantity, but they drew attention to the 'marked monotony' of diet in many cases.[43] This was their main criticism when they visited Denbigh, and they suggested providing a less predictable cycle of menus. A dietary scale for rate-maintained patients was provided in the annual report for the Denbigh hospital for 1925–6, showing the allowance of different items per patient, and the 'formula' used for soups and stews. Another scale was provided for private patients, which of course included the service patients. Private patients had twice as much meat for dinner and superior breakfasts.

Private Patients and Relatives

Thirty women patients were classed as private in 1935 and eighty-one men, although of these sixty-one were service patients. After the First World War the Ministry of Pensions had agreed to accept financial responsibility for ex-service cases where it could be shown that their illness was 'attributable' to the war. The remaining private patients were paid for by their families. The correspondence files of the asylum include a number of letters from distressed relatives who found the cost of maintenance over a long period an enormous drain on their resources. They wrote to the hospital administrator seeking either a reduction of the charge, or transfer of the patient to the rate-maintained category. Mr Barker, the clerk, contacted the public assistance officer of Llangefni, for instance, regarding the circumstances of a man who was paying for his wife to be cared for as a private patient. The committee had already granted a reduction in the fee but, as Barker explained, 'This gentleman is a grocer in a small way, and, owing to

competition, is earning a bare living only'. The committee now suggested
that the woman be transferred to the rate-aided class where the charge was
18s. 1d. The husband or father of a rate-aided patient had to be assessed and
might have to contribute in full to the cost, but the charge was materially less
than the 2 guineas or more for a patient in the private class. There are letters
from a widow about her son. The prognosis was very bleak and the burden
of maintaining him on the proceeds of a small post office was proving a
crippling financial burden for her, so that this, in addition to her feelings of
grief for a son who was seriously ill, weighed heavily upon her.[44]

Relatives were still encouraged to visit the hospital. For some the journey
was prohibitively long and the transport facilities inadequate. Special buses
were provided and, in addition, the hospital management approved the
purchase of a car, both for the use of the medical superintendent and for the
purpose of taking small groups of patients on trips and on home visits. A
smart new Daimler was acquired, the arrival of which outside a terraced
house in Bethesda or Blaenau Ffestiniog must surely have signalled to all the
neighbours a visit from an asylum patient. Unfortunately, when returning
across the Denbigh moors from one such home visit, the car went off the
road. It was found to be beyond repair, and a far more modest vehicle
replaced it.

Often relatives did manage to maintain contact, even over many years in
the case of chronic patients. Amongst the files remaining in the hospital at
closure there were scores of letters from patients' relatives, some thanking
the staff for their support, others sending small sums of money so that their
sibling, parent or child might have 'extra comforts'. Sometimes they tell of
observing a deterioration in the health of the patient, sometimes they
inquire about the prognosis. One man wrote from south Wales inquiring
after his brother called John Davies and enclosing a 10s. note for him. The
staff had difficulty in identifying the patient as they had so many patients of
that name. Many relatives seem to have visited on a monthly basis, but there
were always some patients who had no visitors at all.

The separation of the sexes was maintained throughout the inter-war
years, although, as the number of patients and staff increased, and the
number of buildings proliferated, policing such a system became increasingly difficult. It was a matter which concerned the commissioners, and in
1925 A. Rotherham reported that, whilst visiting the laundry during his
annual inspection, 'the question of the possible mixing of the sexes was
discussed, and Dr Jones promised to make certain alterations, so that in
future, it will be practically impossible for the sexes to meet'.[45]

Apart from the enforced sexual divide, there were attempts to relax some
of the rules. Following a recommendation by the Board of Control inspector,
several of the male patients were allowed to stay up until 9 or 9.30 p.m. and
were said to 'enjoy the privilege very much'. They would play cards and

listen to the wireless.[46] Patients, both male and female, were granted parole within the hospital grounds and in 1927 the medical superintendent extended this to allow suitable male patients their liberty beyond the grounds during the daytime. 'After giving their promise not to misbehave in any way, they can go out and come in just as they please during daylight.'[47] They all acquitted themselves well that year, and some were subsequently discharged. But, for all its sense of liberalization of rules, this was still the language of custodial care. During the same year one female patient escaped and was absent for twenty-two and a half hours before being 're-captured'.

For patients entering the hospital in the inter-war years there was little privacy. In order to avoid the problem of having patients lock themselves into the toilets, or attempt to commit suicide behind their closed doors, the hospital had adopted the strategy of not fitting doors at all. This policy was criticized by the commissioners, who in 1934 urged placing doors on toilets, especially on the women's side, expressing the opinion that 'we think this want of privacy may be very distressing to some patients'.[48] Nor did patients have any private space to keep their belongings. The commissioners drew attention to the practice in the more progressive hospitals of providing private lockers. In many of the wards there simply was not space to place a locker, with beds packed so closely together that patients had to climb in from the bottom of the beds at night, and store their possessions underneath. This may not have been true in all wards, but many staff and patients recall instances of such overcrowding.

Between 1914 and 1931 the average recovery rate of patients admitted to the Denbigh asylum was 40.0 per cent, which compared favourably with the mean rate throughout the mental hospitals of England and Wales of about 32 per cent. This was calculated as a proportion of annual 'direct admissions', and did not include transfers from other institutions. A recovery rate of 40.3 per cent on direct admissions in 1930–1 represented only 5.2 per cent of the total number under treatment.[49] Comparison between asylums was always difficult because of the different methods of calculation adopted by various hospitals, a point noted by the Board of Control. (Some asylums, for instance, calculated recoveries only on the basis of the number of 'recoverable' cases admitted!)

The year 1929 saw 'an unusually large number of applications for discharge', most of which were acceded to, under section 79 of the 1890 Lunacy Act. This permitted a patient to be discharged under the order of two 'visitors' if a relative offered to take responsibility for the patient. The committee of visitors surmised that this increase reflected a growing awareness amongst the public of this facility under the Act. Also it was thought to indicate 'an increased interest in the patients and a sense of responsibility for their care at home, where practicable'.[50] Perhaps this was an outcome of the publicity given to the debates about standards of care and newspaper coverage of the reports concerning the future of mental hospitals.

Individual Patients

Some patients who had been admitted to the asylum before the outbreak of the First World War remained under care throughout the inter-war years. One such patient was W.R., who had been admitted aged twenty-nine in 1902 suffering from melancholia. He was a farm labourer from Llanfaethlu, in the Holyhead union, and a Calvinistic Methodist. He had been threatening to drown himself. His medical certificate explained that he had contracted venereal disease some time previous to the onset of his mental affliction, and that he had been treated and cured by a 'Medical man'. W.R. denied that he was cured, and this 'preyed upon his mind'. He was in fact clear of the disease, but feared that he had 'done some great sin and that he cannot possibly live long'. He remained in the asylum, diagnosed as suffering from 'hypochondria', throughout two world wars, as well as the entire inter-war period, and died in the hospital in 1945.[51] Events outside the hospital bypassed him, a man imprisoned by his own inner anxieties and by a system that perpetuated the long-term incarceration of patients.

Many other patients were suffering from delusions and a sense of persecution. Some thought that their food was poisoned, others could not sleep at night for fear that someone would murder them. A woman claimed to hear witchcraft in the telephone wires. Others heard voices from the ceiling. One man would often have a chat ('sgwrs') with his dead mother and brother. A woman insisted that she was in communication with the politician, Sir Rufus Isaacs. A married woman with five grown-up children, Jane W., stated that her 'real' husband was a black man from India who lived in Dundee. She insisted upon the truth of this and believed that this man was the only person in the world with the mark of India, and that this mark was now imprinted all over her body. After being admitted she conversed perfectly sensibly upon all points but this one fantastic idea. Sometimes the nurses had to remove the bedstead from her room, as she thought the black man was hidden under it, and that poison was stuffed in the mattress. She was discharged in less than two years, but she still had the same delusions.[52] If family members were willing to accept the patient home on trial, and the arrangement worked, the doctors were willing to agree to discharge. However, some of the delusional patients who were diagnosed as suffering from dementia praecox were still in the hospital thirty years later.

A farmer from Trawsfynydd took to going out at night to turn out the livestock and cut the corn. He frequently beat his wife. Admitted to the asylum, he was found to be suffering from arterio-sclerosis, and had oedema of the ankles. His memory was impaired and he was very confused. At first he was very loud and garrulous, rambling and disconnected. A year later he believed that one of the attendants was having an amorous relationship with his wife. He took to decorating himself with flowers. But the next year he gave this up, and said that the talk about his wife's affair was all 'lol' (nonsense). He became quieter and happier and, with his health improved, he was sent home on trial and then discharged, having spent nearly two years in the asylum.[53] It was not often that elderly patients made any recovery. Many of them were suffering from senile dementia and experienced a steady deterioration, and so remained in the asylum until death freed them.

Patients suffering from epilepsy continued to arrive at the hospital and, despite improved knowledge and medications, the condition could be extremely disabling. Frequent and heavy seizures led to deterioration in mental capacity. There was always a risk of injury, and one patient was scalded when a fit commenced as she was lifting a tea urn. Relatives sued the hospital for the injury.

Treatments varied, and sometimes involved no more than careful attention to diet and sleep. Occasionally more active efforts were made, and a variety of ingenious methods adopted. John T. was admitted to the hospital in March 1922 aged thirty-five. He was a banker from a quarrying town, but was admitted as a pauper (rate-aided) patient. Taken to the police station after attempting to cut his throat, he informed the inspector that he had been detained in military asylums during the war. He had also been in Denbigh, having been discharged eighteen months previously. He had two brothers in the asylum. (It was not uncommon for more than one member of a family to be in the asylum at the same time.) He claimed he had committed sins, and that his career was ended. He persistently refused food and in the end 'had to be fed per stomach tube'. Over the next few months he became progressively worse. By midsummer he had to be kept under a strong hypnotic 'practically the whole time . . . If not he stands in the corner of the room night and day without any clothes on and strongly resents any interference.' His feet would swell terribly from standing so long. The situation continued through to the autumn.

> He has to be fed generally once a day, but occasionally every other day. Within 15 minutes of being fed together with a sleeping draught he calls for food and for the next 24 hours will take his food exceptionally well and sleep in the interval, then when the effect of the draught begins to wear off he gets out of bed, stands in the corner and cries bitterly the whole time, stating that he has been a traitor to his King and Country and there are people outside crying for his blood. He will remain in this pitiable state until next fed.

He began to get worse, raving at times, and had to be 'carefully watched'. Tried on paraldehyde, he became even more noisy and boisterous. The

following April, over a year after his admittance, he was showing no improvement, but was 'very troublesome and strikes out at anyone approaching
him'. As summer arrived Dr Sidney Davies decided to try a new strategy:

> A fortnight ago when the weather had become warmer, he was forcibly
> dressed in the morning, and placed in charge of two attendants (in relays)
> all day, and allowed to make all the noise he liked all night. He struggled
> and fought for some days without ceasing and without taking a mouthful of
> food or drink. On the morning of the 5th day, however, he became quieter
> and in the evening took his tea. For the next six days his condition was
> erratic, one day being quiet and taking his food, perhaps two meals,
> whereas on the next he would be violent and refusing everything. For the
> last three days he has improved a great deal, taking his food regularly and
> giving no trouble. Today he spent almost the whole day on the bowling
> green.[54]

His progress was satisfactory, if somewhat unsteady, and he was kept on a
caution card to guard against suicide for many more months. In December
1924, two and a half years after his admittance, he began to appear fairly well.
In January a great improvement was observed, and he was now at work
assisting in the clerk's office. By April he was allowed out every day on parole
in the asylum grounds.. The following month he was passed for discharge and
was merely waiting for a medical board. He was then allowed full parole and
'plays golf on the Denbigh links every day'. At the end of the month he was
out on trial and in July he was signed 'off the books'. This story well illustrates
the persistent efforts made by the medical staff to aid a patient's recovery, and
the utilization of a wide armoury of therapeutic aids. Such treatment could be
extremely labour-intensive. If there was room for optimism the hospital could
provide an environment where a patient could regain health and be discharged. Not all of the suicidal patients were so fortunate.

A patient admitted to the hospital suffering from melancholia was actively
suicidal at the beginning of his stay and so was put on a 'caution card'. He
was then taken off the special watch, as he seemed to have recovered, and
was later discharged only to commit suicide a few weeks later. He was a coal
miner from Rhos, Wrexham, and suffered delusions of sin and unworthi-
ness. He had fearful dreams and could not sleep. He drowned himself at
Christmas.[55]

A Writer's Tragic Inspiration

The collision of social change and personal life history invariably provides the
substance of good literature. So it is in the story of one woman's descent into

insanity, graphically depicted by her son, Caradog Prichard, in one of the finest novels written in the Welsh language during the twentieth century, *Un Nos Ola Leuad*.[56] In it a number of the characters are committed to the Denbigh asylum, and the work is partly autobiographical. According to critic Katie Gramich, the novel, which 'revolves around madness, anguish and oppression', is about 'dissolution, the fragmentation of a society, of relationships within it and of the individual psyche'.[57] Caradog's mother had struggled to bring up her three sons on very little money, and like many other widows admitted to the asylum she had taken in washing, and gone 'charring'. Her youngest son Caradog was born in 1904. The family was then living at 24 Penybryn, Bethesda, and Margaret's husband John recorded his trade in the Register of Births as 'Quarryman'.[58] Within a few months, in April 1905, the name of her husband was recorded in the Register of Deaths. He had been killed in an accident at the quarry. Margaret spent the next eighteen years of her life bringing up their children alone. They moved to live more cheaply at Bryn Teg in the shadow of the quarry, the scene of the novel. Even this proved too expensive and Margaret was forced to move again to a tiny one-bedroomed house in a terrace on Glanrafon hillside. Caradog recalled that here they lived 'ar y plwyf' (on the parish) in receipt of 5*s.* a week – 'yn dlawd ymhlith tlodion ond yn gyfoethog mewn gobeithion a breuddwydion' (in poverty amongst the poor, but rich in hopes and dreams).[59] In the novel Caradog describes a neighbour, Catherine Jane, locking herself in the coal-house following an eviction and 'screaming the place down'. Hours later she was still locked in the coal-shed mewing like a cat and was sent away to the Denbigh asylum. When the young man in the novel finally accompanies his mother to the asylum he describes her too as crying like a cat.

In his autobiography, *Afal Drwg Adda*, Caradog skips hurriedly over the crisis leading up to his mother's committal to the Denbigh asylum, instructing his readers to turn to the novel for an account. Yet the fictional portrayal renders it difficult to pick out the sequence of events as the chronology does not fit the admission date recorded at the asylum. Scholars continue striving to differentiate fact from fiction in the writings of Caradog Prichard, especially with regard to the events associated with his mother's committal to the Denbigh asylum, experiences that had such a profound impact upon his emotional and creative energies.[60]

On 14 November 1923, Margaret Jane Pritchard was admitted to the Denbigh hospital, where she was to remain for the next thirty years, until her death in 1954. She was classified as a 'direct admission' on 26 November 1923, which means that she was admitted from home, and not sent via a workhouse or other institution. She was further detained under a series of continuations of this first reception order.[61]

From Caradog's description in the novel we know that on arrival at the hospital his mother was taken into a reception room, where she had to remove her clothes and put on hospital garments. Her own clothes were then wrapped in brown paper and handed to her son to take home. This handing over symbolized the change of status, a transfer of ownership, not just of property, but of person. With certification, Margaret's future was no longer her own to decide. There were already a number of other women patients in residence who had been sent from Bethesda by local practitioner Dr William G. Pritchard, women who would have shared the same background. One was Catherine E., a housekeeper, from 33 Tanybwlch, Douglas Hill, Bethesda, admitted in July 1903, who remained there until her death in 1941.[62] Former members of staff recall Margaret as someone who was 'very quiet' and 'not much trouble'. The act of accompanying his mother to the asylum clearly left her son with an abiding sense of guilt and resentment. When she died he would not allow any flowers upon the coffin – 'Mewn ffit o'r hen lid, yr oeddwn wedi gwrthod cael yr un blodyn ar arch Mam'.[63]

During the inter-war years dramatic changes were taking place in north Wales as the old primary and extractive industries that had hitherto been the mainstay of employment fell into serious decline. The numbers employed in the quarrying industry shrank, and the coal industry went through periods of falling demand and acute foreign competition. The General Strike came and went, affecting the asylum only in so far as it pushed up the price of coal supplied when its ample stocks finally ran low. North-east Wales was particularly badly affected by the Depression, if not as much as the south Wales valleys. In attempting to explain the high numbers of patients admitted from Flintshire, which was the only county in north Wales significantly and consistently exceeding its quota of patients during the 1930s, the medical superintendent noted that a social cause might be part of the explanation for the pattern. 'I find', he said, 'that unemployment in Flintshire is considerably higher than in other counties.' The less densely populated counties of north-west Wales also suffered, not only from the slump in quarrying and maritime trade, but from the effects of the agricultural depression, particularly the fall in livestock prices. Farming, rural industries and commercial businesses went through a very difficult time. A general practitioner, who served a large semi-rural community in the Llŷn Peninsula in south Caernarfonshire, wrote of the adverse effects which the 'underlying economic worry' had on the general health of both tenant farmers and the working classes during this period.[64]

During their visit to the hospital in May 1935 the commissioners observed that the number of actively suicidal patients was equal to 5 per cent of the total patient population. This was considerably above the average of 2.1 per cent for mental hospitals in England and Wales. In discussion with the medical superintendent they learned that 'an unusually high proportion of newly admitted patients are of the depressed type'.[65] They advised that there was scope for a scientific investigation to ascertain the factors

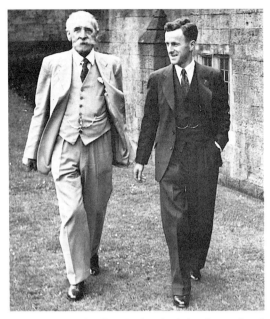

12. Photograph of William Barker, the clerk and steward, and his assistant and successor, Sidney Frost. The photograph was taken in 1939 for the purpose of producing identity cards.
Denbighshire Record Office

contributing to this unusually high level of mental depression amongst incoming patients. It would have been interesting had such an investigation been carried out.

For most patients within the asylum there was little real sense of optimism, and the prognosis for the majority was bleak. The medical super-intendent of the NWCMH reported in 1937 that, out of a total of 1,359 patients, he regarded 1,308 as incurable. He believed that only ten men and eleven women were likely to be cured, and that a further fifteen of each sex just might have some chance of recovery.[66] The number of incurable cases continued to accumulate, year by year.

In 1939 a new assistant and deputy clerk and steward was appointed. Mr S. L. Frost had previously been employed at Runwell, a hospital opened in June 1937 serving East Ham and Southend, and had experience of asylum administration.[67] In 1940 when Mr Barker retired, after serving for fifty-two years as clerk and steward to the Denbigh hospital, Sidney Frost was ready to succeed him. An era had come to an end, for Mr Barker was only the second clerk and steward to have held office since the asylum was opened in 1848. He had followed closely in the footsteps of Mr Robinson his predecessor so that effectively there had been a continuity of administrative office for over ninety years. As Britain once again faced war, the management at the Denbigh asylum had custody of a largely static population of patients, employed a large well-disciplined workforce and was commencing the introduction of a new range of therapies.

✵

The Second World War

Following lengthy negotiations with the Board of Control an agreement to enlarge the hospital on the existing site had finally been reached, and architects' plans for a £200,000 extension submitted for approval to the Board and the Ministry of Health.[1] Abruptly, as Britain moved into a war economy, the hospital management was informed that the application for loans to carry out new building works could no longer be entertained. Although disappointed at this reversal, the committee of visitors was relieved that it had not already entered into any liabilities prior to receiving the news. However, the pressure on bed space was to increase when the institution was added to the list of emergency war hospitals. The management was required to relinquish the new reception ward to the military authorities immediately, and so early in 1940 Gwynfryn was vacated to make room for 120 war casualty cases if required.[2] Subsequently the mental hospital was again allowed use of the reception ward on condition that it could be evacuated within twenty-four hours if necessary. Not long after this the Denbigh hospital was redesignated as a centre for the treatment of service mental cases.

Emergency air-raid protection measures were quickly adopted, with a blackout enforced, and both staff and patients issued with gas masks. Eighty attendants and nurses undertook training in anti-gas procedures, and some were taught to use a special decontamination station erected in the garden. Twelve men were also taught to deal with incendiary bombs and high explosives.[3] A crow's nest was rigged up on the top of the clock tower, and this provided an excellent view of all the roofs of the main building. In 1940, a hospital section of the Home Guard was formed, but was soon disbanded on the recommendation of the Board of Control, 'who felt that Staffs of Mental Hospitals should remain available for the care of the buildings and the patients in the event of air-raids or combatant action'.[4] The internal arrangements of the hospital were radically altered, so that those who suffered from limited mobility, including the sick and the elderly feeble patients, could sleep in wards located on the ground floor, allowing quicker evacuation in the event of attack. Patients themselves contributed to the war effort, those engaged in occupational therapy producing 2,000 special air-raid protection lampshades and 2,000 sand bags, and those involved in outdoor work helped to increase productivity on the land to ensure greater self-sufficiency of food for the hospital.[5]

War mobilization was soon presenting logistical difficulties throughout the entire hospital system in England and Wales, and in 1940 eighty-five male patients and one female were transferred to the NWCMH from the Mid-Wales Counties Mental Hospital, Talgarth, Breconshire, when that hospital was requisitioned for military purposes.[6] These patients remained for the duration of the war. In order to identify existing capacity within what was essentially a ramshackle system of local authority, charitable, private, occupational and trade union hospitals, a complete survey was undertaken of all hospital services in England and Wales. The report for north Wales, published in 1942, showed that the NWCMH was by far the largest establishment in the region, outnumbering in terms of bed space the total number of hospital beds in any one county in the region.[7] Indeed, setting aside Flintshire, the mental hospital had almost the equivalent capacity of all hospitals in the other four counties combined.

The war caused considerable disruption to the normal running of the hospital, complicated by shortages of supplies, transport problems and the transfer of many skilled and experienced staff, including the engineer. All of this resulted in a heavy reliance upon temporary, untrained replacement personnel. On the whole standards were maintained and in 1943 the committee of visitors was gratified to report that the administration, 'based on practices well established during the course of nearly a century of the Hospital's existence, has been able so far to weather the storm of War as well as it has'.[8]

Although no extension was built during the war years a number of essential improvements were carried out in the kitchens and laundry. At the suggestion of the Board of Control a staff canteen was introduced, and this proved to be a successful, and indeed a profitable, venture.[9] When the cinematograph equipment was renewed following receipt of a bequest from the relative of a patient, the canteen profits were used to provide a weekly show throughout the winter months. In 1942 the profits were used to purchase a second cinematograph projector, obviating the need to interrupt the show to change reels of film. The entertainment of patients remained a priority, the usual concerts and whist drives were regularly held and additional billiard tables were provided for the men's wards. A central library was established through the donation of books from libraries in the region. Small improvements such as these helped to retain some sense of progress and attention to patient care throughout the war. Members of staff were also encouraged to take advantage of the facilities for an active recreational life.

Dr Roberts believed it was vitally important 'that the staff should be as happy as possible'.[10]

In such ways the routine running of the hospital continued during the war years, with a minimum of interference from outside. Dolly Owen, who began work as a shorthand typist at the hospital in 1930, recalled the endless instructions which arrived from Whitehall.

> There were so many directives from H.Q. about the procedures to be adopted, – alterations, deletions, additions to Sections and Sub-Sections, paragraph this and paragraph that, that a hard-pressed staff could not possibly cope with all the amendments. So everything received was put into an ordinary Box File and importantly labelled 'War Matters'. Such was the tenuous link between us and the War Office.[11]

Staff Changes and Workforce Issues

In 1940 Dr Frank Jones retired as medical superintendent having held that post for twenty-seven years and served the hospital for thirty-nine years. Dr J. H. O. Roberts succeeded him having served as deputy for the previous eight years. In May 1941 Dr Robert Scott Wilson of the Warwickshire and Coventry Mental Hospital was appointed to the vacancy.[12] Although he had retired, Dr Frank Jones continued as a consulting physician and to conduct outpatient clinics.

The matron, Miss Price, who had served the hospital for twenty-eight years, retired in 1941. Remarkably, when this post was advertised it attracted twenty-seven applicants. The committee decided to appoint two ladies from this shortlist, who were both Welsh-speaking and had excellent experience. Miss B. Hughes, deputy matron at Runwell Mental Hospital, Essex, was appointed to the post of matron, and Miss E. G. Griffith, deputy matron at Haywards Heath Mental Hospital, Sussex, assumed the post of deputy matron.[13] This was the first time in the hospital's history that a deputy matron had been appointed.

The demand for labour generated by the war economy was to have a significant impact upon staffing levels in mental hospitals throughout England and Wales. The payment of war bonuses commenced in 1940 and was not sufficient to stem the tide of staff leaving the service, and so more draconian measures were adopted. In 1941 the Mental Nurses Employment and Offences Order was introduced, making it an offence to leave the service without the permission of the hospital. In order to secure the cooperation of the labour force, the Minister of Health insisted 'upon the observance of agreed hours of employment, rates of remuneration, and conditions of service generally'.[14] The committee of visitors agreed to adopt the new rates of pay and conditions of service agreed by the Joint Conciliation Committee of the Mental Hospitals' Association and the Mental Hospitals' and Institutional Workers' Union, and these were implemented on 1 January 1942.[15] This arrangement proved the value to hospital management of negotiating with a mature trade union organization, capable of securing an agreed national settlement.

Standards of Care

With the enormous pressure on staff and resources there were fears that standards of health, nutrition and hygiene would fall. The commissioners of the Board of Control continued their regular inspections and kept a close eye on relevant standards. On the whole they were warmly appreciative of the efforts of the staff and management committee, but were concerned when they visited the hospital in 1942 to discover that there had been 133 deaths during the previous year. This represented a death rate of 11.5 per cent on the average number of residents, considerably in excess of the 7.6 per cent death rate of the previous year. It was feared that this sharp rise might signal a permanent trend, mirroring the continuous rise in death rates that had occurred during the First World War. However, the rate declined again in the following year and, in line with other hospitals, remained steady for the remainder of the war. Previously the Denbigh hospital had prided itself on the very low rate of death amongst patients in comparison with other establishments. The increase in 1941 was partly attributable to a large number of deaths from tuberculosis – twenty-seven in all. To step up efforts to contain this problem, extra vigilance was taken in examining patients for early signs of the disease and the pathologist instigated a rigorous screening process. A blood sedimentation test was performed on all patients in the hospital, as well as on all new admissions, and in cases where this test showed positive (which could be for any one of a number of reasons) the patient was given a radiography test. A specialist in tuberculosis, Dr H. M. Williams of the King Edward VII Memorial Association, assisted in interpreting the radiographs. If patients were found to be harbouring tuberculosis they were immediately isolated and placed in the specialist wards, where they could be nursed by highly skilled staff and benefit from open-air facilities. Following these strenuous efforts by the pathologist and nursing staff, the problem was brought under greater control.

During the war staff carried out a systematic reclassification of all patients and reorganized the hospital. To begin with, all of the male wards and the female sick wards were rearranged 'with the object of eliminating cross classification and improving the facilities for the control of infectious diseases'. Secondly, all of the disturbed patients were removed from the oldest central block, which was considered unsuitable, and instead each of the three floors were formed into a self-contained ward, suitable for housing 'the better patient in homely comfort'.[16] A new set of gradations was introduced, headed by the private patients, the best parole patients, and the good patients (that is, those who were generally quiet and well behaved, with intermediate patients being divided into two levels), and then the disturbed and very disturbed patients each being housed separately. The visiting commissioners had recommended such a policy over a number of years, and the hospital was at last complying with their official guidelines.

New Treatments – The Emergence of ECT and Neurosurgery

Despite the hold on investment in the mental hospital system, the constraints on staff and the general shortages of resources, especially drugs, scientific advances began to play a more enhanced role. Radical changes occurred in psychiatry during the Second World War. However, unlike the experiments of the First World War, the changes were all based on a biological rather than a psychoanalytic approach to treatment. Doctors at the NWCMH were quick to embrace the new somatic innovations.

Initially the outbreak of war had put a brake on the utilization of new treatments. Insulin shock treatment was potentially dangerous and required skilled nursing in intensive care. Early in the war this treatment was abandoned, since 'its proper execution made too great demands on our curtailed wards and staff'.[17] However, within a year staff began using a modified form of the technique, 'whereby the dosage given has just been short of that needed to produce coma, resulting only in the milder shock symptoms'.[18] This modified insulin shock treatment 'proved useful', especially in cases where the patient was not sufficiently strong to withstand cardiazol treatment, which continued to be the preferred drug in most cases of induced shock treatment. Cardiazol and triazol convulsive treatment had become the standard treatment for schizophrenia, as well as being used in certain types of depression. During 1940 twenty-seven cases were treated by this method, of which fifteen were deemed either recovered or sufficiently improved to leave hospital.[19]

In the 1930s, Professor Ugo Cerletti at Rome began investigating the application of electricity to give a shock to the brain directly through the skull. With Lucio Bini he devised a means of providing a non-lethal dose of electrical current that would induce a convulsion, using a machine capable of applying a controlled voltage for a fraction of a second.[20] The technique was first successfully applied in 1938. It was soon to revolutionize 'shock treatments' throughout both Europe and North America.

At this time, new psychiatric practices were being disseminated rapidly, partly as a result of the movement of refugee doctors through Europe to

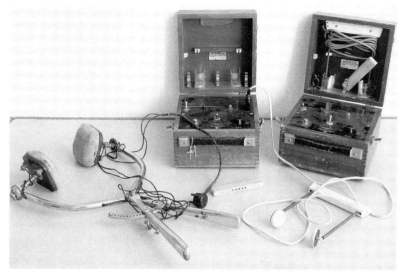

13. Early ECT equipment. Crown copyright: Royal Commission on the Ancient and Historical Monuments of Wales

Britain and North America. Lothar Kalinowsky, a Jewish doctor, fled Germany for Italy in 1933, where he witnessed early experiments with ECT (electroconvulsive therapy). Later, he helped to introduce ECT to France. He then moved to England and worked with Sanderson McGregor at the Netherne Hospital in Coulsdon, where he again promoted use of ECT. He sought to popularize this technique with a British audience through a paper in *The Lancet* in December 1939.[21] Already psychiatrists based at the Burden Neurological Institute in Bristol had published a report of their trials on the use of electrically induced convulsions on five schizophrenic patients, concluding that the effects were the 'equivalent of those of cardiazol'.[22] Their successful application of this revolutionary technique reassured psychiatrists in Britain that the method was relatively safe. ECT treatment was introduced at the Maudsley Hospital in 1940,[23] and was rapidly taken up throughout Great Britain.

It was adopted in the Denbigh hospital in July 1941, when the committee of visitors authorized the purchase of an Ediswan electric convulsion therapy apparatus. The new member of staff, Dr Wilson, already had experience of this machine, and so was able to instruct his colleagues in its use. The therapeutic principle embodied in this technique was the same as that of utilizing shock inducing drugs – to produce a bodily convulsion, which appeared to have a healing effect upon the mind. The medical super-intendent explained the advantages of the electrically induced convulsion over that induced by cardiazol: 'First, as there is immediate loss of consciousness, it is not unpleasant. Secondly, it is milder so that mishaps are less liable to occur and its use can be extended to older patients. Thirdly, it is more convenient.'[24] The change it brought to therapeutic practice was dramatic and within a year Dr Roberts was able to report that, 'As a result of these relative advantages, treatment by cardiazol has been to all intents and purposes completely suspended.'[25]

In this way one treatment immediately superseded another. Berrios has argued that ECT was perceived at the time of its adoption as essentially a modified form of convulsive therapy.[26] The rationale provided by doctors at the Denbigh hospital for using this technique confirms this interpretation. The convulsive therapies were based on the notion that epileptic patients were much less likely to suffer from schizophrenia, and that there was there-fore an inherent 'neurobiological opposition between epilepsy and schizo-phrenia'.[27]

However, although ECT was initially advocated for use in cases of schizophrenia, within a year Denbigh's medical superintendent was reporting that experience had quickly shown that 'its chief field of usefulness is amongst the Depressions'.[28] This conclusion was probably based upon observations of patients, on a reading of current medical literature and attendance at conferences. In 1941 Hemphill and Walter published an account of their use of ECT treatment with over 200 patients, from which they concluded that 'manic-depressive and involutional melancholics respond best to treatment'.[29] In the same issue, Freudenberg published an account of trials conducted at Moorcroft House in Middlesex, where he concluded that the affective psychoses responded better to shock therapy.[30] The practice at Denbigh certainly indicates that members of the medical staff were keeping fully abreast of current developments in a rapidly advancing field.

The treatment was administered on an increasingly regular basis at the NWCMH during the war years; forty-seven patients received ECT in 1941, 192 in 1942, and 158 in 1943. In 1944 Dr Roberts reported that cardiazol and triazol had been totally discarded and that the 'electrically induced convulsion has been used exclusively'. He emphasized the positive out-comes, particularly in cases of severe depression.

> While Convulsive Therapy is of value in Schizophrenia and Mania, the best results are obtained among the Depressives. The Melancholia of middle life nearly always responds and an illness, which formally dragged on for months or years, can now be brought under immediate control, and untold suffering cut short.[31]

The introduction of electric shock treatment to the NWCMH was reported in the local press, and by 1948 there was press coverage of the 'Amazing' number of cures being effected at the hospital.[32] This celebratory approach to the positive outcomes offered by these new treatments, ECT in particular, may have encouraged many more people to seek advice for their mental health problems, for there was a sharp rise during the post-war years in attendance at outpatient clinics.

During the first years of its use ECT was administered without either anaesthetic or muscle relaxants, and staff who were present at these early applications of the treatment recall having to stand close by the bed to prevent patients being hurled to the floor. Some patients incurred fractured bones from the force of their jerks during the fit, and some gnashed their teeth so hard that they fractured their jaws. It is testimony to the awfulness of cardiazol treatment that patients preferred ECT shock treatment to that experience. Technologically, the early ECT machines were crude by comparison with modern apparatus, so the power of the shock applied was fairly standard, and often far in excess of that required to ensure a therapeutic outcome. Nonetheless the results were dramatic enough in many cases for patients and, on their behalf, relatives to request the treatment. However, there is little to suggest that patients participated in giving fully informed consent to ECT. Most were certified patients, not voluntary, and so their consent was not required.

A pattern soon emerged whereby female patients were twice as likely as male patients to receive electric shock treatment. During the year 1947, for instance, ECT was administered to 165 female patients, but to only forty-three male patients.[33] J. D. Williams, who recalled nursing experiences at the hospital immediately after the war, told the writer that although staff did not like being present at the earliest ECT treatments, nonetheless they found the results quite astonishing. The effectiveness of this treatment was most impressive, he said, in cases of women suffering from post-natal depressions and post-natal psychoses. These patients were immediately transformed by the electrical shock, and could quickly be discharged, whereas previously such cases had been very difficult to manage. ECT has survived as one of the most important methods of treatment still in widespread use today, although in a rather more sophisticated form. There is no full understanding of how it works, and, whilst some patients have found it helpful, other former patients regard its use as a form of abuse.

During the war a number of new pharmacological preparations were adopted. Epanutin, a new drug for the treatment of epilepsy, was introduced to the Denbigh hospital in 1939. It had been introduced to the UK from America in 1938. The medical staff used it with some caution, due to its possible toxic effects.[34] Thirteen of the fourteen patients treated with epanutin showed significant improvement, with a decline in the frequency of fits and an improvement in their mental condition. This was greatly welcomed because, since 'chronic epileptics are amongst the most difficult cases to handle, the benefits accruing from the use of this drug are likely to be considerable'. However, whilst in some cases it proved 'most helpful', in others it produced unpleasant side effects, and whenever patients showed toxic symptoms the treatment had to be curtailed.[35] In 1944 it was said to be 'always worth trying as it occasionally brings about marked benefit', but the standard drug used in most cases was luminal.[36]

Initial experiments with somnifane injections had proved disappointing when administered to patients at the NWCMH. When in 1939 somnifane was employed to induce deep sleep in a patient suffering from mania the outcome was positive and the patient was discharged recovered.[37] A further two patients were treated the following year, and seven the year after. The treatment was considered to be particularly useful in cases 'of extreme excitement and loss of control'.[38] Windholz and Witherspoon claim that by the end of the 1930s prolonged sleep therapy already 'belonged to history', having been superseded by the use of cardiazol to treat cases of schizo-phrenia.[39] Yet here we see it being employed in Denbigh in 1939, and used alongside cardiazol treatment, as a specialized technique found particularly 'useful in some cases'. By 1942 medinal had displaced somnifane as the drug favoured by psychiatrists at the Denbigh hospital, and during that year thirteen patients received the treatment, seven of whom were discharged either recovered or improved. By 1944 Dr Roberts referred to the use of barbitone sodium as the means for securing prolonged narcosis.[40] Whatever medication was chosen it was administered in order to keep the patient asleep for up to fourteen days. Dr Roberts explained to his chairman and committee of visitors that 'its action can be likened to a splint which ensures rest while the natural recuperative powers of the body come into play'.[41] Popularly known as 'deep-sleep' therapy, the aim of this treatment was to assist the mind to make a full recovery, and overcome any tendency towards excitement.

In the 1930s psychiatrists in Europe and America were also experi-menting with neurosurgery. Attending a conference in London in 1935 Egan Moniz heard of the research findings reported by Carlyle Jacobsen and John Fulton of Yale on the emotional changes brought about by cutting the frontal lobes of the brain of a chimpanzee. Over the next six months Moniz, with neurosurgeon Almeida Lima, operated on twenty patients at the Santa Marta Hospital in Lisbon. He claimed that seven of the patients were cured, seven improved, and that in the remaining six there was no change.[42] American neurologist Walter Freeman also attended the London conference and, in collaboration with a neurosurgeon James Watts, began experiment-ing on developing a similar surgical operation on the brain, which they termed 'lobotomy'. (In Europe the term used was 'leucotomy'.) In 1942 they published a major research monograph which eventually led to widespread practical application of their techniques.[43] By this time pioneering work on the new surgery had already been carried out in the UK at Bristol by Hutton, Fleming and Fox, and the results of their work were published in *The Lancet* in 1941.[44]

The operation was first performed at the NWCMH in April 1942, by local surgeon, Dr D. G. Duff, who was based at the Denbigh Infirmary but acted as consulting surgeon to the mental hospital. In 1943, Dr Roberts announced that three prefrontal leucotomy operations had been performed, 'whereby nerve fibres passing from the prefrontal lobe to other parts of the brain are divided'.[45] This surgical intervention represented, he claimed, 'the latest development in the field of treatment of mental disorder', and was carried out in the hospital's operating theatre by Dr Duff. He reported that two of the three cases were unimproved, but that one case showed 'a marked benefit'. Dr Roberts and his assistants took a keen interest in the development of this technique. Former members of staff recollect that Dr Ernst Schwarz was the doctor most involved with the leucotomy operations, and he selected the patients for this treatment. He worked on the male side of the hospital, and, whereas more women than men received ECT treatment, more men than women in the Denbigh hospital were given leucotomies. By 1948 sixty-one men and thirty-seven women had received leucotomy operations.[46] The initial results were sufficiently encouraging for medical staff at Denbigh to continue experimenting with the technique. The operation posed a considerable risk from haemorrhaging, and therefore was only considered suitable for use on long-term patients who had failed to respond to all other forms of treatment. During the following year a further nine operations were performed, and four of the patients appeared to make 'good recoveries'. In 1945 it was reported that, of the thirteen men and three women treated by leucotomy since 1942, five had left the hospital recovered and eight were steadily improving within the hospital. Two remained unimproved and there had been one fatality. The visiting commissioner found the results interesting, and observed that 'The patients chosen for this operation have been of the schizophrenic and chronic depressive types, all had long histories of mental illness and all had failed to respond to the less heroic methods of treatment'.[47] The medical superintendent claimed that 'the results have been remarkable, and, to our minds, the procedure constitutes a further definite advance in the treatment of serious mental illness'.[48] The following year Dr Duff published a report in *The Lancet*, describing his technique and the new surgical instrument which he had devised to perform this delicate task. As a rule he conducted the operation using only a local anaesthetic, and remarked that 'the patients are usually cooperative and unworried about the operation. Trephining has often a soporific effect.'[49] He described how he would push a bradawl through the anaesthetized scalp, and prepare a hole in which to insert the half-inch trephine, after which an

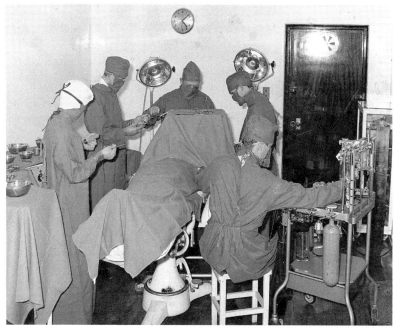

14. In the operating theatre: performing a leucotomy operation (a 'mock up' for the purposes of the camera). Denbighshire Record Office

incision 3.5 cm. long is now made sagitally through the puncture mark, the pericranium stripped back, and the self-retaining retractor inserted. The trephine is operated with a brace; and, when the bone button is removed, a puncture place near the centre of the exposed dura is chosen which will provoke the least meningeal haemorrhage.[50]

He designed a special instrument in collaboration with his colleagues at the Denbigh hospital, and Dr Wilson arranged for a Birmingham steel manufacturer to produce a prototype of the implement.

Interested observers wondered how Dr Duff could have learnt the techniques, since operating inside the cranium involved considerable risk. According to Dr Ceinwen Evans, Dr Duff did not attempt the operation on a live patient without first of all having some practice. Whenever she had a 'suitable cadaver' (that is, a patient who had died, and who had no relatives interested in claiming the body) she would telephone the surgeon, and he would visit the mortuary and practice drilling into the cranium and probing the frontal lobes.[51] His innovation was to devise a new type of leucotome with blunt edges, which would not cut blood vessels. He attached a piece of snare wire to project from the leucotome, but which could be retracted inside the device until it touched the orbital plate of the frontal bone. The snare wire could then be extended and the instrument swept outwards to cut through the white matter in the oval centre of the brain's two front lobes. Dr Duff explained that, as the wire loop passed close to, or even cut into, the thin, usually uniform layer of grey matter, 'the patient sometimes winces slightly as a sensitive area is touched'.[52] At that point, he claimed, the transformation was miraculous. Dr Duff found the experience energizing, 'for it is a thrill (on occasion) to see the lines of anxiety disappear and the patient suddenly become extrovert and interested for the first time in his surroundings just as the second hemisphere is cut'.[53] And all of this was achieved by what he considered a 'comparatively easy' operation.

Prefrontal leucotomy was widely seen as a treatment of 'last resort', and yet huge claims were made for its success. Ernst Schwarz experimented with this type of psychosurgery for a number of conditions. In 1945 he published a paper on the use of leucotomy as a treatment for Parkinsonism, where he described how one Denbigh patient with distressing symptoms of Parkinsonism, chiefly unilateral, was given a contralateral hemileucotomy with 'very encouraging results'.[54]

Ever since the rise and subsequent decline of this particular form of psychosurgery controversy has raged about the value of such a drastic intervention, and its place in the history of psychiatry.[55] Valenstein has labelled the treatment as 'bizarre' and as a form of 'mutilation'.[56] He has emphasized the extent to which the development and popularization of psychosurgery served the career ambitions of the psychiatrists who experimented with it. Pressman, however, argued that the experiment with psychosurgery played an important role in the development of a more scientific and methodologically sophisticated approach in psychiatry.[57]

Dr Duff left Denbigh in 1946 to become surgeon-superintendent at the Belford Hospital, Fort William.[58] In 1947 his successor Dr Lewis performed seventy such operations. The introduction of leucotomies brought about other changes in the Denbigh hospital, including the development of more methodical clinical assessments of patients, and the enlargement of case files. The need to carry out IQ tests both prior to and after the leucotomy operations resulted in the part-time appointment in 1944 of a Hungarian psychologist, Dr Martha Vidor. In 1947 she was given an established full-time position, and her professional role became more mainstream within the hospital, and included work for outpatients clinics and the child guidance teams, to which Dr Schwarz increasingly turned his attention.[59] During the post-war years considerable efforts were made to rehabilitate the post-leucotomy patients, through the use of group therapy. As some of the patients grew older and their hair began to recede it exposed the two indentations on the head where the bone had been drilled, creating a rather alarming appearance. In order to avoid leaving new patients with this embarrassing legacy, a small adaptation was made to the procedure. Before closing the scalp a plastic button, the exact size of the trepanned hole, was inserted to plug the gap and the skin was then placed carefully over and stitched.[60]

The use of ECT and of surgical methods had the effect of both shortening the length of stay in the mental hospital and making the institution look less custodial and much more like a general hospital. These 'drastic' treatments thereby had the surprising effect of persuading more patients to seek treatment voluntarily. During 1944 the number of new admissions to the North Wales Counties Mental Hospital was 356, an increase of roughly 50 per cent on the pre-war rate of admission. This was not believed to be due to any increase in the rate of insanity, but to the 'greater willingness of people suffering from the less serious degrees of mental illness to enter this hospital'.[61]

David Crossley, who had access to the Denbigh case files of patients who received leucotomies, suggests that the results were variable. There was a known risk of epilepsy and three of Dr Duff's patients subsequently developed seizures. Dr Martha Vidor reported that one female patient 'looked very aged and broken' after the operation. 'I could hardly recognise her', she said. The wife of another patient who was discharged after the operation claimed that 'The operation had very bad results . . . he turned out to be a sex maniac, using filthy language to everybody.' He was subsequently readmitted to the hospital as a forensic (that is, criminal) case, with a diagnosis of hypomania.[62]

However, medical staff continued to view the surgical operation as a useful treatment. Specialists from Liverpool would travel to Denbigh to perform the operation during the 1950s. The practice of performing leucotomies became well established at Denbigh and continued until the closure of the operating theatre in 1966, long after many other hospitals had abandoned the practice.

Besides the introduction of new forms of treatment, a number of important social changes had occurred during the war, some affecting the status of women. They became more visible as they took on new roles and the old divisions between the male and female sides of the hospital began to break down. Two members of the Women's Land Army would each day take a party of twenty female patients to the farm and gardens to undertake light work such as hoeing, collecting fruit, etc. The 'innovation' was hailed as a great success, and the sight of women working in the fields and gardens became an accepted part of the new hospital scene. Generally in Wales women's confidence and expectations were raised during the war, but as Deirdre Beddoe has pointed out, 'in essence the post-war world was as male-dominated and as patriarchal as ever'.[63]

The war created many casualties, and staff at the hospital recollected poignant cases of patients whose lives had been changed irrevocably by the experiences of the conflict. One service patient, invalided home after a serious battle, was beyond verbal communication with either staff or visitors. Yet the staff observed that he listened avidly to the news reports on the radio and followed every detail relating to the whereabouts of his brother's regiment. Another would write screeds of Welsh poetry on hospital toilet paper. Using a spoon at meals, he would invariably take the wrong end, stuff the handle into his mouth and become very angry if staff tried to help. He had been a very intelligent man and was the brother of a distinguished Welsh academic. Many of the male staff had a deep respect for the service patients produced by the Second World War, just as they had for veterans of the First World War.

✻

Chapter Twelve

Welfare State Years – A New Dawn?

At the end of the war the health services faced major change, as plans were laid to establish a unified, centralized system, funded through taxation to provide free treatment to patients. The establishment of the National Health Service had important implications for mental hospitals, until then the responsibility of local government.[1] The central authority with overall responsibility for the mental health services throughout the United Kingdom was to be the Ministry of Health. The Board of Control was to retain its quasi-judicial powers and duties, which it would continue to exercise independently of the Minister.

NHS Structures

The hospital was to be administered by a new hospital management committee, whose members were appointed by the Welsh Regional Hospitals Board.[2] The structure of authority was therefore radically different from the old system whereby members of the committee of visitors represented the interests of five counties. The new hospital management committees were allowed a considerably degree of autonomy, 'although they will necessarily be subject to regulations, and to directions, both from the Minister, and from the Regional Hospitals Board on whose behalf they are performing most of their functions'.[3] The budgetary allocations would henceforth be decided by central government. This affected not only the meeting of patient costs, and of administration, but also staff appointments and conditions of service.

The restructuring of the health services had an immediate impact on estate and other assets of the Denbigh hospital. According to section 13 of the Act, 'the entire resources of the existing local authority and voluntary hospitals are to be transferred to the Minister', with effect from 5 July 1948. The transfer of ownership of the Denbigh hospital took place on the appointed day. The property valued at a sum exceeding one million pounds was transferred, but in addition the Minister of Health demanded a contribution towards the costs of established staff.[4] A number of details remained in dispute over the coming months, including the future of the various charitable trusts attached to the old asylum. Finally it was agreed that the funds of the Ablett Trust, which for nearly a century had provided financial help to patients on their discharge from hospital, were not transferable and could be retained by the hospital in order to fulfil the aims attached to the bequest.[5] Other funds all had to be transferred to the Minister of Health's Endowment Fund.

In the immediate post-war years of economic austerity expenditure was stringently curbed although over the longer period more resources became available. Many individuals on the staff have remarked that, with the coming of the National Health Service, the 'old parsimonious regime' was replaced by an era of plenty as the penny-pinching ways of make do and mend gradually disappeared. There was a decisive change of culture in the institution following nationalization. This cultural transition, however, appears to have been gradual and incremental rather than sudden. Many of the former members of the management committee were reappointed by the Welsh Regional Hospitals Board to the new committee, which took up office in 1948. This ensured continuity in the short term.

Two members of the old committee of visitors to the NWCMH were appointed in 1947 to sit on the Welsh Regional Hospitals Board. Dr Roberts, the medical superintendent, became a member for his special knowledge of mental treatment. Mrs Jones Roberts, of Merionethshire County Council, was selected for her interests both in mental health and especially in women's health and child welfare. In earlier life she had acted as personal secretary to Ernest Jones, the Welsh psychoanalyst and biographer of Freud. The chairman of the committee of visitors, Alderman David Evans of Holyhead, welcomed the appointments and said that 'It certainly put the North Wales Counties Mental Hospital "on the map" and gave it recognition as one of the country's most progressive Mental Hospitals'.[6]

One of the immediate management issues of the post-war years was the rapid rise in costs. Delays in the payment of government grants to fund two major salary increases, resulting from national pay awards, caused some short-term financial problems in 1946.[7] By the following year the cost of maintaining patients in the asylum had risen rapidly so that, whereas the fixed rate of maintenance paid by the counties amounted to 31*s.* 7*d.* per head per week, the actual cost of maintaining them was closer to 34*s.* 2*d.* The provisions expenditure was increasing but so too were the general running costs of the hospital. Also, the appointment on 'high salaries' of 'specialist staff', such as the new chef and a male occupational therapist, was described as 'a new departure' for the institution.[8]

At the July meeting of the committee of visitors in 1947, the medical superintendent referred to the recent meeting of the British Medical-

Psychological Association at Eastbourne, where the hope had been expressed that closer collaboration would develop between general hospitals and mental hospitals.

> Er mai ystrydeb oedd dweud bod iechyd corfforol a meddyliol yn cydfynd a'i gilydd yr oedd diffygion wedi codi yn nhriniaeth y naill a'r llall oherwydd y gwahanfur rhwng y ddau fath o ysbyty. Dylai gosod y ddau fath o ysbyty o dan un awdurdod rwyddhau'r ffordd i uno'r ddwy gangen o feddygaeth. Yn y dyfodol fe ddylai fod yn haws i'r meddyg cyffredinol fynd i mewn i'r ysbyty meddwl ac i'r meddyg meddwl fynd i mewn i'r ysbyty cyffredinol. Fe wneir hynny eisoes yn America ac ar y Cyfandir. Fel y deuai'r bobl i sylweddoli'r cysylltiad rhwng y ddwy gangen fe ddeuai hefyd yn haws i berswadio'r rhai sy'n dioddef oddi wrth afiechyd meddwl gymryd triniaeth mewn pryd.[9]

It was anticipated that, as a result of nationalization and the bringing together of the health services, the mental hospitals would achieve equal status with general hospitals. The drive to introduce new treatments was changing the whole emphasis of this branch of medicine, and psychiatrists wanted to be regarded as a specialism like any other within the broader medical profession.

Bed Space and Staffing

The major problems faced by the North Wales Mental Hospital at the end of the war were those which had dogged it for many years – overcrowding and shortages of staff. In 1946 the forty-nine patients evacuated from Brecon and Radnorshire were returned to Talgarth, and in 1947 nineteen patients from the Cardiff County Mental Hospital were returned too; but with a rising number of new admissions the accommodation was insufficient. Even without the above 'out of counties' patients, the hospital was overcrowded to the extent of about 20 per cent, according to the standards of the Board of Control.[10]

The hospital was still housing about 200 mental deficiency cases, and there were renewed calls for the establishment of a 'Colony for Mental Defectives'.[11] Meanwhile, it was necessary to take in yet more new cases, 'because North Wales is woefully short of appropriate accommodation'.[12] The commissioners were losing patience with the region's failure to make suitable provision, observing that the mental defectives 'ought really to be in an institution for their own kind'.[13] Following this report, renewed efforts were made to find alternative accommodation, and by 1952 there had been a significant reduction, although some fifty to sixty 'mental defectives' were

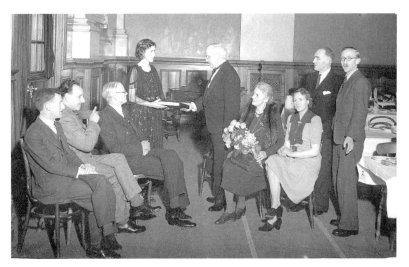

15. Dr E. H. Hutton's retirement presentation. In the centre standing: Dr Ann Ceinwen Evans presents a retirement memorial to Dr Hutton. Seated from left: Sidney Frost, clerk and steward; Dr Wilson, deputy medical superintendent; Dr J. H. O. Roberts, medical superintendent; Mrs Hutton; Matron Blodwen Hughes. Standing on right, Thomas John Davies, chief male nurse; far right, Dr Schwarz, assistant medical officer.
Denbighshire Record Office

still taking up beds in the hospital.[14] In 1954 the medical superintendent reported that he hoped that Oakwood Park would take a number of the remaining mental defectives, and their transfer was finally accomplished in 1958.[15] They had long been regarded as an anomaly within the institution, but, as the nature of the hospital changed to one where active treatments were employed, and greater emphasis was placed on early discharge, the presence of these 'mentally defective' patients had become ever more incongruous.

The shortage of medical staff in relation to the number of patients had been a persistent problem. In 1946, with nearly 1,500 patients in the hospital at any one time, there were only six medical staff. In 1947 Dr Eustace Hutton retired as assistant medical officer after thirty-one years' service. 'His popularity with the patients was unique', wrote Dr Roberts, 'no doubt because of the unfailing courtesy and kindliness which characterised all his dealings with them.'[16]

The Welsh Language Dimension

Given the expansion of psychiatry and the increasing number of patients admitted each year, additional qualified medical staff were urgently required. The growing emphasis on outpatient work made it all the more important to employ Welsh-speaking staff, since in order to work effectively 'in the community' it was essential that the psychiatrists were able to speak the first language of much of the local populace. According to the 1951 census, 30 per cent of the inhabitants of Flintshire and Denbighshire remained Welsh-speaking, and over 74 per cent of those living in Anglesey, Caernarfon and Merioneth were Welsh-speakers. Yet, despite active efforts, the hospital failed to recruit a Welsh-speaking medical officer. Indeed, it proved difficult to recruit a new medical officer at all. Advertisements were placed in the *North Wales Times* in 1946, and then in the *Lancet* in April and again in June 1947. The commissioners noted with concern, when they visited the hospital in July 1947, that there were now only four medical officers. The fact that the entire day of two medical officers was taken at each of two weekly clinics, and the time of another medical officer at each of two other clinics, meant that in effect there were only three medical officers available to treat 1,450 inpatients.[17] Chronically understaffed and with holiday time approaching, the medical superintendent offered the appointment to a non-Welsh candidate, who promised to acquire the language. Soon the 'man-about-town' columnist of the *North Wales Times* printed news of the latest development in his 'Denbigh Jottings':

> I understand that a non-Welsh speaking doctor has been appointed on the staff of the North Wales Mental Hospital to succeed the only Welsh-speaking member of the medical staff – apart from the Medical Superintendent (Dr Roberts) and a lady doctor. The Chairman of the Committee of Visitors stated following the appointment that the new doctor had 'promised to learn Welsh'. Similar promises have been made in the past, and I should like to know how many of those members of the staff who knew no Welsh when they were appointed have made any progress at all in their study of the language of a large number of the patients? The ability to say 'Iechyd da' and ' 'S'mai' would not be of much use to a doctor who wanted to inquire into a monoglot patient's mental health. Many people have observed that every Welsh-speaking officer who leaves the Mental Hospital is replaced by a non-Welsh-speaking officer, and the posts which are not strictly medical have also been similarly filled. Is this the policy of a committee of Welshmen?[18]

With the political temperature raised, the appointment was blocked by the finance committee, which voted that advertisements be again placed for a Welsh-speaking medical officer. The medical superintendent attended their next meeting to report 'that no applicant had been forthcoming'.[19] The committee insisted on the need for a Welsh-speaking doctor, 'particularly having regard to the nature of the work at clinics in predominantly Welsh speaking districts' and a subcommittee was appointed to consider the matter further. In the end pragmatism prevailed, and the non-Welsh-speaking medical officer was officially appointed. From this point onwards English-medium appointments were regularly made, although Welsh-speaking psychiatrists were sought whenever possible.

Frequently during the post-war years there were periods when vacancies at the Denbigh hospital remained unfilled. Psychiatry was still not a high-status area of the medical profession and the health service in Wales was considered a professional backwater by many practitioners. During the early years of the NHS, hospitals throughout Wales relied heavily on the recruit-ment of immigrant doctors, a number of whom entered the mental health services. Interviewed for the Millennium Memory Bank in 1999 consultant psychiatrist Farrukh Hashmi recalled his arrival in London in 1953. He sought the advice of a man from the BMA, who pompously and patron-izingly said to him: 'trouble with you boys, you come here, don't contribute anything, if you want a job, go out of London to a non-teaching hospital – Wales – might get a job in a mental hospital, but otherwise no hope for you'.[20]

Following the transfer of the hospital to the Ministry of Health the medical staff were regraded and some improvement took place in the staffing position. In 1949 Dr Roberts had the assistance of two consultants, Dr Williamson and Dr Williams, three senior registrars, Dr Lucy, Dr Edwards and Dr Aspinwall, a registrar, Dr Hannal, and a junior registrar, Dr Monks.[21] His staff had more than doubled in little over a year.

It was also becoming difficult to recruit Welsh-speaking nursing staff, even as trainees. Numerous advertisements and features appeared in the newspapers of north Wales in an attempt to attract new applicants. Emphasis was placed on the career possibilities, as well as on the remunera-tion and the conditions of service. Still the shortage of recruits proved dire, and the hospital took to advertising in Ireland in an attempt to attract trainee nurses, pointing out that the NWMH at Denbigh was the nearest British mental hospital to Dublin.

Opening the Doors

Despite the overcrowding and the staff shortages, the North Wales Hospital was viewed as a 'progressive hospital' by the standards of the 1950s. The commissioners spoke warmly of the efforts of staff – 'Everywhere there was evidence that both the medical and administrative staffs have shown much zeal in overcoming the many difficulties inherent in old and overcrowded buildings.'[22] Gradually the medical superintendent was able to introduce a more liberal and actively therapeutic regime, and adopt an 'open door'

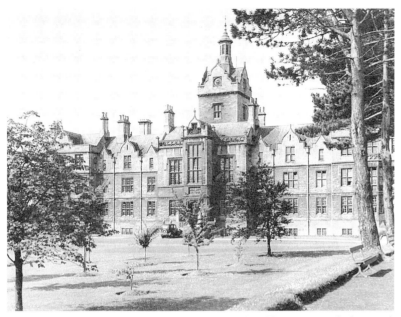

16. The frontage of the main buildings of the Denbigh asylum. The yew trees in the foreground were cut down after the Second World War, because patients and visitors complained that they reminded them of a cemetery. Denbighshire Record Office

policy. Staff remembered that prior to this change a large bunch of keys was required for all of the doors which separated one part of the corridor from the next, and one ward from another. During the post-war years many of the intervening doors were removed, revealing for the first time the full length of some of the corridors. The thick brown paint was stripped off by blowtorch, and whites and bright colours were introduced. Sights and sounds changed, clanking of keys no longer signalled the approach of a member of staff. The wards themselves became brighter and livelier.

By 1954 each ward had not only its own radio but also its own television. For many patients this was a novelty, as they could not afford to buy them for home use. In all aspects the hospital was becoming a more modern institution. A ladies' hairdressing salon, opened for patients in 1948, was such a success that in 1956 a second full-time hairdresser was appointed. Patients also had access to a shop selling confectionery and cigarettes. They could use cash or the tokens given to patients as payment for work. Each week the hospital issued 1,800 tokens to the male patients and 900 tokens to female patients.[23] The shop was run by one of the patients, who even kept the slate.[24]

The abandonment of 'locked doors' heralded a more relaxed approach, with greater emphasis on therapeutic methods. The railings were removed from the outside 'airing courts', and patients given much greater freedom to explore the grounds of the hospital. An increasing number were allowed on 'town parole' – forty-seven men and fifty-two women were allowed outside of the hospital grounds in 1948. The new policy raised concerns amongst senior nursing staff who, having served their apprenticeships under the old regime, had been schooled to watch every patient carefully. It was they who were answerable for any escapes, accidents or for violence against other patients, and for suicides. Expected to maintain the same standards of care but lacking the old sanctions or authority, many of them felt undermined. The commissioners, visiting in 1958, commented that 'This is not an entirely open door hospital and there are still two male and four female locked wards'.[25] The reason for the higher number of locked wards on the female side was a combination of greater staff shortages, more overcrowding and a large number of elderly chronic patients who, being very demented, were liable to wander.

The policy of opening doors was widely adopted in mental hospitals throughout England and Wales during the 1950s. It had been pioneered in a lengthy experiment by Dr Good at the Littlemore Hospital in Oxford during the 1920s, but under pressure of overcrowding and staff shortages was abandoned. It did not seriously re-emerge as a policy option until the 1940s, when the issue of abandoning 'locked doors' was widely discussed in medical and nursing journals. The first completely open institution was the Dingleton Hospital, Melrose, which after three years' transition opened all its doors in 1949.[26] This was followed by Mapperley Hospital, Nottingham, in 1953, and in 1954 by the renowned Warlingham Park Hospital, whose Welsh superintendent, T. Percy Rees, was a powerful advocate of the new system, and had begun the process by unlocking the gates to the institution soon after his appointment in 1935.[27] By implementing the policy during the 1950s the Denbigh hospital was in line with the more advanced mental hospitals in England.

The liberalization of the post-war years was partly a reflection of the changing composition of the patient population. Patients who came voluntarily seeking treatment and cure did not want to be confined under lock and key. These changes in expectation were as much responsible for the change in policy as the introduction of new drug treatments, and the ensuing pharmaceutical revolution, which has sometimes been credited with facilitating the transformation of the closed institution into an open one.

In 1950 the commissioner noted that the number of annual admissions to the Denbigh hospital had quadrupled over the past ten years.[28] The discharge rate too was accelerating, so that many of the extra admissions were transformed into quicker discharges. Nonetheless, without any commensurate fall in the number of long-stay cases, these expanding admissions were bound to swell the overall population of the hospital. During 1949 805 patients were admitted to the hospital, and 669 patients were discharged. The overall numbers kept creeping up, despite the quicker turnover, the re-location of mentally defective patients and the discharge of many of the older chronic cases to local authority homes.

Delivering Services Outside the Hospital

The work of the outpatient clinics expanded rapidly in the immediate post-war years, as the service formed an increasingly important part of the hospital's work. In 1947 the medical superintendent said that he regarded the outpatient clinics as the most fundamental service provided by the hospital.

> Of all cases of mental or nervous disorder within the community only a small proportion require admission to Hospital. The Majority have always been dealt with and will continue to be treated by the general practitioner and it is primarily with the object of providing him with a specialist service to which he can refer cases requiring special investigation or treatment that the out-patient clinics are run.[29]

These clinics provided the opportunity for much closer liaison with general practitioners in the many localities served by the hospital. By 1950 the majority of the intake were patients who had in the first place been seen at the outpatient clinics.[30] This meant that admissions could be planned, and patients persuaded beforehand of the efficacy of entering hospital for treatment on a voluntary basis. Outpatient consultations also enabled the psychiatrists to classify patients before their arrival at hospital, so in 1952, when it became necessary to impose some sort of restriction on the intake of patients due to overcrowding, it was possible more easily to adopt a system of screening applicants. Priority was given to urgent cases, and three separate admission units were set up on both the male and female sides of the hospital. Patients were classified into (a) the aged and infirm, (b) the socially disagreeable and (c) the mild and cooperative. A separate waiting list was maintained to correspond to each of these categories. The commis-sioners commented with approval on the policy: 'By reserving Gwynfryn for the third category a very large turnover is possible and a valuable service is being carried out.'[31] It gave psychiatrists much greater control over the selection of patients, a role denied under the old system of certification. In the beginning the development was slow because of the need to overcome prejudice and to convince general practitioners of their usefulness. Attend-ance rose from 304 in 1944 to 1,167 in 1948 and to 3,630 in 1954. By the end of the decade doctors from the NWMH were offering four sessions per month in Rhyl, six sessions in Bangor, five in Wrexham and one in Dolgellau.

In addition to setting up outpatient clinics, the hospital staff played a leading role in the development of the child guidance service in north Wales. Dr Frank Jones had taken an early interest in this service, and his successor as medical superintendent, Dr J. H. O. Roberts, was equally supportive of the expansion of psychiatry into this area, which he regarded as 'preventative' work. The member of staff most closely identified with the child guidance service was Dr Schwarz, who at the end of the war changed his name to Simmons. In 1947 he studied for the Diploma in Psychological Medicine and Fellowship in Child Guidance.[32] On completion of the qualification he was designated special liaison officer and worked with other providers in the field, such as Flintshire LEA and Caernarfonshire County Council. The normal mode of referral to the child guidance clinics was through the school medical officers. Dr Roger of the Education Department of the University College in Bangor also took a keen interest in the developments, making this into a formidable team, which did much to shape the growth of this professional service in north Wales. Child guidance clinics were held in Rhyl, Wrexham, Colwyn Bay and Flint.[33]

The work of the outpatient clinics was supported and enhanced by the work of the psychiatric social worker, who could spend time investigating the home environment of patients. The social worker also had a valuable role to play in the after-care of the patient, ensuring a smooth re-entry to occupational and family life. The first, Miss Thomas, was appointed in 1945. During 1948 students taking the mental health course at Manchester University each spent a month at the Denbigh hospital for the purpose of gaining experience. During that year 536 home visits were made, 209 visits to schools or other social agencies and 286 interviews were held in hospital or clinics.[34] From these energetic beginnings the social work department soon proved to be an extremely valuable part of the professional team working within the hospital and the community. By 1951 the hospital was employing three trained psychiatric social workers, two social workers and a clerk, and this 'well-organised department' was moved into a self-contained office at the reception unit.[35] At the end of the decade Kathleen Jones referred to the arrangements at the North Wales Hospital at Denbigh as a good working example of a hospital 'which has a well-staffed psychiatric social work department' and 'undertakes after-care in the surrounding area in lieu of the local authorities'.[36] The role of the social work department, the psychiatrists and the child guidance team developed further during the 1950s, stimulated by the growing practice of the courts in seeking psychiatric and home assessment reports before passing sentence on young offenders.

The growing pressure on bed space within the hospital indicated the need either to make further substantial additions to the buildings or to find some way of reducing both length of stay and total population over the long term. The overcrowding on the female side, which had been exacerbated by the dramatic rise in female admissions, was eased somewhat by the opening of a new villa in 1956. During the early 1950s there were still many long-term patients who had been resident in the asylum for twenty or thirty years or more. As the hospital tried to move away from the notion of a custodial regime, the intention was that patients would not in future stay in the hospital for such a lengthy duration, and that the rise in numbers would begin to show a reversal. Increasing emphasis was put on efforts to 'rehabilitate' patients. A new fifty-bedded villa for male patients, Bryn-hyfryd, built in the hospital grounds, was opened in 1957, and within two years had been designated as the 'rehab centre'. J. D. Williams, who started working at the hospital in 1947, recalled the setting up of the rehabilitation centre. The emphasis was on group work, and patients, especially those with 'depraved habits', would be sent there for 'habit training'. Sometimes patients would 'sit and chew their slippers'; others would turn up their trousers and fill them with faeces from the toilets. The staff tried to teach appropriate habits so that patients would be more readily accepted outside the hospital. The focus was primarily on the group as a whole, and there was very little individual attention. All of the men in the 'rehab ward' were provided with a suit, which they were expected to wear each day. The supplies were bulk-purchased so they all received similar clothes, including a fawn cardigan. There was little accommodating for individuality although, as J. D. Williams explained, Dr Roberts, the medical superintendent, a man of progressive ideas, was trying to introduce innovations. Percy Rees had pioneered methods of 'habit training' at Warlingham Park, in association with his open-door policy.[37]

One group of long-term patients, the ex-servicemen, received special attention. In 1947 a psychiatric social worker, Miss Sonia Drynan, was seconded from the National Association for Mental Health to the North Wales Hospital to take over the work with these cases. Her role was to liaise with families and outside agencies and to implement a care plan for each individual case. These patients received an official inspection each year to check on progress and to monitor care standards. When T. Owen visited on behalf of the Board in 1954 he remarked upon the cordial relationship which existed between the service patients and the nursing and medical staff. In 1957 medical inspector W. A. Collins visited fifty certified and seven voluntary service patients. He interviewed the patients and found them all 'quite contented'. Several had been given a leucotomy, but only one patient appeared to be making progress following the operation.[38] On his visit the following June he observed that 'Many of the patients are very demented and need general care and attention'.[39] In other years the inspectors commended the hospital upon the excellent recreational facilities, both at the main hospital and at the annexe at Pool Park, where some of the service patients were placed. Many of them were allowed out of the hospital both into town and to visit relatives, and the inspectors applauded the standard of clothing issued, and the fact that it bore 'absolutely no distinguishing features by which the wearer should be recognised'.[40] Following the Mental Health Act of 1959 the system of classification for patients was changed, as a result of which twenty-eight of the service patients were redesignated as informal patients, four as 'voluntary' and nine only remained classified as 'certified' insane. Several of the service patients were employed in making toy telephones for an outside manufacturer. This was regarded as a form of occupational therapy. The service patients all received a government allowance of 10s. per week to enable them to purchase 'extra comforts'.

By the mid-1950s official policy was undergoing a change, and the cost of state-funded mental hospitals was coming under the close scrutiny of central government. The Audit Office began to take a particular interest in the financial affairs of hospitals, and guided by their advice the Board of Control in 1955 came to the conclusion that asylum farms were no longer appropriate to the needs of a modern hospital. Instructions were issued that all asylum farms were to cease operation, and the land sold. There was an outcry from staff and committee members at the Denbigh hospital, and a submission was prepared requesting exemption from the ruling. The farm had for well over a century been a central feature of the asylum and the patients, many of whom were from agricultural and rural backgrounds, fitted happily in to the farming routine. The farm management committee had recently invested in a new herd of Friesian cattle, purchasing additional stock from the Runwell Hospital in Essex.[41] During the wartime years and the post-war period of rationing, the produce from the farm had played a vital role in maintaining dietary standards in the hospital. Board of Control inspectors agreed to carry out a special investigation, and received a deputation, but remained adamant that the decision be adhered to, despite some obvious sympathy for the protesters. 'One would have liked to humour these conscientious, well-intentioned people but we must be realistic and there can be no doubt that a case for regarding this farm as therapeutically essential has not been shown to exist.'[42] They therefore concluded 'reluctantly' that the ruling laid down by the Ministry had to apply, as it did to all other mental hospitals in the UK. The farm ceased operation and the land was sold. A private housing estate was built on some of the fields.

Although the loss of the farm was a blow to the institution, in other ways the creation of the NHS provided a boost to its ancillary services. The number of artisan staff was increased. The tailors' shop continued to produce hospital clothing, the kitchens were kept busy catering for the growing number of staff and patients on site, and a new printing department was established. It was run by charge nurse D. J. Jones, a qualified printer, to

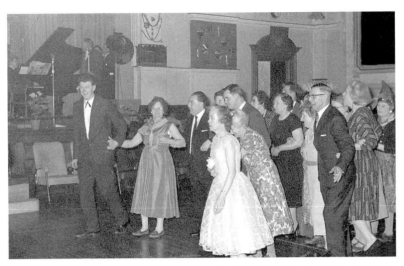

17. The Hospital Ball. Dai Bryn Jones takes the hand of the lead lady for the Grand March. Third from the left is Dr Elwy Owen, a member of a local Denbigh family who later became medical superintendent at the Talgarth Mental Hospital. Denbighshire Record Office

provide patients with the opportunity to try a new form of occupational therapy. It produced supplies of hospital stationery and the quarterly hospital magazine. The administrative burden of processing so many new patients, combined with the bureaucratic requirements of the new NHS, required an enlarged secretarial staff, so that incrementally a great number of additional jobs were created during the 1950s.

The disposal of the farm, however, meant a loss of work opportunity for the patients. In order to provide alternative outdoor work the hospital embarked on a new scheme to extend the recreational facilities, and the patients helped to create new gardens, new playing fields and a splendid sports ground. An excellent sports pavilion, overlooking both the cricket ground and the football field, was completed in 1960.

The patients continued to have a good choice of entertainment. Besides the long-established sporting facilities, there were trips to flower shows, dog shows, sports days, fêtes, coach tours and picnics on the beach at Rhyl and Pensarn in the summer. In 1959 the hospital began organizing week-long holidays, booking an entire guest house for the use of hospital patients. There were concerts and choirs, drama productions and whist drives. The reception hospital had its own more 'middle class' social life, including a mixed social once a week, and a brains trust each Sunday evening. The Christmas Ball remained the social event of the calendar for patients, staff and the people of Denbigh and tickets were always in hot demand. Some of the leading big dance bands of the day played at the hospital. In such ways the hospital was possibly at the pinnacle of its social life and achievement.

Occupational therapy suffered a setback during the war, due not only to shortages of staff, but to scarcity of craft materials. By 1948 there were three occupational therapy centres on the male side of the hospital and three on the female, and each was under the charge of a nurse. On the male side one of the nurses had trained as an occupational therapist, and provided overall supervision, and on the female side Mrs Howe Thomas continued to attend on a part-time basis. The value of OT continued to be emphasized by the commissioners, who in 1951 expressed their satisfaction with the 'extensive and careful organisation of the patients' activities'. They noted that 'Indoor crafts are taught in several different centres allowing suitable classification of patients to be maintained'.[43] During the 1950s art therapy and creative crafts were developed. The new occupational therapy centres and the employment of trained staff enabled the work to be taken more seriously. In 1958 the hospital decided to invest its own accumulated resources in a purpose-built pavilion for OT on the Gwynfryn site. This greatly enhanced the provision for chronic patients and made it possible to commence 'industrial' occupational therapy. Over the coming years work was extended to include light assembly and packing work.

Treatments

More experience was being gained with new treatments introduced during the war, and some refinements taking place in their application. In 1949 electroconvulsive therapy was administered with the aid of curare, a muscle relaxant, and had already become the most commonly used therapy in the hospital. By 1951 about one hundred patients with more persistent forms of mental illness had received a leucotomy operation, and about 33 per cent of these had been discharged. On the whole, however, the success rate with the chronic cases of long duration was not greatly improved. As the turnover of new patients increased, the long-term population came to be seen as a separate cohort, with an increasing proportion of elderly patients.

ECT was by far the most important treatment in use during the early 1950s, as shown by the table. There is an interesting gender pattern, in that far more women than men were receiving ECT. Alcohol aversion therapy had only just been introduced and was given to two male patients only, as was subconvulsive stimulation and hormonal treatment, the latter to suppress testosterone levels. More women than men were now receiving surgical treatment in the form of prefrontal leucotomy. A similar number of women were receiving narcoanalysis. The first mention of the use of psychotherapy in the hospital was in 1947, when it appears in the list of

Treatments administered to patients at the North Wales Hospital, Denbigh, in 1953

No. treated by various physical methods	Male	Female	Total
Electric convulsive therapy	261	417	678
Modified ECT	51	29	80
Deep insulin	21	16	37
Modified insulin	51	76	127
Partial narcosis	10	3	13
Ether or CO_2 abreaction	2	3	5
Alcohol aversion therapy	2	0	2
Prefrontal leucotomy	5	12	17
Narcoanalysis	4	12	16
Subconvulsive stimulation	8	0	8
Hormonal treatment	5	0	5

treatments provided by the medical superintendent in his annual report. There was no discussion of the introduction of this method. It is possible that it was introduced in conjunction with narcosis, a combination already practised in Swansea. It was believed that deep sleep therapy made the mind more receptive to psychotherapy and that the value of narcosis as a treatment was significantly enhanced if the 'talking treatment' followed it.

During the 1950s a revolution in treatments began to occur with the introduction of new drug treatments. Largactil was introduced and was one of the first drugs widely used by mental hospitals to treat schizophrenia. It was effective in controlling some of the more extreme symptoms of schizophrenia, and radically changed the problems of patient management. Increasingly patients were admitted to hospital and prescribed a medication, and, once their condition had stabilized under the influence of the drug treatment, they were discharged home to continue life on the medication. In the early years patients suffered a range of side effects. However, by 1970 it was reported that these were fewer with the latest drugs and that it was no longer necessary to administer an anti-Parkinsonian agent alongside the psychotropic medication. By this time 75 per cent of patients discharged from the hospital were on a pharmacological treatment for their psychiatric condition.[44] Yet strangely there is very little discussion of this in the annual reports of the Board of Control, which have been the main source available at the time of researching and writing this book. The first pharmacist had been appointed in 1943 and combined the work with that of taking X-rays. By 1948 there were three full-time dispensers working in the hospital.

The development of outpatient clinics alongside a range of new therapies undoubtedly inspired a new attitude towards receiving treatment in a mental hospital during the post-war years. People in Wales became more willing to talk frankly about their illness and actively to seek treatment. It is no surprise that a man who had been imprisoned for his ideals during the First World War, represented the University of Wales as a Christian Pacifist Member of Parliament 1923–4 and worked for a Quaker settlement in south Wales during the Depression years, should have been willing to seek treatment and speak honestly and openly of his illness. Burdened by the legacy of the horrors of Auschwitz and Belsen, Dachau and Buchenwald and by the devastating effects of the atomic bomb on Hiroshima and Nagasaki, he remained fearful for the international situation and especially the future of the peace movement. Perhaps he felt these concerns more acutely than most. He wrote to his brother in a private letter: 'We have a heavy heritage of despondency in our family.'[45] In 1948 he entered the York Retreat (a Quaker hospital for the treatment of the mentally ill) and was administered electric shock treatment.[46] He returned home in time for Christmas but continued to suffer from a deep despondency and in February was admitted as a voluntary patient to Gwynfryn ward at the North Wales Hospital.[47] After receiving treatment for his condition he was discharged home in April. During the summer he met many old friends and even managed to attend the National Eisteddfod at Dolgellau. Then by the autumn his condition had deteriorated and in October he was readmitted to the Denbigh hospital. He drew solace from listening to classical music and was grateful to Dr Lucy for allowing him to enjoy his wonderful recordings of works by Schubert.[48] On the morning of 16 December 1949, staff found him behind the door to his room, with a dressing gown cord around his neck. He had secured one end to the shutters of the window and attached the other to the door.[49] The immediate cause of death was a heart attack, but at the inquest the coroner concluded that it was caused by shock from hanging. Dr Williams, the consulting psychiatrist, stated that his patient was 'mildly depressed and had ideas of guilt, believing that his motives were unworthy'.[50] Whether this was the ultimate destiny of a cyclothymic personality or of the conscience of the Welsh people will remain amongst the many enigmas of one fondly known as 'George M. Ll.', a man whom some still consider 'un o'r dynion mwyaf a welodd yr ugeinfed ganrif'.[51]

By the end of the decade the change which had occurred in this sector of the health service was plain for all to see. In 1960 the hospital was visited by one of Wales's finest photographers, Geoff Charles, who had been commissioned to do a feature for *Y Cymro*.[52] The collection of photographs published on a full double-page spread showed various aspects of asylum life. The accompanying article was partly a recruiting drive to persuade more young people to join this modern hospital, in a pioneering branch of modern medicine. 'Psychiatry', it claimed, 'has changed the whole outlook of hospitals such as this. It is the spearhead of medical advance.' Most importantly the hospital was anxious to recruit Welsh-speaking students, and called upon them to serve their country: 'Dyma Cyfle Chwi – Merched a Meibion Cymru i wasanaethu Cymry mewn Gyrfa fodern ac anturus – gyrfa a dyfodol disglair iddi, a manteision eang.'[53]

The future looked bright, but in that same year the policy towards large-scale mental hospitals such as these was facing a sea change.

※

CHAPTER THIRTEEN

New Directions

Legislative Change

The Royal Commission on the Law Relating to Mental Illness and Mental Deficiency, known as the Percy Commission, was appointed in 1954 and reported in 1957. It was established in response to widespread concern about the chronic overcrowding in mental hospitals across the country and the acute shortage of nursing staff and junior doctors. The Mental Treatment Act of 1930 had introduced changes to the law, but not a complete reform and much of the 1890 Lunacy Act still remained in force. The Macmillan Commission of 1925 had made recommendations for an even more radical overhaul, yet there had been no major parliamentary debate upon the issue of mental health legislation since the readings of the 1930 Bill.[1] The Percy Commission's report reflected the change of thinking that had meanwhile taken place in regard to mental illness. One of its basic premises was that 'those suffering from mental disorder should, as far as possible, be treated in the same way as those suffering from physical illnesses and that compulsion and custody should be used as little as possible'.[2] Hence the Mental Health Act 1959 which arose from the Percy Report reversed many of the principles embodied in preceding mental health legislation. A new approach was enshrined in a term that signified a broad spectrum of illnesses of many gradations, namely 'mental disorder'. This was intended to cover all forms of mental ill health including what the Act described as 'mentally ill patients', 'psychopathic patients' and 'severely subnormal patients'. This signalled an abandonment of the concept of 'mental deficiency' and the terminology adopted – 'severely subnormal patients' – was intended to refer to those whose level of disability prevented them from living an independent life. In future no differentiation of legal status would be applied to anyone in terms of mental capacity if they were able to live independently. Mental illness was henceforth to be seen as a purely medical rather than a legal category. The Board of Control was to be abolished, and its monitoring functions handed to the Ministry of Health.

The inspection of individual hospitals disappeared, the Ministry instead being more concerned with the overall resourcing of mental health services. (From the point of view of the medical historian this signifies the end of those wonderfully detailed annual reports on each hospital.) The LEAs were to be responsible for dealing with severely subnormal children, and the welfare services for assisting elderly mentally ill people. This would necessitate better integration of services at regional level. Whereas the establishment of the NHS in 1948 signified the triumph of centralization, the 1959 Act implied a movement towards decentralization and greater emphasis on local authority and community-based provision.

Kathleen Jones has argued that the 1959 Act represented a complete reversal of the administrative principles established in 1845. Whereas the aim of the earlier legislation 'was to separate out the "insane" from the poor and the sick and the criminal, to provide a special service for them, and to centralize', now, as the pendulum swung back, the mentally disordered were to be again dispersed.[3] The concept of integration and the abolition of any distinct legal separation of the sane from the insane were the new hallmarks of policy.

One crucial change introduced by the 1959 Act was the principle that the decision to admit a patient to a mental hospital was primarily a medical one, transferring responsibility away from magistrates to medical staff. The change in admittance procedures enhanced the influence of medical superintendents and their professional staff. Psychiatrists now had even greater power to choose their patients.

Widening Participation

As the number of people willing to use the mental health services on a voluntary basis expanded, so the wider public became ever more accepting of mental illness. A psychiatric neurosis, it was argued, was 'as common as the common cold' and need no longer instil fear. Large institutions with long corridors and vast wards now seemed less appropriate to something so personal and intimate. Pressure groups like the National Association of Mental Health were beginning to influence public opinion, stimulating a popular debate about the nature of psychiatric care and provision.[4] By the 1950s there were widespread objections to what were colloquially referred to as 'loony bins'. A reappraisal of the role of the old long-stay mental hospitals was now climbing higher on the political and policy agenda. The modernization of mental hospitals had enormous resource implications. As television journalist Robin Day suggested, in an interview with the Minister of Health, Derek Walker Smith, there were some questions that the 1959 Bill did not address. One of these related to resourcing and current underfunding of mental hospital provision. The cost of medical attention was estimated to be about £3. 3s. 0d. per week per patient in a general hospital, but nationally the cost of funding a patient in a mental hospital was calculated at only 5s. a week. Similarly, in terms of research, the mental health services were the poor relation and received only 4 per cent of the Medical Research Council's investment.[5] There were demands for a greater equality of status.

Policy Changes

It was within this context of ongoing public debate that the newly appointed Minister of Health, Enoch Powell, visited the North Wales Hospital in October 1960. He was in the area to address the Welsh and English NHS Executive Councils' Conference in session at Llandudno. Having first called at a local GP's surgery and hailed such community-based provision as the backbone of the health service, he then moved on to the Denbigh hospital. During a tour of wards and facilities he apparently made clear to staff present his disapproval of this type of institution. They had hoped to impress on him the need for more beds and resources and so had taken him to see some of the crowded, long-term chronic wards. Apparently he was appalled, and visibly cringed at some of the sights and smells. His agenda would not be to commit more funding to such institutions.. He reserved his praise for the liaison work between the hospital and the local authority and told reporters that he was 'particularly interested in a course, provided for mental welfare officers of local authorities in preparation for the operation on November 1st of the new Mental Health Act'.[6] In his address to the conference the following day he spoke of the new attitude to mental illness and the dramatic possibilities for reform of the mental health services. 'One had to achieve the transition as rapidly as possible from one concept of a hospital's function to a quite different one', he said. Within less than six months Powell was to announce a total restructuring of mental health services and the abolition of the old-style mental hospitals.

In March 1961 Powell delivered another speech before an audience of the National Association for Mental Health, outlining his vision for the future of the mental health services. In colourful and emotive language, he poured scorn upon the mental hospitals of England and Wales: 'There they stand', he declaimed, 'isolated, majestic, imperious, brooded over by the giant water tower and chimney combined, rising unmistakable and daunting out of the countryside.' Now they were to be phased out. No money would be available for upgrading, and future provision was to be in the form of a combination of community facilities and general hospital wards. This policy was to be operationalized in the new Hospital Plan of 1962.

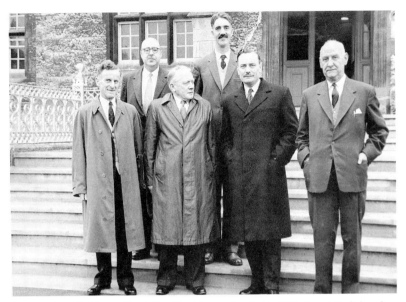

18. Photograph taken on Enoch Powell's visit to the hospital in 1960. From left: Sidney L. Frost, hospital secretary, E. Deakin, finance, ? Tudor, A. H. Lucas, supplies officer, Enoch Powell, Minister of Health, R. Glyn Pritchard, engineer. Denbighshire Record Office

The 1962 Hospital Plan for Wales forecast a reduction in the number of long-stay hospital beds, with a shift of resources towards the development of psychiatric wards in general hospitals. Projections were based on the assumption that all long-stay patients would have either died or been discharged by 1975. The number of beds provided by the North Wales Hospital was projected to fall to 800.

The rundown of large-scale mental hospitals was an international pheno-menon, pioneered in Italy and the USA.[7] The concept of 'deinstitutional-ization' or 'decarceration' gained tremendous support and there was a strong popular reaction against the negative and oppressive aspects of psychiatric care in large-scale mental hospitals. There is lively debate as to whether new drug therapies, economic forces or simply changing public attitudes were primarily responsible for instigating this new direction in policy. The influence of the anti-psychiatry movement provided an intel-lectual justification for the movement to run down and close many long-established institutions and the new policies found support from a wide political spectrum from the radical right to the radical left. There is not room in terms of this institutional/regional history to address this major issue, but simply to provide an account of the process of deinstitution-alization in north Wales and describe some of the many associated changes.

Rising Admissions

At the time that the Hospital Plan was published it was hard to see how such a vast reduction in the number of beds could be accomplished. The growing number of patients entering mental hospitals for treatment was putting increasing pressure on their resources rather than reducing patient demand. Of course, within the overall pattern there were geographical variations and that in north Wales may have differed somewhat from other regions. The number of annual admissions to the Denbigh hospital at this time was

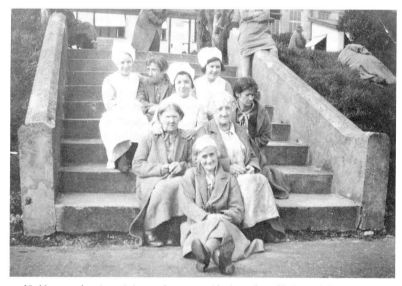

19. Nurses and patients sitting on the steps outside the asylum. Clothes and shoes were still made in the asylum. Many of the chronic patients cared for in the hospital during the 1950s had been there since the 1930s. Denbighshire Record Office

steadily upward, from 828 in 1950 to 1,026 in 1955 and reaching 1,515 in 1960 (see Figure 20). An increasing number of those admitted were success-fully treated and discharged within a short time. The patient population of the hospital peaked in 1956 when 1,523 were resident at the end of the year. Over the following three years the total number of patients in the institution declined, assisted perhaps by the introduction of new drug treatments and by some vigorous rehabilitation work on the male side of the institution. Then in 1960 this trend faltered. The majority of chronic patients still remained in the hospital, and each small addition of new patients who failed to achieve rapid and lasting recovery added to their number. Although the process of accretion had slowed down, it had never gone into reverse. What was more, an increasing number of the annual admissions were patients who were being readmitted to the hospital for further treatment. Whereas the number of 'first admissions' rose from 156 in 1939 to 767 in 1964, the number of readmissions (that is, of patients who had been discharged but who subsequently needed to be readmitted) rose from 51 in 1939 to 904 in 1964.[8]

In addition to the increasing proportion of readmissions, a clear demographic shift was taking place, which did not augur well for the recovery and discharge pattern. The superintendent pointed out that an increasing proportion of patients were over the age of sixty-five. During the period 1949–62 the annual admission of male patients over sixty-five years of age had almost doubled, while the female admissions in this age group had quadrupled. The increasing number of elderly patients admitted was swelling the group of ageing patients already in the institution so that this age group was becoming proportionately larger within the hospital. In 1962 the over-sixty-fives constituted 36 per cent of the population compared with only 26 per cent in 1950. He warned that, if the overall trend of accumulation continued, then, far from being reduced as envisaged by the Minister of Health, the bed complement would have to be increased.[9]

A Reversal of Trend

However, the pattern was about to change. Between 1964 and 1970 the number of patient beds at the Denbigh hospital declined by about 250. The average daily bed occupancy declined still more dramatically, falling by almost a half, from 1,349 in 1964 to 749 in 1970. This meant that there was less pressure on beds than formerly, bringing about a radical change in the spatial density of the hospital. As Dr T. Gwynne Williams wrote: 'Wards which formerly housed eighty people now treat about thirty patients. This is a reasonable number if there is to be a high standard of care.' He explained the implications for the type of treatment required. 'It should be understood', he remarked, 'that the patients now in Denbigh are much more demanding of medical and nursing skill than the quietly stabilized schizophrenics who were our former residents and who probably contributed more to the hospital than they required from us.'[10]

The reduction in numbers was achieved despite a continuing steep rise in annual admissions. In 1970 the total number of admissions was 1,948, a dramatic increase when compared to the figure of 207 patients admitted in 1939, and more than double the number of patients (904) who were admitted in 1964 (see Figure 20). To have secured such a marked reduction in the patient population while treating twice the number of admissions was an astounding achievement.

How was this dramatic reversal finally accomplished? First, the turnover of new patients admitted to the hospital was becoming ever more rapid.

Patients admitted on a voluntary basis, or on short-term (three-day) orders, could be given modern treatments, and as soon as they responded positively they were quickly discharged. It was believed that any tendency towards institutionalization would thereby be avoided. Secondly, the reversal in trend was brought about by the discharge of long-stay patients. Nearly 5 per cent of the patients discharged between 1965 and 1970 had been in hospital continuously for two years or more, and therefore fell into the category of 'long-term chronic' patients.[11] They numbered only 504 out of a total of 10,366 patients discharged during that same period. The significant point is that these were chronic patients, who had traditionally accumulated year on year. This was the one group that successive medical superintendents had tried to relocate outside of the asylum. It was only by reducing this core population of long-stay patients that a reversal in trend could be attained. Thirdly, some of the elderly chronic patients simply died.

A psychiatric social worker based at the hospital, M. Rolf Olsen, showed a keen professional interest in the new discharge policy and undertook an in-depth investigation of the patterns of patient accumulation and discharge.[12] He found that 65.5 per cent of the inpatients resident in July 1964 had been hospitalized for more than two years. He analysed the patterns of discharge for the period 1939–64, and discovered that out of a total of 1,536 patients discharged only forty-four had been in the hospital for two years or more.[13] The figures clearly proved that patients who remained resident for this period were extremely unlikely ever to be discharged. To reduce the in-patient population significantly, this was the group that would have to be targeted.

Olsen attributed the sharp reversal in policy to the appointment in December 1964 of a new consultant psychiatrist who had clinical responsi-bility for almost all of the 700 or so long-stay female patients at the hospital. Soon after his arrival Dr Dafydd Alun Jones began screening all the chronic patients with a view to discharge. Prior to his appointment to this post Dr Jones had conducted a survey in Anglesey, sponsored by the Nuffield Trust, into the prevalence of mental disorder in the community.[14] The investigators asked local general practitioners to screen their caseloads for patients with psychiatric symptoms that family doctors regarded as being 'outside of the normal'. Most GPs regarded mild anxiety states and periods of depression as being 'normal' and no more serious than a head cold, but outside of this they identified 1,988 'cases' who were 'active' during 1960, the equivalent of about 4 per cent of the population. Only 195 of these were in hospital or some form of residential accommodation and the remainder, a total of 1,793, were in the community. These findings convinced Dr Jones of the community's ability to absorb large numbers of people with a psychiatric condition. As he explained in an address delivered to the annual conference of the National Association of Mental Health in 1970:

Over 700 had fairly substantial problems. Only a little over 100 were long-stay patients at the North Wales Hospital. However, we found many individuals in the community who were clinically indistinguishable from many in hospital and it seemed clear that there were factors other than medical which determined who was there. In terms of actual numbers the proportion of the total load which was carried by the hospital was comparatively small. Halving the hospital population would add only one-twentieth to the community numbers. It certainly does not suggest flooding of the community by completely different ex-patients. On the other hand, the impact of such a reduction in the hospital would clearly be enormous.[15]

The level of family support was found to be critical in deciding whether a patient became a long-stay case in the Denbigh hospital. The study established that there was 'little hope of family support for the chronic institutionalised patients, and little readiness to accept the patient at home'.[16] It was the lack of family support that appeared to be the critical element in deciding the fate of the long-stay patient.

The message of these research findings was that some alternative option to family care must be provided to enable these patients to leave hospital. Local authorities had failed to provide the additional accommodation required by the rundown in long-stay hospital beds. Private landladies were encouraged to fill the breach, and to make accommodation available on a commercial basis for former long-stay patients. The boarding house schemes were established 'mainly through the initiative of the hospital consultant staff'.[17] The discharge of long-stay patients began.

Within about eighteen months of the launch of this scheme letters of opposition began to reach local councillors and the local press seized upon the issue. Residents of Abergele rural district objected to the use of a farmhouse in the area as a boarding house for a group of former patients who, it was alleged, 'roam the countryside and frighten people'.[18] The county medical officer of health appealed for a 'little practical Christianity', and 'sympathy and understanding for people less fortunate than oneself'.[19] The *Western Mail* reporter was told that the Denbigh hospital had arranged similar accommodation in Rhyl, Anglesey and Wrexham. A Welsh Board of Health spokesman explained that throughout Britain people who no longer needed mental hospital care and who did not have homes were being helped to find such accommodation in hostels and halfway houses. Anyone could convert a house to multi-occupation and take in ex-patients, since there was no system of registration in operation. Rhyl and District Trades Council expressed concern about this lack of regulation, and the fact that homes were being operated by unqualified staff, free of any monitoring or inspection.[20] Former patients were provided with a minimal allowance of 25*s.* a week from the Ministry of Social Security, but little else. Without any system of social support many of them, it was claimed, were vulnerable to exploitation or neglect. It was alleged that in one boarding house a landlady misappropriated patients' pocket money.

When the discharge policy began, regular multi-disciplinary case conferences were held on each client, but after about a year these came to an end. When patients were discharged they were no longer the responsibility of mental hospital staff. Without the local authority assuming the duty, the former patients were effectively left without support. There was no overall coordination of the scheme, no systematic transfer of information between the hospital and the local authority, and no after-care arrangements were made.

Some professional observers were critical of the discharge policy. One psychiatric social worker in north Wales claimed that

> patients were simply thrown out of the hospital without preparation. Buses and coaches collected them and they were crammed into boarding houses, dumped on landladies. One group of patients was placed with a woman whose own children were in care. It was a travesty of a service for vulnerable, frightened people.[21]

Denbighshire County Council became concerned about reports of over-crowding in some boarding houses, particularly in properties which were not properly adapted or equipped with fire doors and smoke alarms. The chief fire officer of Denbighshire and Montgomeryshire was quoted in both local and national newspapers as saying that some patients were living in 'death traps'.[22] He had already written to the hospital, warning of the danger of placing patients in a boarding house at Marchweil.[23] The local authorities believed that the best way to uphold standards would be to register all of the boarding houses as nursing homes, under section 19 of the Mental Health Act 1959, which applied to residences accommodating two or more mentally disordered persons. Registration under this clause would impose certain obligations on the landladies, not only in terms of registration and compliance with building and fire regulations, but also in regard to providing patients with access to clinical, social and occupational therapy. The hospital consultants argued that former patients had been discharged 'recovered' and no longer required support of this nature. Use of the term 'nursing home' would, they protested, only serve to stigmatize the patients and perpetuate their dependence.

Public disquiet escalated to the level of public scandal when a general practitioner called at one boarding house to examine a patient who was suffering from pneumonia, and discovered other residents in the same home suffering from anaemia, severe under-nourishment and scabies. The affair received headline coverage in the *News of the World* and *The Sunday Times*, as well as the north Wales press.[24] Mr Tom Ellis, a local MP, tabled a parliamentary question, and in reply Peter Thomas, Secretary of State for Wales, stated that in future local authorities intended to 'maintain a close watch' on all of the boarding houses.[25] Finally a system of registration was established, and most landladies agreed to cooperate.

In 1969 a preliminary examination of all long-stay hospitals in Wales was conducted. Subsequently, in 1970, a team was appointed by the Welsh Hospital Board to carry out a more detailed investigation of the North Wales Hospital. During their survey 'it became apparent to the team that there were certain aspects requiring more urgent consideration than others' and so they proceeded to prepare a two-part report. Certain management problems surfaced during the inquiry. There was a lack of consensus amongst staff as to whether the hospital operated as a 'whole unit' with all available beds being pooled, or whether certain wards were the prime responsibility of a particular consultant and designated for a certain type of patient. The policy of allocating particular categories of patients to specific wards, adopted during the Second World War, was by now a long-established practice. Some wards, for instance, provided care exclusively for elderly female patients. The situation regarding admissions was complicated by the fact that, in addition to this spatial division within the hospital, there was also a division of responsibility amongst consultants for the geographical catchment areas allocated. North Wales was divided into three regions for the purpose of outpatient provision. In order to ensure continuity of care a patient seen at a clinic would remain with the same consultant during their in-stay period. This sometimes cut across the division of responsibilities within the hospital and had the potential to create a somewhat chaotic situation. The survey team reported that

> nursing and junior medical staff have informed us that the diversification of clinical responsibility in a particular ward is difficult for them to operate, and nursing staff in particular considered that it was a contributory factor to their complaint of insufficient medical cover.

There was no overall responsibility in such a situation, and often patients were not seen regularly by any consultant. Nursing staff claimed they were left in charge of patients for whom there was no treatment plan and in some cases not even a diagnosis.

The survey team identified a number of problems associated with the rapid reduction in patient numbers. Whilst affirming that consultant psychiatrists had demonstrated beyond doubt that a unit of 1,500 beds, 'providing primarily custodial care, is capable of evolving into an active treatment unit', the team indicated that this had 'not been achieved without causing problems'. Currently there appeared to be no clear policy regarding the number of beds that were available, or likely to be available after the refurbishing and upgrading of wards. Indeed there was a marked lack of agreement. According to the Welsh Hospital Board's statistics there were 1,096 beds available, but on investigation it appeared that there were approximately '600 beds which could be described as being available to accommodate patients'.[26] The survey team detected a lack of executive responsibility. The rapid decarceration began presenting more problems as some patients who had been discharged to boarding houses were readmitted to hospital. Medical staff made efforts to resist this trend. In January 1971 Dr D. O. Lloyd raised the problem of the 'recent influx of patients from Boarding Houses which had proved unsatisfactory'.[27] The superintendent suggested contacting the psychiatric social worker for Denbighshire to discuss the problem, and pointed out that it had already been agreed that no Flintshire patients would be readmitted unless there was a serious doubt as to their suitability for a boarding house.

The status and welfare of patients discharged to boarding houses re-mained a source of ongoing concern. In March 1970 Dr D. O. Lloyd visited the Talardy Boarding House and found that a number of patients had left without his knowledge. He expressed worries regarding the likelihood of follow-up care, since most of these patients were, he considered, only able to care for themselves 'to a very limited extent'. Dr Williams echoed these con-cerns, and referred to the case of another former patient, M.W., as an instance of someone who had been disturbed in the community for 'quite a long period' before the mental welfare officer took action.[28] The situation appears to have improved somewhat as, following criticisms, the hospital paid more attention to resettlement of long-stay patients. There were improvements too in community facilities and in social work support following the reorganization of social services in 1971.

Choosing Patients

To maintain the reduction in patient numbers it was vital to ensure that a new cohort of long-stay patients did not build up. The persistent reappear-ance of 'undesirable' patients led to discussions amongst medical staff concerning the type of clientele for which the hospital should cater. Medical staff argued that the hospital should avoid being used to house socially deviant individuals. Some patients were persistent returners. In May 1968 Dr D. O. Lloyd raised concerns about two in particular, who had been recurrent readmissions and who 'could or should be presented as policy problems rather than psychiatric'.[29] Medical staff decided to make it 'clear to the Mental Welfare Officers that they should advise the Police to the effect that anti-social behaviour, drunkenness and aggression were matters for the Police to deal with, rather than the psychiatric units'.[30] Dr Lloyd said that he did not mind colleagues phoning him at home concerning such patients and their readmission, should it be deemed necessary. This provides some indication of how seriously the matter was viewed by senior consultants.

From October 1968 a list of problem patients, accompanied by brief clinical notes, was lodged with the switchboard operators. Although inclusion of a patient on the list 'did not necessarily preclude admission', nonetheless it was clearly aimed at effecting better gatekeeping. A list of former Afallon patients was also provided, with the instruction that any question of readmitting any one of them should first be discussed with Dr D. A. Jones.[31] Afallon ward was currently designated for patients with personality disorders.

Alerting staff to the possible reappearance of undesirable patients remained a standard practice. In October 1969 Dr T. G. Williams insisted that a patient should not be readmitted unless he displayed 'undoubted evidence of psychotic illness'.[32] At the end of the month Dr Craig asked that lists of problem patients be given to medical staff, so that they could easily be consulted when telephone calls were received requesting admissions of patients to hospital. It was agreed that the list would be brought up to date and circulated.[33] In these and other ways medical staff sought to control the intake of patients.

Control of Sexuality

Changing attitudes towards sexuality and the more liberal regime introduced by the open-door policy led staff to confront anew the ethical problems raised by the free association of the sexes. Male patients were able to fraternize with female patients to an extent never previously possible. The difficulty that arose was the degree to which male patients would 'prey upon' or 'pester' vulnerable female patients. Once movement in and out of villas and wards and about the hospital grounds became relatively unrestricted, it became difficult to observe and monitor personal interactions. In terms of medical care and responsibility the old division between the male and female sides of the hospital continued. Many of the patients did not so much transgress, as simply ignore, the old boundaries. The dilemmas posed are illustrated in some of the discussions that took place during the weekly staff meetings. Medical staff clearly continued to feel a paternalistic or perhaps a patriarchal responsibility towards the protection of vulnerable female patients. In May 1968 doctors talked about the effectiveness of Stilboestrol in suppressing the sexual potency of male patients, or whether it would be ethical to administer the contraceptive pill more liberally on the female side. Faced with such complex moral issues the consensus of the meeting was that 'it was difficult to know how to restrict breeding without restricting companionship in the hospital'. Many of the medical officers found it hard to decide 'where our province lies', but felt fairly certain that 'one must protect a psychotic female from exploitations'.[34]

Difficult ethical issues also arose in relation to same-sex relationships, although here there seems to have been less hesitation about the need to repress such activities. In March 1968 Dr Owen asked the medical superintendent what measures had been taken regarding a patient who had been transferred from the high-security mental hospital at Broadmoor, and who 'was involved in homosexual activity'. In response Dr. Williams explained that the patient had been transferred to male 6 ward, where he could be kept under closer supervision, and put on Stilboestrol injections.[35]

Stilboestrol was by this time being used liberally for its calming properties. Opinion seems to have been divided amongst the medical staff concerning its 'effect on male sexual drive'. The superintendent physician was clearly in no doubt about its efficacy, but he did acknowledge that there were limitations to its use. He told his colleagues that 'Stilboestrol in effective doses, taken regularly, was usually satisfactory, but it would be pretty ropey to put a patient on a section simply for the purpose of administering Stilboestrol'.[36] (It was only by putting a patient 'on a section' that medication could be administered without the patient's agreement.)

In December 1969 staff were alerted to a circular sent out by the Committee on Safety of Drugs, which gave advice that in future only those brands of contraceptive tablet which contained less than 50 mg of Stilboestrol should be used.[37] There was concern about the side effects of this medication as, over the long term, some of the male patients who were given the drug developed enlarged breasts, or experienced impotency or other bodily changes, with grave implications for their sexual identity.

Dr Williams consulted a colleague in Cardiff, Dr Rawnsley, concerning the ethical aspects of the protection of female patients to prevent conception. He advised that if the 'male subjects refuse to take Stilboestrol' it would be outside of the medical staff's legal province to force them to do so. In his hospital 'the intra-uterine coil was used to a great extent', and he suggested this was a useful alternative.[38] Oral contraceptives were prescribed to female patients, but there were certain rules of medical etiquette regarding prescription. If a patient who was admitted to hospital was already taking an oral contraceptive, then she should continue on that particular pill, and continue to pay for it. If necessary a hospital doctor could write a private prescription. If, however, a patient was admitted and then prescribed oral contraceptives, the medical staff were instructed to prescribe Ovulen or Norinyl–1, which the hospital would provide.[39]

In July 1968 Dr Lloyd reported that 'some nuisance' had been caused to nursing staff by male patients visiting female wards, and asked Dr D. A. Jones if he could verify this. Dr Jones replied that 'there were dangers involved when immature or inadequate short-stay patients met others of similar personality'. He had grave reservations about the mixing of such people, and felt that, ideally, short-stay patients such as those admitted to Bryn Hyfryd, should be segregated. This prompted the superintendent to point out that, with adequate staffing, 'the dangers of undesirable attachments could be discussed with the patient'. Whereupon Dr Lloyd retorted that 'patients can meet anywhere.' Consensus on such delicate matters was hard to find and, although a lengthy discussion followed, 'no decisions were reached regarding the extent to which segregation of the sexes was desirable in hospital'.[40] Now that there was no longer an acceptance of rules preventing sexual relationships between patients, the issue inevitably began to absorb an increasing amount of time, and the ethical considerations associated with the decision of whether or not to intervene were raised again and again.

Sexual misdemeanours were still a cause of anxiety, particularly when allegations were made against staff. In 1970 a chronic alcoholic patient accused a male nurse of attempting fellatio with him. Prior to any inquiry, a doctor reminded colleagues that it was vitally important that the patient was not given ECT or other treatment which might affect his short-term memory, since this could be interpreted as suppression of evidence. Staff could no longer simply be asked to resign, and both patients and staff had the right to a fair hearing.

In the wider society, the sexual liberation of the 1960s led to a more open acceptance of premarital sexual relationships and greater freedom of expression. It did not, however, lead to the disappearance of prejudices concerning same-sex relationships. During these years aversion therapy was used in the hospital not only for gambling and alcohol abuse, but also in order to 'cure' gay men of their sexual orientation. Author and sexual health worker John Sam Jones recalled his own experience of growing up in north-west Wales during the 1960s and discovering his sexual identity. 'It was the age of peace, free love and tolerance', he said. And yet he faced only intolerance. The religious prejudices and insidious homophobia of Welsh society caused him to experience feelings of guilt, fear and confusion. At the age of eighteen he tried to commit suicide. He was admitted to the Denbigh hospital, and having confessed to homosexual activities he was given electric shock aversion therapy. 'I was shown pornography and given shocks', he explained. 'It was the only treatment available and I hated myself so much that I didn't resist. But it screwed me up even more.' It took him a long time to overcome the psychological and emotional trauma, and during the years of self-healing and recovery he took the unusual step of training to become a

Methodist minister. He now campaigns against the homophobic attitudes
that so nearly cost him his life.[41] Electric shock therapy is no longer used as a
medical device to repress homosexuality.

Drug Treatments

The greatest change to take place between 1950 and 1970 was the
introduction of a growing number of drug treatments for a range of
illnesses. By 1970 75 per cent of all patients were discharged on a pharmacological regime for their psychiatric condition.[42] Since the 1950s there had
been significant improvements in many of the drugs, so that they gave fewer
side effects and it was longer necessary to regularly administer an anti-
Parkinsonian agent. A wide array of new drugs was constantly becoming
available and the hospital pharmacist regularly updated staff on their availability. In June 1968 it was reported that a supply of Melleril, a substitute for
Largactil, was in the pharmacy and that it had fewer side effects.[43] In
January 1969 there was some discussion of the relative advantages of
Modicct over Moditen Enanthate and doctors increasingly had to be
cognizant of contra-indications.[44] Dr Siddiqui pointed out the hallucino-
genic properties of mandrax, reminding colleagues that like many sedatives
it was addictive. This introduction of new drugs continued apace in the early
1970s. Anafronil, a tricylic anti-depressant to be administered by intra-
venous infusion, was tried at the hospital in November 1970.

The use of a wider variety of medications and the sheer number of
prescriptions had cost implications. Dr Williams expressed concern that
expensive drugs were being prescribed for twenty-eight days at a time, a
practice that should be strictly reserved for routine treatments.[45] Between
January and mid-September 1968, prescriptions of one drug alone, Moditen
Enanthate, cost £879. In the hospital it was possible to make use of a multi-
dose bottle, but when the drug was administered to patients visiting the outpatient clinic, it was necessary to use an ampoule, and these were only
provided in 25 mg doses. If a patient required only half of this dose, the
other half was wasted. In September 1969 the pharmacist highlighted the
price of Genticin, which was costing 19*s.* 6*d.* for each injection. It was noted,
however, that such advice was intended 'purely to inform and not in any way
to control the prescribing doctor, whose responsibility was final'.[46]

With the growing turnover of patients, the relaxing of rules and the
greater freedom of movement in the hospital, the need to ensure the security
of drugs and medications became more pressing.[47] The increasing number
of patients with drug addiction problems exacerbated the problem, and on
occasion medications were stolen from insecure cupboards. Jurisdiction over
drugs was a potential source of friction within the institution. Some drugs

needed to be kept in medicine cupboards in the wards for emergency use when the pharmacy was closed. If the pharmacist found that practices were becoming too lax, he insisted that measures of good practice be observed.

The common practice of continuing drug treatments after patients were discharged home or to boarding houses raised further issues of safety and monitoring. In January 1970 the pharmacist expressed concerns about the condition of a patient who had returned to the hospital from a boarding house in the Rhyl area, having been given 'a large prescription of several varieties of tablets'. The medical superintendent suggested that when patients left hospital their medication should be simplified as far as possible. There were obvious dangers for patients who were no longer under medical supervision when self-administering powerful drug treatments.[48]

The language used to discuss individual 'cases' changed profoundly with the shift towards a greater dependence on pharmacological treatments. The patient became objectified as the symptomotology of mental conditions was described in more technical and scientific terms. Alongside this altering discourse, the gulf between perceptions of the medical staff who monitored bodily and psychiatric symptoms and the nursing staff responsible for the daily care of patients grew. This change may have been partly responsible for the changing relations between nursing and medical staff within the hospital.

The growing plethora of drug treatments meant that a large part of the doctor's work now revolved around making assessments and prescribing medications. Drug therapies replaced most of the other treatments introduced during the Second World War. The last leucotomy seems to have been carried out in 1964. It resulted in haemorrhaging from the skull and the patient's death. The one treatment that remained in regular use was ECT. Thousands of patients had now received this treatment, and the equipment, which had been purchased years before, was beginning to deteriorate.

Financial stringency and ageing equipment meant that the hospital was not well served by its technical machinery. At a meeting of the medical officers committee in November 1968, a complaint was heard from Dr R. R. Hughes that the present EEG machine was obsolete. It appeared that the cost would be 'greater than the amount of money available in the next financial year for equipment'.[49] A month later the question of the ECT equipment was discussed, this too being regarded as obsolete.[50]

In September 1969 the medical superintendent asked his staff to consider the proposition of centralizing ECT so that all treatment would take place at one location. Some staff expressed misgivings, fearing lest patients 'should lose personal contact with members of the medical and nursing staff whom they knew during treatment', and because it would involve having their treatment in unfamiliar surroundings. It was anyway to be some time before this proposal was put into effect.

Meanwhile some of the ageing equipment was causing concern, and in July 1969 it was reported that certain ECT machines were producing burns. Staff generally agreed that only one of the machines on the female side of the hospital could be used satisfactorily. Dr Williams passed the problem to the hospital secretary, asking him to contact the manufacturers.[51] The manufacturers replied to the effect that minor burns were possible using mains electricity if the electrodes were not properly placed, but that burns could not be caused when the battery was used. Dr D. A. Jones advocated that the battery charge only should be used, but it was generally felt that it was not possible to apply this rule to all wards. Much dissatisfaction was expressed over the replies from the manufacturers. It was even suggested that the Medical Defence Union should be approached to take up the issue. Finally it was agreed that the secretary of the medical staff committee write to the senior administrative medical officer expressing the unanimous concern of the medical staff and their dissatisfaction with the position.[52] By the following week, however, the seriousness of the discontent had already escalated, following a burn sustained by a patient receiving ECT, prompting the hospital secretary to communicate directly with the Welsh Hospitals Board. Dr Williams felt it would be advisable to convert all ECT machines for use off the mains supply to ensure that the patients were receiving an adequate convulsive shock, 'but that such apparatus should then be used for only a brief one-second shock with adequate muscular relaxation'. The problem was that only two of the machines in the hospital were adapted for use on mains only, whereas all of the others were battery operated. The techniques required for administering the mains shock differed from that used on the battery model. Hence, it was once more emphasized that ' the shock should be applied with the mains only machine for a period of no more than 1–3 seconds, whereas with the battery apparatus it was necessary to apply the shock until a fit was actually observed'.[53]

In February 1970 complaints of patients receiving burns from ECT treatment were still being raised. The problems were gradually solved as improved ECT equipment was purchased and operated and maintained centrally, rather than being available for use on individual wards. This allowed for greater staff expertise to be developed. However, debates associated with this changeover, and the problems experienced with the machinery, reveal a certain level of amateurishness in dealing with the application of shock therapy. When it was suggested at one point that patients be given 50–100 mg of Phenergan by mouth some four hours before their ECT treatment, some members of staff held that Phenergan was incompatible with mono amine oxidase inhibiting drugs. It was suggested the pharmacist write to the firm concerned for advice. It was fortunate that this precautionary enquiry was initiated, since Mayer & Baker, the makers of Phenergan, advised against, making it clear that no assurance could be given that simultaneous administration of these medications would be safe.

The use of new medications, and of electric shock therapy and the increasing rate of admission and discharge were placing greater demands on the medical staff. So, too, was the increase in non-traditional work within the hospital. Two new groups of patients rapidly expanded during the late 1960s and 1970s – the patients with drug problems, and young women seeking abortions.

The admission of a growing number of patients with drug-related problems also had implications for hospital management. The needs of these patients were very different from those of the traditional categories of patients with which staff were familiar. Some of them, usually quite young patients, could be disruptive, particularly of the routines on wards operated along traditional lines.[54] Many staff believed that patients with drug-related problems required skilled and specialized treatment, and that it was not in their interests, or in the interests of other patients, to mix them together. The problem was that no adequate provision existed in the region, and so the North Wales Hospital became, in the view of many staff, a 'dumping ground' for this new social phenomenon. Nursing staff believed that the majority of these patients were not suffering from a psychiatric illness, and could not benefit from the regimen of a hospital designed to cater for nervous and mental diseases.

Monitoring of drug addicts was required, both by central government and at ward level within the hospital. In July 1968 the medical superintendent reported that the Welsh Hospitals Board had asked for the number of drug addicts admitted each month to be reported. It was decided that each individual doctor should decide which of their patients fell into the categories of 'drug addict' or 'alcoholic', and the numbers should then be returned to the chief male nurse's or matron's offices. The question was raised as to whether the number of outpatients falling into these categories should also be recorded, but it was decided not to do this unless clear instructions were forthcoming from central government.[55] In November 1968 a directive was received from the Home Office concerning heroin addicts, who might present themselves at the hospital complaining of withdrawal symptoms. Full details of such patients, including physical characteristics that would allow them to be clearly identified, along with the medication they were on, needed to be forwarded immediately to the Home Office, which offered a twenty-four-hour service. The central register could then be checked to ascertain whether they had previously received treatment and medication at other hospitals, or whether they were new patients. This would allow the Home Office to maintain up-to-date information, and to monitor the situation on a countrywide basis.[56] The hospital thereby took on a new role as an agent of state surveillance.

Monitoring drug-related problems meant that doctors had to comply with a growing list of official procedures in administering medications. In

May 1971 their attention was drawn to a circular stating that dexedrine, mandrax and some other items were put on Section A. This ruling had previously only applied to morphine and heroin addicts. Henceforth only certified addicts could be issued with these drugs, and only two approved consultants at the hospital, Dr Gwynne Williams and Dr Parsons, were allowed to prescribe them.[57]

Within the hospital, monitoring of addiction cases was built into operational procedures. In July 1968 the medical superintendent drew attention to a 'difficult case who might be an amphetamine addict', and suggested that the special observation card should have the categories 'drug addiction' and 'alcoholism' added, and this was agreed.[58] In October it was announced that the special observation cards would no longer constitute 'Caution Cards', and would therefore bear no special instructions. Their main advantage was that they would be a means of communicating to nurses information about patients, and would be of assistance both in deciding the appropriate ward and in overcoming any possible breaks in nursing continuity. They were to be renamed 'Special Information Cards'.[59]

Although the hospital had dealt with many alcoholic patients over the years, the growing number of drug addicts was an entirely new pheno-menon, and even in north Wales it was of growing proportions. In January 1971 Dr Dafydd Alun Jones drew the attention of the medical committee to the 'marked increase in the abuse of drugs in this area over the last 12 months'. This prompted a general discussion about the hospital's policy towards drug-related problems, but no definite guidelines were agreed upon.[60]

The hospital was taking on other new functions in relation to the wider changes in society which were a feature of the 1960s. The Abortion Act of 1968 permitted an abortion to be carried out under the NHS if it could be shown that a continuation of the pregnancy was detrimental to the mother's health. As a result, an increasing number of patients were referred for psychiatric assessment, since it was now possible to obtain an abortion under the NHS if a psychiatrist was prepared to sign a recommendation that to proceed with the pregnancy could damage a patient's mental health. Obviously these cases needed to be dealt with promptly, since time was of the essence. In June 1969 Dr D. A. Jones reported that he had made arrange-ments for a consultant obstetrician to examine patients first. If a termination 'was not surgically contra-indicated' following this assessment, then Dr Jones would see the patient from the psychiatric point of view. Other psychiatrists expressed concerns that abortion reports were time-consum-ing, and appeared to be 'taking precedence over normal clinical cases'.

In addition medical staff were now being required to produce reports for the justice system. Psychiatrists were under increasing pressure to respond to the needs of probation officers and legal officers in providing evidence for court reports. This growth in demand coincided with the repercussions in terms of workload arising from the Abortion Law reform. Medical staff proposed that probation officers be advised that clinical priority should take precedence over social and that such cases should take their turn on the out-patient lists. Following some discussion of the legal implications of this, it was suggested that if a report was urgently required, then 'a proper fee for making a special report out of the routine clinical hours' should be paid, since such work could be very time-consuming.

The nature and orientation of psychiatric work was changing alongside the policy shift and as the hospital reduced its bed space many changes took place. As the hospital was gradually reduced in size the central gravity of work shifted toward other sites.

CHAPTER FOURTEEN

The Final Years

Launched in 1989, the Welsh Mental Illness Strategy promoted the development of locally based mental health services, in conjunction with psychiatric units based in general hospitals. A closure programme was prepared for the North Wales Hospital, necessitating a rapid acceleration in the relocation of remaining patients. The emphasis on community care of the mentally ill could not fully obviate the necessity for secure accommodation for patients who represented a risk. In 1994 planning permission was obtained for a purpose-built twenty-five-bed medium secure unit at Bryn y Neuadd Hospital, Llanfairfechan.[1] Bryn y Neuadd was still operating on a limited scale providing accommodation for patients with learning difficulties in cases where it was difficult to locate them elsewhere. Its main building was in use as an administrative centre for Gwynedd Health Authority. There had been widespread local opposition to the proposal to locate a medium secure unit on this site, whereas the town of Denbigh had become very accustomed to having a psychiatric hospital on its doorstep, and accepting of the presence of mental hospital patients in its community. As staff pointed out, the hospital was viewed as Denbigh's 'bread and butter'. This was not the case in some of the towns that were originally proposed as sites for a medium secure unit. In Rhyl residents successfully opposed hosting a medium secure unit, and similar responses were met with elsewhere.

The process of closing and dismantling the services of the Denbigh hospital was a complicated and protracted affair. The remaining few wards had to be decommissioned, and the patients found alternative accommodation. This was a difficult time, and the procedure required careful and thoughtful management. There was a danger that, with staff morale running low, standards would slide. Keeping staff and patients informed could be difficult when the power to take decisions lay beyond the hospital. Finding places for the last of the patients proved troublesome. Over the previous decade, with growing experience of patient's needs within the community, a great deal of care had been taken in matching patients to suitable accommodation. The remaining patients were those very ones for whom it had been most difficult to find suitable placements. Ultimately, these reloca-tions became a matter of urgency. A skeleton nursing and administrative staff continued to function, with the patient records department remaining in the building almost to the last. Certain functions of the institution had to remain as long as a small staff remained on site.

Ward after ward was cleared and equipment and furniture removed. As rooms and cupboards were emptied more and more records and artefacts were discovered, and the question arose as to what to do with them. Original plans of the hospital were discovered in the boiler rooms, nurses' day and night ledgers were turned out of ward offices and stock-taking lists were found in the old stores. The mountain of papers grew and grew. It filled male ward 5, spilling over into adjoining wards. Skips were parked outside the hospital and each day they were filled with debris. Vast quantities of administrative records were shredded. All patient records, which are subject to legal controls, were secured by the health authorities. It was quite im-possible to retain all of the other records but there was a keen awareness of the value of many of these papers. The history group within the asylum had always received enthusiastic support from amongst the nursing, artisan and administrative staff. Anything that looked as if it might be of historical interest was sent to the 'history collection'. The county archives had already accepted a large quantity of hospital records, and were willing to take more, but space was limited. A selection process had to take place. This in itself was a time-consuming process, and members of the staff history group gave generously of their time. If their influence is written large in this book it is only because of the many long hours which the writer spent in their company, rescuing what could be found of the lives of generations of patients and the succession of employees and of the life of the institution itself.

Amongst the last activities to finish was occupational therapy. The workrooms remained in use to the end, and the garden and greenhouses, always so popular with some of the patients. During the late spring of 1995 tomato plants were on sale, and flowers were still being cut that last summer. A sense of finality loomed as the corridors became emptier, and staff numbers dwindled. The kitchens continued to provide meals for the remaining patients and staff, but the number of dishes served became fewer and fewer. When the ceiling fell in on the canteen, fortunately without causing injury, it somehow seemed to many remaining staff symbolic of the hospital's final demise. With the chapel no longer required, its altar, pews, chairs, vases and crucifix were transferred to the Denbigh Infirmary. The commemorative stained-glass windows were removed, the apertures boarded up and the doors sealed.

Given the wealth of history locked within the hospital walls, it seemed important to keep a record of the very buildings themselves. The Royal

Commission on Ancient Monuments for Wales was contacted and agreed to send a photographer and architectural historian to complete an emergency recording of the architectural heritage of the site.[2] They arrived on an extraordinarily fine summer day, and staff brought out a jug of ice cold water with lemons, as we all sat on the hot steps at the front of the asylum, and planned the task ahead. This involved making a careful photographic record of buildings and artefacts and copying architectural drawings, so that the sometimes fragile originals could be retained within the main collection of hospital documents.

Until the last days of operation the women at the reception desk continued to take telephone calls from families anxiously seeking advice on whom to contact for assistance for distressed and sick relatives. The Denbigh asylum was widely known and, although the number had long since stopped being the simple Denbigh 7, it was still the one port of call which many knew and to which they would turn when desperation took hold.

The hospital and its 120-acre site was put on the open property market. A national and international marketing campaign was conducted by property agents Knight, Frank and Rutley, but despite pursuing a vigorous sales drive for a year or more no serious bidders materialized. Then, in 1996, a London-based property company took out an option to buy the site, primarily to develop residential housing, involving an investment of between six and eight million pounds.[3] They submitted a plan to convert the 1848 building into 100 flats and to erect hundreds of other houses in the grounds. Planning permission was refused, as was a second application, following opposition from local councillors.[4] This time the company withdrew. By 1997 various local groups were anxious to develop a museum and use the hospital for community facilities. The sums of money quoted for purchase and conversion were enormous and seemed out of reach. There was also talk of plans for a prison, an army barracks, tertiary college, folk museum and hotel. Then a plastics firm from Halifax expressed an interest. They had an ambitious scheme, including a research unit in the main hospital linked to energy and conservation, further and higher education facilities with residential provision, new business units and teletrade centre, high quality housing, conference, leisure and amenity facilities. It was claimed that 350 jobs would be created and work could begin the following spring.[5] The company took out an option on the estate before submitting outline redevelopment plans, but, when approval was not immediately forthcoming, appealed to the Welsh Office against the failure of Denbighshire County Council to reach a decision within the statutory eight-week period.[6] The planning issue was a difficult one, as the proposals conflicted with the Glyndwr District Local Plan and with Clwyd County Structure Plan. The company's residential development was opposed because there was no indication of 'local need'. It was thought that such a large addition to the local property market could only lead to more second homes, and the attraction of incomers to the area, to the detriment of the local economy and Welsh-language culture. The deal, believed to worth over one million pounds, collapsed. Meanwhile the listed buildings and site were costing the North Wales Health Authority £100,000 a year to secure against theft and vandalism. With the hospital now having been on the market for five years, an increasingly desperate health authority finally agreed to a 'profit share' proposal from Lancashire businessman, Gerald Hitman and his wife. The price paid for the entire site was £155,000. A spokesman for the North Wales Health Authority said it had 'a statutory obligation to dispose of property surplus to NHS requirements'.[7] When news of the deal broke, the chief executive of Howell's School protested that in the past the school had had a substantially higher offer refused.[8] Rod Richards, Welsh Assembly Tory leader, called for a public inquiry, and claimed that the sale was a 'scandal'.[9] The district auditor began an investigation.[10] Three plots of land were auctioned and raised £253,000. Mrs Hitman claimed that the proceeds would go only 'some small part of the way' towards the costs of maintenance and security.[11] A scheme for a training workshop for potters was then launched and, with local feelings still running high, 300 Denbigh residents turned out to hear this latest proposal for the old hospital site.[12] It appeared that these plans were in their infancy and that they would be dependent on securing grant aid. Residents were more concerned about the proposals for 160 houses. Rumours abounded that the intention was to build low-cost social housing designed to exploit the DHSS claimant market.[13] Gerald Hitman denied this and offered to sign a legal agreement to provide only high-quality properties, stating he and his wife had already developed a similar site at Brockhall Village in the Ribble Valley. Further properties on the Denbigh hospital site were sold, raising a further £88,000, but no progress was made on the ambitious plans for redevelopment. The county council again rejected plans for a housing estate. Without these, the owner claimed, the scheme for light industry and educational uses was unviable. In 2000 Mr Hitman 'accused the authority of being obstructive and said he had no further plans for the site'.[14] At the time of writing the outlook is bleak. In March 2001 thieves stole the historic clock, donated by Mrs Ablett in memory of her husband, and all the brass door handles and fixtures disappeared. Thieves have removed doors and lead flashings, and vandals have broken windows and damaged the roofs. The hospital that was once overcrowded and had insufficient room for all the beds required now lies empty and deserted.

❋

Conclusion

This book began by exploring the situation of the mentally ill in north Wales in decades prior to the establishment of the Denbigh hospital. It has ended with the closure of the hospital and the return to community-based systems of care. The new arrangements are of course located within the very different context of welfare state provision.

There has been a tendency for historians to stress the social control function of the old-style mental hospitals. This study, however, has chosen to emphasize the care and treatment provided by the institution and to look more closely at the work of the staff and the interactions of patients. The founders conceived of the asylum as providing nursing care and curative custody that would reform as well as heal the patients who came within its orbit. Visions of an ordered and structured regime informed the early efforts to assist the mentally ill. Within the context of the asylum the notions of curing, protecting and correcting could acquire a contradictory unity. Larsson has drawn on the theoretical ideas of Norbert Elias to argue that the development of institutional care for the mentally ill constitutes part of a 'civilizing process' and that this humanitarian task simultaneously embraced a form of disciplinary control.[1] He maintains that the civilizing and disciplinary functions are contradictory manifestations of a unitary whole.[2] This study has shown how therapeutic intervention often entailed disciplinary control of aberrant behaviour and how concern for the protection of female patients privileged patriarchal control. The contradictory tensions inherent in the institution came sharply to the fore during the post-Second World War years as many prevailing assumptions were challenged. It was not simply the introduction of new drug treatments but the changing ideas of the optimum of care and treatment that were to lead to the demise of the hospital. Changes in the social representation of mental illness, and particularly a reconceptualization of the role of professional psychiatry, were instrumental in bringing about the restructuring of provision and the collapse of the large institution.[3] However, this study also recognizes the crucial role of political decision-making at central government level in determining the path of hospital closures.

The transfer of the hospital to the National Health Service in 1948 brought the benefit of central government funding and with it many other changes. The sense of continuity was threatened as the farm was sold off and old styles of management disappeared. The number of patients treated increased rapidly while the long-stay population decreased. Yet long-established institutional values survived, sustained by many of the nursing staff. When Patrick Thomson, a Scotsman, moved from Swansea to Denbigh as principal nursing officer in the 1970s he was much impressed by the high standard of patient care, regarding it as one of the hallmarks of the institution. This quality of nursing reflected an institution that for much of its history had been forward-looking on many fronts, including its provision of recreational opportunities and pioneering of after-care and psychiatric social work.

Apart from the aforementioned, probably the most defining characteristic of the Denbigh hospital was the emphasis placed upon the Welsh language. The priority accorded to use of the Welsh language by patients and staff in its earliest days was quite remarkable. This commitment continued until after the Second World War. Despite the new legal status accorded to the Welsh language in the late twentieth century, the recent history of the North Wales Hospital charts a declining role for the language, rather than a strengthening. The need for people, particularly in periods of distress and suffering, to be able to communicate through their first language was acknowledged by the founders and early staff of this institution and should not be forgotten today.

A recurrent theme in this history has been the issue of how to provide appropriate care for those suffering from long-term chronic illness. Medical officers repeatedly bewailed the fact that many of the patients sent for treatment were unlikely to recover and would require continuing care. It would seem that expeditious hospital treatment, followed by swift return of the patient to the outside world, has overcome the problem of a long-stay population. Since the closure of the North Wales Hospital at Denbigh, mental health services in north Wales have been based on community mental health teams and a number of psychiatric inpatient units. At the beginning of the new millennium there was a total of 441 psychiatric hospital beds in north Wales, dispersed in different locations.[4] The ideal of a community-based service with units for the treatment of acute cases of mental illness sited in each of the four counties of north Wales[5] has been realized and the number of long-term chronic beds has been minimized.

However, closer scrutiny does raise some interesting questions, pointing to some complexity in the present picture. The psychiatric units in general hospitals are designed to provide treatment for acute cases, while care for the chronically ill is now provided in the community. The level of usage of the acute services has continued to increase. A recent comparison between the number of admissions from north-west Wales to the Hergest Unit with admissions from the same catchment area to the Denbigh hospital a century before, showed that from roughly the same total population there were fifteen times as many admissions in 1996 as in 1896. Although the majority of admissions are on a voluntary basis, it revealed that there were three times as many enforced committals in 1996 as there were a century previously. The same audit showed that out of 737 admissions that year only 25 per cent were admitted for the first time.[6] A roughly equal proportion was readmitted during the same twelve-month period. Out of the total of 572 individuals in the study as many as 60 per cent had a previous admission. A large proportion of this group of readmissions (294) suffered from severe mental illness (SMI). Of these, 76 per cent had up to three previous and/or up to three subsequent admissions and some were referred to support-bed facilities after discharge. This suggests that there is still a large cohort of patients suffering from long-term chronic illness requiring recurrent admissions for hospital treatment. The long-stay hospital has closed but the need for care, treatment and support over the long term continues. Chronically ill patients have not disappeared; they are simply being dealt with in a different way.

As the Denbigh hospital prepared for closure a residue of long-term patients had to be relocated. In the later stages of resettlement during the 1980s and 1990s, the experience gained from earlier failures and successes together with greater investment in social services and voluntary provision led to a better service. For many patients the move from hospital to community represented an improvement in the quality of their lives.[7] For Enid and Jo, Ellen May and others the move to sheltered housing, aided by support services in the community, offered greater freedom of self-expression and a new feeling of independence. When resettlement involved careful patient assessment and a care plan was implemented, the transfer to community care was a success. It could allow patients to 'live life to the optimum which they are capable of'.[8] As one support worker put it, 'jyst cael y lle iawn a'r bobl iawn' and community care can bring positive benefits for the individuals involved.[9] Emlyn for one was quite adamant that he never wanted to go back to Denbigh – 'dwi ddim eisiau mynd yn ôl yno!'[10]

Those who recall the Denbigh hospital have expressed contradictory opinions and a deep sense of ambivalence. Groups of patient 'survivors' still meet to reflect upon the harrowing recollections of confinement. For some it was an agonizing episode in their lives and many can see nothing of value in the treatment they received. Some people have said to me simply 'Pam, it was awful'. Others have responded more positively and even admitted frankly that 'Denbigh saved my life'.[11] In her study of Severalls hospital Diana Gittens noted a similar level of contradiction in people's retrospective assessment of the institution.[12]

What then of the specifically Welsh and regional context of this institution? One dimension that has become evident throughout is the importance of social and cultural context in shaping the patient *experience* of mental illness. The social background of class, gender, language, religion and family structure profoundly influences the pattern and impact of illness. Social tensions and crises of unemployment, industrial conflict, religious revivalism and war shape the individual experiences that are associated with mental illness. The interrelationships between the personal and social, and the personal and political are highly complex. Only through a much greater research emphasis upon personal narratives of illness will we begin fully to comprehend the social experience and meaning of mental illness for patients and sufferers.

This book has provided a survey of provision for the mentally ill in north Wales over two centuries, 1800–2000. Rather than accepting that the system of care and treatment developed during the nineteenth and twentieth centuries represented a 'monumental injustice' it has reached the view that the many shifts in policy and provision have embodied genuine attempts to address the needs of patients. It is appropriate, then, to close with a quotation from Charles Webster, the official historian of the NHS, who has concluded that the mental health services as a whole, despite being 'underfunded and generally unappreciated', have nevertheless 'performed a colossal humanitarian task'.[13]

Notes

PREFACE

[1] L. Stanley and S. Wise, *Breaking Out Again: Feminist Ontology and Epistemology*, London, Routledge, 1993. Extracts from pp. 152–63 reprinted in Ian Marsh (ed.), *Classic and Contemporary Readings in Sociology*, London, Harlow, 1998, 339.

ARCHIVAL SOURCES

[1] Prior to the most recent reform of local government in Wales this was a branch office of Clwyd Archives Services.
[2] This means that some of the source materials utilized in this book are not fully referenced.
[3] For a full discussion of the certification process and the use of certification papers as a historical source, see David Wright, 'The certification of insanity in nineteenth-century England and Wales', *History of Psychiatry*, 9, 1998, 267–90.
[4] For a full discussion of the use of medical case notes as historical sources, see Jonathan Andrews, 'Case notes, case histories and the patient's experience of insanity at Gartnavel Royal Asylum, Glasgow, in the nineteenth century', *Society for the Social History of Medicine*, 11, 2 August 1998, 255–81. Also, see S. Swartz, 'Shrinking: a post-modern perspective on psychiatric case histories', *South African Journal of Psychology*, 26, 1996, 15–156.
[5] Peter Tyor and Jamil Zainaldin, 'Asylum and society: an approach to institutional change', *Journal of Social History*, Fall 1979, 44.

INTRODUCTION

[1] Kathleen Jones, *Lunacy, Law and Conscience, 1774–1845*, London, Routledge & Kegan Paul, 1955; Kathleen Jones, *Mental Health and Social Policy*, London, Routledge & Kegan Paul, 1960; Kathleen Jones, *Asylums and After: A Revised History of the Mental Health Services from the 18th Century to the 1990s*, London, Athlone, 1993.

2   Andrew Scull, *Museums of Madness: The Social Organization of Insanity in Nineteenth-Century England*, London, Allen Lane, 1977; Andrew Scull, *The Most Solitary of Afflictions: Madness and Society in Britain, 1700–1900*, London and New Haven, Yale University Press, 1993; Andrew Scull, Charlotte McKenzie and Nicholas Hervey, *Masters of Bedlam: The Transformation of the Mad-Doctoring Trade*, Princeton, Princeton University Press, 1994; Andrew Scull, 'From madness to mental illness: medical men as moral entrepreneurs', *European Journal of Sociology*, 16, 1975, 218–61.

3   Andrew Scull, *Decarceration: Community Treatment and the Deviant – A Radical View*, New Brunswick, NJ, Rutgers University Press, 1984, 2nd edn. Andrew Scull, *Social Order/Mental Disorder: Anglo-American Psychiatry in Historical Perspective*, Berkeley, University of California Press, 1989; Andrew Scull, 'Asylums: utopias and realities', in Dylan Tomlinson and John Carrier (eds), *Asylums in the Community*, London, Routledge, 1996, 7–17.

4   Michel Foucault, *Madness and Civilisation: A History of Madness in the Age of Reason*, London, Routledge, 1971, 1967 (trans. Richard Howard).

5   Colin Jones and Roy Porter (eds), *Re-Assessing Foucault*, London, Routledge, 1994.

6   Andrew Scull, in a review of developments in the history of psychiatry over the last quarter of the twentieth century, spoke merely of a 'geographical extension of focus' to encompass 'England's Celtic Fringe'. Andrew Scull, 'A quarter century of the history of psychiatry', *Journal of the History of the Behavioural Sciences*, 35, 3, Summer 1999, 239–46, 243. However, two edited collections of recent research emphasize that this extension of gaze offers an increasingly complex picture. See Peter Bartlett and David Wright, 'Community care and its antecedents', in Peter Bartlett and David Wright (eds), *Outside the Walls of the Asylum: The History of Care in the Community 1750–2000*, London, Athlone Press, 1999, 1–18, 5–9. Joseph Melling, 'Accommodating madness: new research in the social history of insanity and institutions', in Joseph Melling and Bill Forsythe (eds), *Insanity, Institutions and Society, 1800–1914: A Social History of Madness in Comparative Perspective*, London, Routledge, 1999, 1–30, 20–2.

7   Tom Walmsley, 'Psychiatry in Scotland', 294–305, Mark Finnane, 'Irish psychiatry, part I: the formation of a profession', 306–13, David Healy, 'Irish psychiatry, part 2: use of the Medico-Psychological Association by its Irish members – plus ça change!', 314–20 – all in German E. Berrios and Hugh Freeman (eds), *150 Years of British Psychiatry, 1841–1991*, London, Gaskell, 1991. T. G. Davies, 'Mental mischief: aspects of nineteenth-century psychiatric practice in parts of Wales', 367–82, David Healy, 'Irish psychiatry in the twentieth century', 268–91, Pauline Prior, ' "Where lunatics abound": a history of mental health services in Northern Ireland', 292–308, all in Hugh Freeman and German E. Berrios (eds), *150 Years of British Psychiatry, 2 The Aftermath*, London, Athlone, 1996.

8   R. A. Houston, *Madness and Society in Eighteenth Century Scotland*, Oxford, Clarendon Press, 2000; Lorraine Walsh, ' "The property of the whole community": charity and insanity in urban Scotland: the Dundee Royal Lunatic Asylum, 1805–1850', in Joseph Melling and Bill Forsythe (eds), *Insanity, Institutions and Society, 1800–1914*, London, Routledge, 1999; Jonathan

Andrews, 'Raising the tone of asylumdom: maintaining and expelling pauper lunatics at the Glasgow Royal Asylum in the nineteenth century', in Melling and Forsythe, *Insanity*; Harriet Sturdy and William Parry-Jones, 'Boarding-out insane patients: the significance of the Scottish system 1857–1913', in Peter Bartlett and David Wright (eds), *Outside the Walls of the Asylum*, London, Athlone, 1999.

9 Mark Finnane, *Insanity and the Insane in Post-Famine Ireland*, London, Croom Helm, 1981. Elizabeth Malcolm and Oonagh Walsh, '"The designs of providence": race, religion and Irish insanity', in Melling and Forsythe, *Insanity*, 223–42. Oonagh Walsh, 'Asylums, gaols and workhouses: lunatic and criminal alliances in nineteenth century Ireland', in P. Bartlett and D. Wright (eds), *Outside the Walls of the Asylum: Historical Perspectives on 'Care in the Community' in Modern Britain and Ireland*, London, Athlone Press, 1999, 132–52, 301–4. Nancy Scheper-Hughes, *Saints, Scholars and Schizophrenics: Mental Illness in Rural Ireland*, London, University of California Press, 1979. Pauline Prior, *Mental Health and Politics in Northern Ireland*, Aldershot, Avebury, 1993. Also various conference papers delivered by Elizabeth Malcolm at Wellcome symposia.

10 T. G. Davies, 'Bedlam yng Nghymru – datblygiad seiciatreg yn y bedwaredd ganrif ar bymtheg', *Transactions of the Honourable Society of Cymmrodorion*, 1980, 105–22; T. G. Davies, 'An asvlum for Glamorgan', *Morgannwg*, 37, 1993, 40–55; T. G. Davies, 'Cyfundrefn y tlodion fel gofalydd seiciatregol yng Ngorllewin Morgannwg yn ystod y bedwaredd ganrif ar bymtheg', *Cennad*, 13, 1994, 78–93; T. G. Davies, 'Wales' contribution to mental health legislation in the nineteenth century', *Welsh History Review*, 18, June 1996, 1, 40–62. T. G. Davies, 'Judging the sanity of an individual: some south Wales civil legal actions of psychiatric interest', in *National Library of Wales Journal*, 29, 1995–6, 455–67. T. G. Davies, *A History of Cefn Coed Hospital*, Swansea, West Glamorgan Health Authority, 1982. Russell Davies 'Inside the "House of the Mad": the social context of mental illness, suicide and the pressure of rural life in south-west Wales, *c.*1860–1920', *Llafur*, 4, 2, 1985, 20–35. Kerry Davies, 'Sexing the mind': gender and madness in nineteenth-century Welsh asylums', *Llafur*, 7, 1, 1996, 29–40.

11 T. G. Davies, 'Lewis Weston Dillwyn and his doctors', *Morgannwg*, 32, 1988, 70–89, 79.

12 William Parry Jones, *The Trade in Lunacy: A Study of Private Madhouses in England in the Eighteenth and Nineteenth Centuries*, London, Routledge & Kegan Paul, 1971, 73. Vernon House continued to operate until 1895, but Amroth Castle was closed in 1856 when the licence was withdrawn.

13 T. G. Davies, 'Of all the maladies', *Journal of the Pembrokeshire Historical Society*, 5, 1992–3, 75–90.

14 House of Lords, *Report of the Metropolitan Commissioners in Lunacy to the Lord Chancellor*, London, Bradbury & Evans, 1844, 200.

15 T. G. Davies, 'An asylum for Glamorgan', *Morgannwg*, 37, 1993, 40–55.

16 In 1839 Shropshire magistrates wrote to the Quarter Sessions of Denbigh, Flint, Montgomery, Worcester and Hereford, inviting each to unite in building an asylum, but received no positive reply. They proceeded to erect their own asylum,

which was opened in March 1845. In January 1846 magistrates in Montgomery-shire voted to unite with Shropshire, and in June an agreement was reached over the terms of joint funding. Shropshire County Record Office QA/7/1/1 Quarter Sessions, October 1839 and QA/7/1/4 Reports of Visiting Justices of the Salop County Lunatic Asylum, General QS 31/10/1845, 29/6/1846.

[17] This was an issue considered by Visiting Justices in Shropshire in 1846: 'as about one third of the Inhabitants of Montgomeryshire speak Welsh it will most probably be necessary to procure the assistance of Attendants who are acquainted with the Welsh language'. Shropshire County Record Office, QS122/183/4. My thanks to Len Smith for drawing my attention to this source.

[18] Geraint Jenkins, Richard Suggett and Eryn White, 'The Welsh language in early modern Wales', Geraint Jenkins (ed.), *The Welsh Language before the Industrial Revolution*, Cardiff, University of Wales Press, 1997, 45–122. W. T. R. Pryce, 'Welsh and English in Wales, 1750–1971: a spatial analysis based on the linguistic affiliation of parochial communities', *Bulletin of the Board of Celtic Studies*, 28, 1, November 1978, 1–36. W. T. R. Pryce, 'Language zones, demographic changes, and the Welsh culture area, 1800–1911', in Geraint Jenkins (ed.), *The Welsh Language and its Social Domains, 1801–1911*, Cardiff, University of Wales Press, 2000, 37–80.

[19] W. T. R. Pryce, 'Welsh and English in Wales', 27.

[20] D. Trevor Williams, 'Linguistic divides in north Wales: a study in historical geography', *Archaeologia Cambrensis*, 91 (1936), 207.

[21] W. T. R. Pryce, 'Language areas in north-east Wales *c*.1800–1911', in Geraint Jenkins (ed.), *Language and Community in the Nineteenth Century*, Cardiff, University of Wales Press, 1998, 21–61. Whereas Wrexham and Mold were strongly anglicized, the industrial community of Rhosllanerchrugog remained intensely Welsh in language and culture.

[22] Colin Williams, 'Questions concerning the development of bilingualism in Wales', in Bob Morris Jones and Paul Ghuman (eds), *Bilingualism, Education and Identity*, Cardiff, University of Wales Press, 1995, 47–78, 69, notes that hitherto little attention has been paid to the issue of language usage in the health sector in Wales.

[23] A. H. Dodd, *The Industrialisation of North Wales*, Cardiff, University of Wales Press, 1971; Wrexham, Bridge Books, 1990.

[24] Neil Evans, 'Regional dynamics: north Wales, 1750–1914', in Edward Royle (ed.), *Issues of Regional Identity*, Manchester, Manchester University Press, 1998, 201–25.

[25] Alwyn D. Rees, *Life in a Welsh Countryside*, Cardiff, University of Wales Press, 1950; Trefor Owen similarly found that 'Family and kin relationships pervade the whole life of the community and supply a basic system of personal contacts between the inhabitants', in Elwyn Davies and Alwyn D. Rees (eds), *Welsh Rural Communities*, Cardiff, University of Wales Press, 1960, 187.

[26] K. O. Morgan, *Rebirth of a Nation: Wales 1880–1980*, Oxford, Oxford University Press, 1982, 17.

[27] George Eliot, *Felix Holt, The Radical*, London, Virtue, 1866, vol. 1, chap. 3, 72.

[28] Michael Ignatieff, 'Total institutions and working classes: a review essay', *History Workshop*, 15, Spring 1988, 167–73. John Walton, 'Casting out and bringing back in Victorian England', in W. F. Bynum, R. Porter and M. Shepherd (eds), *The Anatomy of Madness*, ii, London, Tavistock, 132 64.

[29] Bill Luckin, 'Towards a social history of institutionalization', *Social History*, 8, 1983, 87–94, 89.

[30] Virginia Berridge, 'Health and medicine', chapter 4 in F. M. L. Thompson (ed.), *The Cambridge Social History of Britain, 1750–1950*, iii, *Social Agencies and Institutions*, Cambridge, Cambridge University Press, 1990, 15.

[31] Anne Digby, 'Perspectives on the asylum', in Roy Porter and Andrew Wear (eds), *Problems and Methods in the History of Medicine*, London, Croom Helm, 1987.

[32] Susan Sontag, 'Illness as a metaphor', *New York Review of Books*, 27 January 1978.

1 The Insane Poor

[1] M. MacDonald, *Mystical Bedlam. Madness, Anxiety, and Healing in Seventeenth-Century England*, Cambridge, Cambridge University Press, 1981. Roy Porter, *Mind-Forg'd Manacles: A History of Madness in England from the Restoration to the Regency*, Cambridge, MA, Harvard University Press, 1987. P. Rushton, 'Lunatics and idiots: mental disability, the community and Poor Law in north-east England, 1600 1800', *Medical History*, 32, 1988, 34–50. P. Rushton, 'Idiocy, the family and the community in early modern north-east England', in D. Wright and A. Digby (eds), *From Idiocy to Mental Deficiency: Historical Perspectives on People with Learning Disabilities*, London, Routledge, 1996, 44–64. R. A. Houston, *Madness and Society in Eighteenth Century Scotland*, Oxford, Clarendon Press, 2000. These authors based their research on diaries, legal papers and poor law records. All of these sources exist for Wales and await research. *The Diary of William Jones*, abridged and ed. R. T. W. Denming, Cardiff, South Wales Record Service, 1995, for example, provides numerous illustrations of the condition of lunatic parishioners in eighteenth-century Glamorgan.

[2] A. H. Dodd, 'The Old Poor Law in North Wales', in *Archaeologia Cambrensis*, 81, 1, June 1926, 2nd series, 6, 111–32

[3] G. Nesta Evans, *Religion and Politics in Mid-Eighteenth Century Anglesey*, Cardiff, University of Wales Press, 1953, 176.

[4] Ibid., 179, in which she acknowledges the advice of Prof. R. T. Jenkins; Trefor Owen, *Welsh Folk Customs*, Cardiff, William Lewis, National Museum of Wales Welsh Folk Museum, 3rd edn, 1974 – see esp. chapter 5, 'Birth, marriage and death'.

[5] Evans, *Religion and Politics in Anglesey*, 177.

[6] S. A. Williams, 'Care in the community: women and the old poor law in early nineteenth century Anglesey', *Llafur*, 6, 1995, 30–43.

[7] *Report from His Majesty's Commissioners for Inquiry into the Administration and Practical Operation of the Poor Laws*, PP 1834(44) XXIX, p. 177 – quoted in David Llewelyn Jones, *Walcott a'r Wyrcws: Tlodi yng Ngogledd Cymru yn Hanner Cyntaf Y Bedwaredd Ganrif ar Bymtheg*, Aberystwyth, University of Wales Centre for Advanced Welsh and Celtic Studies, 1997, 7.

8   PP (Lords) 1844, vol. xvi, *Supplemental Report of the Metropolitan Commissioners in Lunacy Relative to the General Condition of the Insane in Wales*, August 1844, 11.

9   17 Geo. III; Kathleen Jones, *A History of the Mental Health Services*, London, Routledge & Kegan Paul, 1972, 25–8; Clive Unsworth, *The Politics of Mental Health Legislation*, Oxford, Clarendon Press, 1987, 53–4; Kathleen Jones argues that the 1774 Vagrancy Act, as opposed to that of 1714, did add the notion that they should be 'cured' and thereby implied a commitment to treatment.

10   In 1818 an Anglesey farmer wrote that, whereas in past years only 'the aged, the infirm, or a neighbour in case of sickness' would approach their door for help, over the last the year the distress had 'broken through every barrier', so that, had magistrates enforced the vagrancy laws strictly, not even 'Beaumaris gaol and castle together' would have held 'the swarm of tramps and beggars'. *North Wales Gazette*, 5 and 19 February 1818, quoted by A. H. Dodd, *The Industrial Revolution in North Wales*, Cardiff, University of Wales Press, 1971; 3rd edn, Wrexham, Bridge Books, 1990, 384.

11   Gwenfair Parry, 'Gweinyddiaeth deddf y tlodion yng Ngorllewin Meirionnydd, c. 1800–1894', unpublished Ph.D. thesis, University of Wales (UCNW, Bangor) 1995, 201.

12   DRO, PD/63/1/56, Vestry Book 1802–1814, Llangollen, 84, 92a, 134a–136a, 142a, 151a.

13   DRO, PD/63/1/55, Llangollen Vestry Records, 76a.

14   DRO, PD/63/1/55, Llangollen Vestry Records, 40, 54.

15   From Poor Law Commission figures reproduced by David Llewelyn Jones, *Walcott a'r Wyrcws*, 3.

16   For an analysis of surviving records for parishes in Denbighshire for the period 1828–58 see David Hirst and Pamela Michael, 'Family, community and the lunatic in mid-nineteenth-century north Wales', Peter Bartlett and David Wright (eds), *Outside the Walls of the Asylum*, London, Athlone, 1999, 66–85, 285–9.

17   R. A. Lewis, 'William Day and the Poor Law Commissioners', *University of Birmingham Historical Journal*, 9, 1964, 163–96. Pamela Michael and David Hirst, 'Establishing the "rule of kindness": the foundations of the North Wales Lunatic Asylum, Denbigh', in Joseph Melling and Bill Forsythe (eds), *Insanity, Institutions and Society, 1800–1914*, London, Routledge, 1999.

18   R. A. Lewis, 'William Day and the Poor Law Commissioners', *University of Birmingham Historical Journal*, 9, 1964, 163–96, 184. D. Williams, *The Rebecca Riots*, Cardiff, University of Wales Press, 1955, 138–47.

19   C. Flynn Hughes, 'Aspects of Poor Law administration and policy in Anglesey, 1834–1848', *Anglesey Antiquarian Society and Field Club Transactions*, 1950, 71–9, 79.

20   A. H. Dodd, *Industrial Revolution*, 396.

21   Peter Bartlett, 'The Poor Law of lunacy: the administration of pauper lunatics in mid-nineteenth century England with special emphasis on Leicestershire and Rutland', Ph.D., University of London, 1993, 71.

22   5 Will. IV, c.76, s.45; Leonard D. Smith, *'Cure, Comfort and Safe Custody': Public Lunatic Asylums in Early Nineteenth-Century England*, London and New York, Leicester University Press, 1999.

23   A. Kidd, *State, Society and the Poor in Nineteenth Century England*, Basingstoke, Macmillan, 1999.

[24]   Steven King, *Poverty and Welfare in England, 1700–1850: A Regional Perspective*, Manchester, Manchester University Press, 2000.

[25]   Steven King and John Stewart, 'The history of the Poor Law in Wales: under-researched, full of potential', *Archives*, 26, 105, October 2001, 134–48, 146.

[26]   Peter Bartlett, *The Poor Law of Lunacy*, London, Leicester University Press, 1999.

[27]   Jonathan Andrews, *The Scottish Lunacy Commissioners and Lunacy Reform in Nineteenth-Century Scotland*, Wellcome Institute for the History of Medicine, Occasional Publications, 8, London, Wellcome Trust, 1998.

[28]   Ruth Hodgkinson, *The Origins of the National Health Service*, London, Wellcome Historical Medical Library, 1967, 578.

[29]   The words of F. T. Bircham, Poor Law Inspector, LGB, *Twenty-Fifth Report*, PP 36, 1896, 221, cited by Anne Digby, 'The rural poor law', in D. Fraser (ed.), *The New Poor Law in the Nineteenth Century*, London, Macmillan, 1976, 149–213, 160.

[30]   Digby, 'Rural Poor Law', in Fraser (ed.), *The New Poor Law in the Nineteenth Century*, 160.

2   Investigating North Wales

[1]   Richard Hunter and Ida MacAlpine, *Three Hundred Years of Psychiatry, 1535–1860*, London, Oxford University Press, 1963, 785.

[2]   Ibid., p. vii.

[3]   Sir Andrew Halliday, *A Letter to Lord Robert Seymour with a Report of the Number of Lunatics and Idiots in England and Wales*, London, Thomas & George Underwood, 1829, pp. vi–vii.

[4]   Ibid., 58–66. I have aggregated these statistics.

[5]   Ibid., 73–4.

[6]   David Hirst and Pamela Michael, 'Family, community and the lunatic in mid-nineteenth-century north Wales', in Peter Bartlett and David Wright (eds), *Outside the Walls of the Asylum*, London, Athlone, 66–85, 285–9.

[7]   Halliday, *Letter*, table VI, p. 85.

[8]   A circular, prepared for the purpose of obtaining information on the subject of pauper lunatics, had been submitted to the commission for approval by assistant Poor Law commissioner R. D. Neave in October 1839. Neave preceded William Day as the assistant commissioner responsible for Wales. See PRO, MH/33/4/8293, dated 28 October 1839.

[9]   Anglesey Quarter Sessions, Lunacy Box 1, General File 1842–82. Letter dated 27 October 1841. I wish to thank my colleague Dr William Griffith for providing these references to Anglesey papers.

[10]   T. G. Davies, 'The Welsh contribution to mental health legislation in the nineteenth century', *Welsh History Review*, 18, June 1996, 1, 40–62, 49.

[11]   PRO, MH/19/64, 334D, letter dated 15 December 1841.

[12]   Nicholas Hervey, 'The Lunacy Commission 1845–1860, with special reference to the implementation of policy in Kent and Surrey', Ph.D., University of Bristol, March 1987, 83.

13 Anglesey Quarter Sessions, Lunacy Box 1, General File 1842–82, letters dated 28 and 30 May 1842, 7 April 1843.

14 L. D. Smith, ' "A worthy feeling gentleman": Samuel Hitch at Gloucester Asylum, 1828–1847', in German E. Berrios and Hugh Freeman (eds), *150 Years of British Psychiatry, ii, The Aftermath*, London, Athlone, 1996, 479–99.

15 *The Times*, Saturday, 1 October 1842.

16 Ibid.

17 PP 1844, xi, Poor Law commissioners, *Tenth Annual Report for 1844*, 19–20.

18 Ibid., 20.

19 Andrew Scull, 'A convenient place to get rid of inconvenient people: the Victorian lunatic asylum', in Anthony King (ed.), *Buildings and Society: Essays in the Social Development of the Built Environment*, London, Routledge & Kegan Paul, 1980, 37–59, 38.

20 Andrew Scull, *The Most Solitary of Afflictions: Madness and Society in Britain, 1700–1900*, New Haven and London, Yale University Press, 1993, 26–34.

21 P. Michael, 'Tenant farming in Merionethshire, 1850–1914', unpublished MA thesis, University of Wales, 1978.

22 Neil Evans, 'The urbanization of Welsh society', in T. Herbert and G. E. Jones (eds), *People and Protest: Wales 1815–1880*, Cardiff, University of Wales Press, 1988, 7–31.

23 Only Cardiff, Swansea and Denbigh had established voluntary subscription hospitals.

24 Mark Finnane, *Insanity and the Insane in Post-Famine Ireland*, London, Croom Helm, 1981, 14.

25 Nancy Scheper-Hughes, *Saints, Scholars and Schizophrenics: Mental Illness in Rural Ireland*, London, University of California Press, 1979.

26 Anglesey Record Office, Anglesey Quarter Sessions, Lunacy Box 1, General file 1842–82, letter dated 18 June 1844.

27 Ibid., letter dated 25 June 1844.

28 Ibid., letter dated 24 June 1844.

29 Ibid., letter dated 1 July 1844.

30 *Carnarvon and Denbigh Herald*, 20 July 1844.

31 PP (Lords), 1844, xvi, *Supplemental Report of the Metropolitan Commissioners in Lunacy Relative to the General Condition of the Insane in Wales*, 25 August 1844, London, Bradbury & Evans, 24.

32 Ibid., 8–9.

33 Ibid., 27.

34 Ibid., 32.

35 Ibid., 31.

36 Ibid., 25.

37 Ibid., 36–7.

38 Ibid., 33.

39 Ibid., 35.

40 Ibid., 24.

41 Ibid., 24–5.

42 Ibid., 25.

43 Ibid., 18–19.

[44]   Ibid., 36.
[45]   Ibid., 36–7.
[46]   Ibid., 28.
[47]   Ibid., 45–6.
[48]   Ibid., 54–5.
[49]   Ibid., 19.
[50]   Ibid., 16.
[51]   Ibid., 28–9.
[52]   Ibid., 45–6.
[53]   Ibid., 37.
[54]   Ibid., 38–9.
[55]   Ibid., 39. The published report is different to the original report filed by the commissioners, which was more explicit with regard to the bodily distortions. The original handwritten report states: 'The chest bone protruded forwards five or six inches from the sides of her flattened ribs – Her body was bent into a position which caused an excoriation of the parts about the navel: and the fixed and unchangeable flexion of the legs had produced anchylosis of the knees and brought the heels nearly into contact with the nates or buttocks.' DRO, QSD/AL/3/3. It seems hard to believe that local people did not know of her existence, particularly as, prior to the window being boarded up, she had been heard crying from the window.
[56]   Ibid., 39–41.
[57]   Ibid., 41–2.
[58]   Ibid., 43–4.
[59]   Ibid., 44.
[60]   *Hansard*, House of Commons, Friday, 6 June 1845, col. 186.
[61]   Georgina Battiscombe, *Shaftesbury: A Biography of the Seventh Earl, 1801–1885*, London, Constable, 1974.
[62]   Kathleen Jones, *Lunacy, Law and Conscience, 1744–1845*, London, Routledge & Kegan Paul, 1955, 197.

3   The Founding of the North Wales Lunatic Asylum

[1]   Michael Donnelly, *Managing the Mind: A Study of Medical Psychology in Early Nineteenth-Century Britain*, London, Tavistock Publications, 1983, Leonard Smith, *Cure, Comfort and Safe Custody: Public Lunatic Asylums in Early Nineteenth-Century England*, London, Leicester University Press, 1999, 20–6.
[2]   T. G. Davies, 'The Welsh contribution to mental health legislation', *Welsh History Review*, 18, 1996, 1, 42–3. Gwyneth Evans, 'Charles Watkin Williams Wynn', unpublished MA thesis, University of Wales, 1934.
[3]   County Asylums Act, 48 George III, c. 96; P. Bartlett, *The Poor Law of Lunacy*, London, Leicester University Press, 1999, 10, 33, 36. K. Jones, *Lunacy, Law and Conscience, 1744–1845*, London, Routledge & Kegan Paul, 1955.
[4]   For a comprehensive account of the county asylums built in England following the 1808 Act see Smith *Cure, Comfort and Safe Custody*.
[5]   *Chester Chronicle*, 28 December 1810.

[6] DRO, QSD/AL/3/6, letter from Wynn to Clerk of Denbighshire Quarter Sessions.

[7] Lord Ashley's statement to the House of Commons, *Hansard*, Friday, 6 June 1845, col. 183.

[8] *Carnarvon and Denbigh Herald*, 15 October 1842.

[9] Ibid.

[10] PRO, MH12/16131, letter from John Heaton to Poor Law Commissioners, 8 April 1842. (This letter refers to previous communications.)

[11] Ibid.

[12] Other representations were made by the dean of St Asaph and Sir Henry Browne, see PRO, 12/16131, correspondence between Poor Law Commission, William Day, and St Asaph Poor Law Union, April 1841; also letter from Henry Browne, Bronwylfa, St Asaph, to chairman of Anglesey Quarter Sessions, regarding enquiries into the expense of maintaining lunatics in north Wales for the period 1835–40, Anglesey Quarter Session, Lunacy Box 1, General File 1842–82, letter dated 27 October 1841.

[13] Andrew Scull, Charlotte MacKenzie and Nicholas Hervey, *Masters of Bedlam*, Princeton, Princeton University Press, 1996, 68.

[14] *The Times*, 1 October 1842, letter from Samuel Hitch.

[15] Ibid.

[16] Ibid.

[17] DRO, HD/1/81, minute book of the founders, October 1842–17 November 1848 (includes letters). For a fuller account of this meeting see M. Rolf Olsen, 'The founding of the hospital for the insane poor, Denbigh', *Denbighshire Historical Society Transactions*, 23, 1974, 193–217.

[18] DRO, HD/1/81, minute book of the founders, October 1842, resolution 2. The term 'Hospital for the Insane' was also used in motions forwarded by R. B. Clough (motion 4) and Dr John Williams (motion 6).

[19] Hunter and MacAlpine, *Three Hundred Years of Psychiatry*, 445–6, where they assess the contribution of John Aikin (1747–1822), whose *Thoughts on Hospitals*, London, Johnson, 1771, 65–71, included one of the earliest discussions of lunatic hospitals. The term 'Hospital for the Insane' was subsequently dropped when it became constituted as a joint counties asylum.

[20] DRO, HD/1/81, minute book of the founders, October 1842, resolution 3.

[21] Ibid., motion 5.

[22] Ibid., motion 6.

[23] Ibid.

[24] W. Tydeman, 'Ablett of Llanbedr: patron of the arts', *Denbighshire Historical Society Transactions*, 19, 1970, 143–87.

[25] *DNB*, 1169.

[26] Nicholas Hervey, 'The Lunacy Commission 1845–60 with special reference to the implementation of policy in Kent and Surrey', unpublished Ph.D. thesis, University of Bristol, 1987, i, 94.

[27] Ibid., ii, appendix C, 123.

[28] *The Examiner*, 19 August 1843; *Carnarvon and Denbigh Herald*, 25 August 1843.

[29] NLW, Bathafarn Ms. 359, 26 June 1844. The trustees were Sir Watkin Williams Wynn of Wynnstay, Bart, Robert Myddelton Biddulph of Chirk Castle, Esq and

Edward Madocks of Glanywern. See also Bathafarn Ms. 358, Indenture dated 26 June 1844, which refers to a previous indenture between Charles Potts of the city of Chester, gentleman and Emma his wife, etc. . . . and Richard Lloyd Williams of Henllan Place in the town of Denbigh.

30   Geoffrey Faber, *Oxford Apostles*, Harmondsworth, Penguin Books, 1954, 140. J. A. Venn, *Alumnii Cantabrigiensis*, entries for Luxmoore, Charles Scott, and Luxmoore, John Henry Montague.

31   Herefordshire Archives, S/60/25–6, Hereford Infirmary Records, governors' meetings 1791–1851, entries for 18 October 1793, 19 December 1793, etc.

32   Herefordshire Archives, Hereford Lunatic Asylum minute books, Q/AL/96, 2 July 1838 and 26 September 1838.

33   *Select Committee on Hereford Lunatic Asylum, Minutes of Evidence, 163*, paragraphs 3388–3569.

34   GRO, main branch, D3848/1/1/58, letter from Charles Bathurst, chairman of the visitors, to Hitch, 4 April 1839. GRO, Shire Hall branch, HO22/3/2, house committee minutes, 7 December 1840. My thanks to Leonard Smith for these references.

35   GRO, HO22/3/2, minute dated 21 December 1840 regarding letter received from the dean of St Asaph.

36   For further details on the interventions of the dean of St Asaph see Pamela Michael and David Hirst, 'Establishing the "rule of kindness": the foundation of the North Wales Lunatic Asylum, Denbigh', in Joseph Melling and Bill Forsythe (eds), *Insanity, Institutions and Society, 1800–1914*, London, Routledge, 1999, 159–79.

37   See, for example, *North Wales Chronicle*, 18 October 1842.

38   PP (Lords), 1884, xvi, *Supplemental Report of the Metropolitan Commissioners in Lunacy Relative to the General Condition of the Insane in Wales*, 25 August 1844, London, Bradbury & Evans, 54–5.

39   Ibid., 22.

40   Ibid.

41   Ibid., 14.

42   *Medical Directory*, 1848, 106–7.

43   *Medical Directory*, 1847 and 1856.

44   A meeting of the governors of the Gloucester Infirmary, held on 14 September 1793, voted to establish a general hospital for the reception of the insane. GRO, X11/45/421. Similarly, the governors of the Herefordshire Infirmary met in 1791 as previously observed.

45   University of Wales Bangor Archives: Papers of Hafodwyryd Estate, Dinam Hall MS 26–7, Nannau MS, 3444–3559; J. J. Griffiths, *Pedigrees of Carnarvonshire and Anglesey Families*, Hafodwyryd, Penmachno, 353; DRO, Swayne, Johnson and Wight papers, DD/SJW, Box 29/26, 29/31.

46   Owen Evans, *Dinbych yn ei Hynafiaeth a'i Henwogion*, Denbigh, Gee & Sons, 1907, 54; John Wyn Prichard, 'Bwrdeistref Dinbych a datblygiadau corfforaethol 1835–1894', unpublished M.Phil. thesis, University of Wales Bangor, 1992, 9; *Carnarvon and Denbigh Herald*, 6 November 1847.

47   For a biographical approach to the growth of professional power see Andrew Scull, Charlotte MacKenzie and Nicholas Hervey, *Masters of Bedlam: The*

Transformation of the Mad-Doctoring Trade, Princeton, Princeton University Press, 1996. Richard Lloyd Williams's son of the same name became county architect and was mayor of Denbigh in 1864–6; his son-in-law T. Gold Edwards acted as solicitor to the lunatic asylum and was nominated high bailiff and county court registrar. See John Wyn Pritchard, ' "Fit and proper persons": councillors of Denbigh, their status and position, 1835–1894', *Welsh History Review*, 17, 1994–5, 186–203, 187, 196–7.

48 *Baner ac Amserau Cymru*, 19 March 1862. My thanks to Dr David Hirst for locating this notice of death. 'He will be mourned by relatives and numerous friends, and the poor will suffer an enormous loss by the passing of one of their most generous supporters. He was exceptional in his humanity and his kindness to everyone in adversity and hardship, and he was extremely dedicated for many years to serving the sick poor voluntarily in the Denbigh hospital. He experienced great suffering with Christian fortitude, and we hope that "death to him is gain".'

49 J. A. Venn, *Alumnii Cantabrigiensis*, pt.ii, *1752–1900*, iii. Alan Fletcher, 'Plas Heaton and the Heatons in the nineteenth century', *Transactions of the Denbighshire Historical Society*, 45, 1996, 21–40. DRO, DD/PH/53; DD/PH/313; DD/PH/348.

50 Michael and Hirst, 'Establishing the "rule of kindness" ', 159–79.

51 J. Rhys Williams, 'The growth and development of banking in Clwyd', *Denbighshire Transactions*, 39, 1990, 91–106, 97.

52 John Wyn Pritchard, 'Bwrdeistref Dinbych a datblygiadau corfforaethol 1835–1894', unpublished M.Phil. thesis, University of Wales Bangor, 1992, 9; Pritchard, ' "Fit and Proper Persons" ', 186–203, 187, 196–7.

53 NLW, Dolaucothi Papers, see Ms. 3501a for copy letter from Sir George Grey dated 6 March 1856 'requiring Justices to build an Asylum', and Ms. 2154 for letter from Lord Evelyn to Jones, 19 August 1856, and Ms. 2155, letter dated 3 September 1856.

54 *Carnarvon and Denbigh Herald*, 15 October 1842.

55 Aled Jones, *Press, Politics and Society: A History of Journalism in Wales*, Cardiff, University of Wales Press, 1993.

56 *North Wales Chronicle*, 18 October 1842

57 Ibid., editorial entitled 'Lunacy in Wales'.

58 *North Wales Chronicle*, 25 October 1842.

59 *North Wales Chronicle*, letter from 'Clericus', St Asaph, dated 21 October 1842.

60 *North Wales Chronicle*, letter from 'Homo', dated 28 October 1842.

61 *North Wales Chronicle*, see editorial 15 November 1842.

62 Denbighshire Library, Denbigh Asylum file, leaflet entitled at 'An adjourned meeting of the committee'.

63 DRO, HD/1/81, minute book of the founders, 31 December 1842 and letters dated 12, 21, 29 and 31 December 1842.

64 DRO, HD/1/81, letter Clough to Anson, 31 December 1842.

65 DRO, HD/1/81, minute 20 January 1843.

66 DRO, HD/1/81, minute 4 February 1843.

67 *Carnarvon and Denbigh Herald*, 4 February 1843.

68 DRO, HD/1/81, minute book of the founders, 18 March 1843.

[69]   Ibid., 22 April 1843.
[70]   Thomas Gwynn Jones, *Cofiant Thomas Gee,* Denbigh, Gee a'i Fab, 1913.
[71]   *Carnarvon and Denbigh Herald,* 4 February 1843.
[72]   *Carnarvon and Denbigh Herald*, 11 March 1843.
[73]   Ibid.
[74]   Ibid.

4   BUILDING THE ASYLUM

[1]   DRO, HD/1/81, minute book of the founders, minutes dated 4, 11, 18, 25 February 1843.
[2]   DRO, HD/1/81. The first reference to Fulljames is in a minute dated 4 March 1843.
[3]   GRO, HO 22/1/1, First County Asylum, General Minutes, 1813–51, minute dated 29 July 1831, 339.
[4]   Edward Hubbard, *The Buildings of Wales: Clwyd (Denbighshire and Flintshire)*, Harmondsworth, Penguin and University of Wales Press, 1986, 67, 70, 148, 153.
[5]   Ibid., 66.
[6]   PRO, MH/50/6, Lunacy Commission minutes, 117, 187, 196, 214, 219.
[7]   DRO, HD/1/81, 5 May 1842.
[8]   DRO, HD/1/81, 28 October 1843.
[9]   DRO, HD/1/81, 18 October 1843.
[10] DRO, HD/1/81, 18 November 1843.
[11] DRO, HD/1/81, 4 December1843.
[12] DRO, HD/1/81, letter from Fulljames 13 May 1844, letter to Fulljames 30 May 1844 and resolution, minutes of meeting 31 August 1844.
[13] DRO, HD/1/81, minute dated 7 February 1844.
[14] DRO, HD/1/81, 15 April 1844.
[15] DRO, HD/1/81, 15 April 1844, 30 May 1844.
[16] DRO, HD/1/81, 13 May 1844, and architect's reports read on 31 August 1844, 5 November 1844, 6 December 1844, 17 January 1845.
[17] DRO, HD/1/81, 22 August 1844.
[18] DRO, HD/1/81, 31 August 1844.
[19] Ibid.
[20] DRO, HD/1/81, 27 February 1845.
[21] DRO, HD/1/81, paragraph reporting on March Quarter Sessions following minutes for 27 February 1845.
[22] DRO, Denbigh hospital collection, recent deposit, *The Book of the Subscribers.*
[23] DRO, HD/1/81, architect's report read at meeting held on 26 July 1845.
[24] DRO, HD/1/81, 26 July 1845.
[25] DRO, HD/1/81, 1 May 1846.
[26] DRO, HD/1/81, minutes 7 July 1845, 17 August 1845.
[27] DRO, HD/1/81, 26 August 1845.
[28] DRO, HD/1/81, 21 September 1846, copy of memorial to the Treasury.
[29] DRO, HD/1/81, 21 September 1846, 7 November 1846.
[30] DRO, HD/1/81, architect's report read at meeting 13 November 1846.

31 DRO, HD/1/81, copy of memorial with minutes, 16 September 1846.
32 DRO, HD/1/81, letter dated 2 September 1846.
33 DRO, HD/1/81, 22 October 1846.
34 UWB Archives UCNW Mss 1110/69–77. This is the appellation given by the archivist, Thomas Richards, in the schedule of papers.
35 This sketch is reliant on a thesis by Emyr Hywel Owen, 'Bywyd a gwaith Dr. Owen Roberts, 1793–1866', University College of North Wales Bangor, MA thesis, 1939, 39:5; and Emyr Hywel Owen, 'Dr. Owen Owen Roberts', *Transactions of the Carnarvonshire Historical Society*, 10, 1949, 53–64. See also *Y Traethodydd*, 1940, 95, 151.
36 O. O. Roberts, *A Few Plain Practical Hints on Cholera, its Causes, Prevention and Treatment*, 1848, dedicated to W. T. Thackeray.
37 PRO, MH 51/745, p. 8 of handwritten report.
38 PRO, MH 51/738, Haydock Lodge Inquiry, 6.
39 UWB Welsh Rare Pamphlet, X/LH 77 Pamffled, Petition of O. O. Roberts, 12 July 1846.
40 PRO, MH/51/738, Haydock Lodge, minutes of evidence taken before the Metropolitan Commissioners in Lunacy, 10 July 1846, Pt. i, 8.
41 Ibid.
42 *Carnarvon and Denbigh Herald*, 10 January 1846.
43 William Parry-Jones, *The Trade in Lunacy*, London, Routledge & Kegan Paul, 1972, 277–80, for a discussion of the case.
44 *Carnarvon and Denbigh Herald*, 29 August 1846.
45 The allegations concerning Sir James Graham were reported in *The Times*, 17 July 1846. This was subsequent to the presentation of O. O. Roberts's Petition to Parliament on 12 June 1846. *The Petition of Dr. O. O. Roberts*, University of Wales Bangor, Welsh Library, X/LH 77 Pamffled.
46 *The Times*, 20 June 1846. R. Mon Williams, *Enwogion Mon (Anglesey Worthies) 1850–1912*, Bangor, North Wales Chronicle, 1913.
47 *The Times*, Saturday, 20 June 1846.
48 Thanks to Dr David Hirst for pursuing the outcome of this case. Haydock Lodge is the subject of a jointly authored forthcoming publication.
49 *Carnarvon and Denbigh Herald*, 3 January 1846, 1.
50 *Carnarvon and Denbigh Herald*, 10 January 1846, 6.
51 Ibid., col. 3, p. 7.
52 *Carnarvon and Denbigh Herald*, 5 September 1846.
53 DRO, HD/1/81, minute dated 7 November 1846.
54 DRO, HD/1/81, letter dated 5 December 1846.
55 DRO, HD/1/81, copy of resolution, Dolgelley, 8 February 1847.
56 DRO, HD/1/81, minute book, 61–2; Andrew Scull, 'John Conolly: a Victorian psychiatric career', in Andrew Scull, *Social Order/Mental Disorder*, London, Routledge, 1989, 162–212.
57 DRO, HD/1/81, minute dated 17 August 1846.
58 *Medical Directory*, 1865.
59 DRO, HD/1/81, minute dated 2 June 1847.
60 DRO, HD/1/81, minute dated 16 June 1847.
61 Within eighteen months of the opening of the Carmarthen Asylum in 1865 the

medical superintendent, the matron and the clerk and steward had all been replaced, St David's Hospital Carmarthen, South West Wales Hospital Management Committee, 'St David's Hospital, Carmarthen Centenary, 1865–1965', First and Second *Annual Report of the Committee of Visitors of the Joint Counties Asylum, Carmarthen,* 1865 and 1866.

5 OPERATING THE ASYLUM

[1] Erving Goffman, *Asylums: Essays on the Social Situation of Mental Patients and Other Inmates,* Harmondsworth, Penguin Books, 1961. See esp. 'The staff world', 73–88, and his discussion of 'living in obedience'.

[2] Rules for the Government of the North Wales Asylum for the Insane, Denbigh, 1849, Library of University of Wales Bangor, LH71, 3.

[3] Regrettably none of these journals appear to have survived.

[4] Rules, 1849, 9.

[5] King William's College Register. George Turner Jones, born 28 July 1820, entered the college in 1834 and left in 1836. He trained at St Bartholemew's (MRCS England, 1842). My thanks to Dr David Hirst for identifying this information.

[6] DRO, HD/1/151, minute book, special meeting of the house committee, 27 May 1862; minute for 15 August 1862.

[7] Rules, 11.

[8] Ibid., 13.

[9] Ibid.

[10] Ibid., 7.

[11] Rules, 15.

[12] Joan Busfield, *Managing Madness: Changing Ideas and Practice,* London, Unwin Hyman, 1989.

[13] North Wales Hospital for the Insane at Denbigh, Duties of Attendants, 1849, para. 1.

[14] L. D. Smith, *Cure, Comfort and Safe Custody,* London, Leicester University Press, 1999, 132.

[15] DRO, HD/1/172, the visitors' books for 1849–53, entry for 7 February 1849.

[16] Ibid., entry for 14 March 1849.

[17] Ibid., entry for 16 September 1849.

[18] Cledwyn Fychan, 'Wil Ysgeifiog', *Y Faner Newydd,* 12, 1999, 12–14.

[19] *The Dictionary of Welsh Biography down to 1940,* London, Blackwell, 1959, 199; *Seren Gomer,* 1832, 312, *Golud yr Oes,* 1863, 111–13; Charles Ashton, *Hanes Llynyddiaeth Gymreig, 1651–1850,* 1893.

[20] 2nd AR, MOR, 1851.

[21] 3rd AR, MOR, 1852.

[22] 5th AR, MOR, 1853.

[23] Ibid.

[24] Ibid.

[25] DRO, HD/1/151, minutes 21 December 1860.

[26] 2nd AR, RCV, 1850.

[27] 3rd AR, RCV, 1851, 6–7.

28   15th AR, 1863, RCV.
29   18th AR, 1866, RMS.
30   John Cranmer, *Asylum History: Buckinghamshire County Pauper Lunatic Asylum*, London, The Royal College of Psychiatrists, 1990, 46.
31   17th AR, 1866, RMS, 8.
32   24th AR, 1872, RVC.
33   27th AR, 1875, RMS, 13, 12.

6 Inhabiting the Asylum

1   Malcolm Shifrin, http://www.victorianturkishbath.org
2   3rd AR, RCV, 1851, 5–6.
3   16th AR, 1864, RVC.
4   1st AR, MOR, 9.
5   3rd AR,1851, RCV.
6   4th AR, RMO, 1852, 10.
7   Negus = a liquor made of wine, water, sugar and lemon juice.
8   1st AR, 1849, MOR, 8.
9   1st AR, 1849, MOR, 8.
10   4th AR, 1852, MOR, 10.
11   L. D. Smith, *Cure, Comfort and Safe Custody*, London, 1999, 241–2.
12   Andrew Scull, *Museums of Madness: The Social Organisation of Insanity in 19th Century England*, London, Allen Lane, 1971, illustrations between 144 and 145.
13   DRO, HD/1/305, 18 and 96.
14   HD/1/172, report book of the committee of visitors, 1849–53.
15   HD/1/151, minute book, minutes of house committee, 15 February 1861 and 17 May 1861.
16   Ibid., 11 April 1862.
17   DRO, HD/1/508, date of admission 14 August 1860, 255 and 286.
18   *Journal of Mental Science*, 7, London, 1861.
19   *Cork Examiner*, 27 November 1847; 15 May 1848, cited by J. S. Donnelly, *Land and People of Nineteenth Century Cork*, London, Routledge & Kegan Paul, 1975; R. F. Foster, *Modern Ireland 1600–1972*, London, Allen Lane, 1988, 330.
20   *Journal of Mental Science.*
21   DRO, HD/1/509, date of admission 26 December 1863, admission no. 1091. 'Oh, mam bach' = Oh, little mother (a term of endearment).
22   25th AR, 1873, RCV, 6.
23   Peter McCandless, '"Build! Build!" The controversy over the care of the chronically insane in England, 1855–1870', *Bulletin of the History of Medicine*, 53, 1979, 553–74.

7 1874–1914

1   31st AR, 1879, RMS, 9.
2   26th AR, 1874, RMS, 8–9.

[3]   26th AR, RMS, 10.
[4]   28th AR, 1876, RCV, 7.
[5]   27th AR, 1875, RMS, 12.
[6]   30th AR, 1878, RMS, 8.
[7]   29th AR, 1877, RMS, 9.
[8]   30th AR, 1878, RMS, 9.
[9]   30th AR, 1878, RMS, 9.
[10] 32nd AR, 1880, RCL, 11.
[11] 28th AR, 1876, RMS, 12.
[12] 26th AR, 1874, RMS, 10.
[13] 32nd AR, 1881, RVC.
[14] 31st AR, 1879, RCL, 13.
[15] 32nd AR, 1880, RVC, 13.
[16] 29th AR, 1877, RVC, 14.
[17] 28th AR, 1876, RCV, 15.
[18] 32nd AR, 1880, RMS, 9.
[19] 28th AR,1876, RMS, 13.
[20] 33rd AR, 1881, RCL, 13.
[21] 33rd AR, 1881, RCV, 5.
[22] 31st AR, 1879, RVC, 13.
[23] Askew Roberts, *Gossiping Guide to Wales*, Cardiff, Hughes, 1881.
[24] Beatrix Potter used to visit her aunt and uncle at their large country house, Plas Gwaenynog, situated a short distance from the asylum. It was here that Beatrix apparently drew the sketches for the story of the Flopsy Bunnies, including those of the gardener, immortalizing him as Mr MacGregor.
[25] Potter, 1881, cited by Dewi Roberts, *Visitor's Delight*, Capel Garmon, Gwasg Carreg Gwalch, 1992.
[26] Laurence Ray, 'Models of madness in Victorian asylum practice', *European Journal of Sociology*, 22, 1981, 229–64.
[27] Pamela Michael, 'From private grief to public testimony: suicide in Wales, 1832–1914', in Anne Borsay and Dorothy Porter (eds), *Medicine in Wales, c.1800–2000: Public Service or Private Commodity?*, Cardiff, University of Wales Press, forthcoming.
[28] This information was provided by the late Dr Lewis Lloyd.
[29] 37th AR, 1885, RMS, 17.
[30] 38th AR,1886, RMS, 15.
[31] 37th AR, 1885, RCL, 11.
[32] DRO, HD/1/455/239, removal order for Mary Davies, patient admittance no. 239.
[33] 38th AR 1886, RCV, 7.
[34] 38th AR, 1886, RVC, 11.
[35] 43rd AR, 1891, RCV, 8.
[36] 43rd AR, 1891, RCV, 6–7.
[37] 43rd AR, 1891, RCV, 7.
[38] PRO, MH/51/789.
[39] PRO, MH/51/789, 26038 Denbigh Asylum.
[40] 45th AR, 1893–4, RCV, 6–8.

41 48th AR, 1896–7, RMS, 30.
42 50th AR, 1898–9, RVC, 7.
43 50th AR, 1898–9, RMS, 31.
44 52nd AR, 1900–1, RMS, 21.
45 53rd AR, 1901–2, RCV, 6–8.
46 54th AR,1902–3, RCV, 8.
47 58th AR,1906–7, RCV, 6.
48 57th AR, 1905–6, minutes of a conference on the subject of future accommodation for patients, 4 September 1905, 11–13.
49 DRO, HD/1/175, visitors' book, entry for 12 June 1901.
50 54th AR, 1902–1903, RMS, 26.
51 DRO, HD/1/365, admittance no. 4111.
52 DRO, HD/1/366, admittance no. 4301.
53 DRO, AR 1905, RMS.
54 Eric H. Pryor, *Claybury, 1893–1993: A Century of Caring*, Mental Health Care Group, Forest Healthcare Trust, Woodford, 1993, 71–2, *The Lancet*, 1943, 244, 1943, 1, 6 February 1943, 189; *BMJ*, 1943, 1, 175.
55 Address to the Honourable Society of Cymmrodorion, 1939.
56 Pryor, *Claybury*, 72; on the work of Helen Boyle see Louise Westwood, 'A quiet revolution in Brighton: Dr Helen Boyle's pioneering approach to mental health care, 1899–1939', *Social History of Medicine*, 14, 3, December 2001, 439–58.

8 The First World War and its Aftermath

1 John Davies, *Hanes Cymru*, Harmondsworth, Penguin, 1990, 496. Trans.: 'why Wales did not lose its soul completely in the day of the great madness'.
2 66th AR, 1914–15, RCV, 8.
3 Emile Durkheim, *Suicide: A Study in Sociology*, trans. John Spaulding and George Simpson, London, Routledge & Kegan Paul, 1987 (first published by the Free Press, 1951).
4 Jack Douglas, *The Social Meanings of Suicide*, Princeton, Princeton University Press, 1973, first published 1967.
5 68th AR, 1916–17, RMS, 18.
6 Ibid., 17.
7 66th AR, 1913–14, RMS, 14.
8 Mott used large-scale material provided by the Claybury patients to investigate genetic patterns, and investigated 3,118 patients belonging to 1,450 families. There is no evidence to suggest that the collection of record cards ever approached this scale in Denbigh, nor do the cards appear to have survived.
9 Malcolm Pines, 'The development of the psychodynamic movement', in German E. Berrios and Hugh Freeman, *150 Years of British Psychiatry, 1841–1991*, London, Gaskell, 1991, 206–31.
10 Richard Slobodin, *W. H. R. Rivers: Pioneer Anthropologist, Psychiatrist of the Ghost Road*, Stroud, Sutton Publishing, 1997, revised edn; first published by Colombia University Press, 1978. The novels of Pat Barker have popularized the Rivers/Sassoon story and elevated this encounter to something of a myth. Pat

Barker, *Regeneration*, London, Penguin, 1992; *The Eye in the Door*, London, Penguin, 1993; *The Ghost Road*, London, Penguin, 1996.

11   66th AR, 1914, RMS, 14.
12   67th AR, 1915, 19.
13   68th AR, 1916, 17.
14   70th AR, 1918, RVC, 14.
15   Ibid., 11.
16   70th AR, 1918, RMS, 18.
17   71st AR, 1919, RMS, 16.
18   66th AR, 1914, RMS, 15.
19   68th AR, 1916, RMS, 17.
20   69th AR, 1917, RCBC, 14.
21   Ibid.
22   J. L. Cranmer, *Asylum History: Buckinghamshire County Pauper Lunatic Asylum – St. John's*, London, Gaskell, 1991, 76–7, 113, 126–7. Cranmer alleges a deliberate policy of semi-starvation, resulting in the death of a third of the patient population at the Buckinghamshire Asylum in 1918. Scull cites this as an extreme example, but argues for the existence of a generally punitive policy of providing 'a bare minimum of care' in public asylums, see Andrew Scull, 'Asylums: utopias and realities', in Dylan Tomlinson and John Carrier (eds), *Asylums in the Community*, London, Routledge, 1996, 12–13.
23   J. M. Winter, *The Great War and the British People*, London, Macmillan, 1986; Linda Bryder, 'The First World War: healthy or hungry?', *History Workshop Journal*, 24, 1987, 141–57; Linda Bryder, *Below the Magic Mountain*, Oxford, Clarendon Press, 1988, 109–13; L. Cobbett, *Journal of Hygiene*, 30, 1930, 79–103.
24   66th AR, 1914, 16.
25   Albert Lyons and R. Joseph Petrucelli, *Medicine: An Illustrated History*, New York, Harry Abrams, 1987, 597.
26   66th AR, 1914, RMS, 42.
27   71st AR, 1919, RMS, 16.
28   70th AR, 1918, RMS, 19; and 71st AR, 1919, RMS, 16.
29   Bryder, *Below the Magic Mountain*, 48.
30   70th AR, 1918, RMS, 18.
31   71st AR, 1919, RMS, 16.
32   70th AR, 1918, RMS, 18.
33   66th AR, 1914, 5.
34   73rd AR, 1921–2, RCBC, 14.
35   Ibid., 15.
36   Jonathan Andrews, A. Briggs, R. Porter, P. Tucker and K. Waddington, *The History of Bethlem*, London, Routledge, 1997, 680.
37   67th AR, 1915, RMS, 20.
38   Arthur Foss and Kerith Trick, *St Andrew's Hospital Northampton*, Cambridge, Granta, 1989, 212.
39   66th AR, 1914–15, RCV, 7.
40   Deirdre Beddoe, *Out of the Shadows: A History of Women in Twentieth-Century Wales*, Cardiff, University of Wales Press, 2000, 47–73.

[41] 66th AR, 1914, RMS, 16.

[42] 68th AR, 1916, RVCBC, 12.

[43] 69th AR, 1917, RCBC, 15.

[44] 74th AR, 1922, RCV, 8.

[45] Mari A. Williams, ' "In the wars": Wales, 1914–1945', in Gareth Elwyn Jones and Dai Smith (eds), *The People of Wales*, Llandysul, Gomer Press, 1999, 179–80.

[46] Elaine Showalter, *The Female Malady*, London, Virago, 1987.

[47] Harold Merskey, 'Shell-shock', in G. E. Berrios and H. Freeman (eds), *150 Years of British Psychiatry, 1841–1991*, London, Gaskell, 1991, 245–67.

[48] Sean O'Mahony, *Frongoch: University of Revolution*, Dublin, FDR Teoranta, 1987, 41.

[49] HD/1/382, admission no. 8721, date of admission 10 May 1917.

[50] O'Mahony, *Frongoch*, 110–11.

[51] David Evans, 'Tackling the "hideous scourge": the creation of venereal disease treatment centres in early twentieth-century Britain', *Social History of Medicine*, 5, 3, December 1992, 413–34.

[52] John Keegan, *The Face of Battle*, London, Pimlico, 1991, 306; first published by Jonathan Cape, 1976. Poison gas was first used at Ypres in 1915.

[53] Ibid., 264–5.

[54] Elaine Showalter, 'Rivers and Sassoon: the inscription of male gender anxieties', in M. P. Higgonet (ed.), *Behind the Lines – Gender and the Two World Wars*, New Haven, Yale University Press, 1987; Paul Fussell, *The Great War and Modern Memory*, Oxford, Oxford University Press, 1975; Gervase Phillips, 'Dai Bach Y Soldiwr – Welsh Soldiers in the British Army 1914–1918', *Llafur*, 6, 2, 1993, 94–105.

[55] Michael Hurd, *The Ordeal of Ivor Gurney*, Oxford, Oxford University Press, 1978; R. K. R. Thornton (ed.), *Ivor Gurney: Severn and Somme War's Embers*, Manchester, Mid Northumberland Arts Group, 1987; Anthony Boden, *Stars in a Dark Night: The Letters of Ivor Gurney to the Chapman Family*, Gloucester, Alan Sutton, 1986.

[56] Gwyn A. Williams, *When was Wales? A History of the Welsh*, Harmondsworth, Penguin Books, 1985, 249.

[57] Martha Hildreth, 'The influenza epidemic of 1918–19 in France: contemporary concepts of aetiology, therapy, and prevention', *Social History of Medicine*, 4, 2, August 1991, 277–94. A. Crosby, *America's Forgotten Pandemic: The Influenza of 1918*, Cambridge, Cambridge University Press, 1989.

[58] W. I. B. Beveridge, *Influenza: The Last Great Plague*, London, Heinemann, 1977; Robert Katz, 'Influenza 1918–19: a study in mortality', *Bulletin of the History of Medicine*, 48, 1974. Sandra Tomkins, 'The failure of expertise: public health policy in Britain during the 1918–19 influenza epidemic', *Social History of Medicine*, 5, 3, December 1992, 435–54.

[59] 70th AR, 1918, RVC, 13.

[60] 70th AR, 1918, RMS.

[61] 73rd AR, 1921–2, RVC, 14.

[62] 70th AR, 1918, RMS, 16.

[63] DRO, HD/1/356, admittance no. 9351, date of admission 25 November 1919.

[64] Eric Jones, '"On active service" – the war diary of a Caernarfonshire quarryman', *Caernarfonshire Historical Society Transactions*, 52–3, 1991–2, 87–102.

9 THE INTER-WAR YEARS

[1] M. Stone, 'Shellshock and the psychologists', in W. T. Bynum, R. Porter and M. Shepherd (eds), *The Anatomy of Madness*, ii, London, Tavistock, 1985, 242–71; H. Merskey, 'Shell-shock', in G. E. Berrios and H. Freeman (eds), *150 Years of British Psychiatry, 1841–1991*, London, Gaskell, 1991, 245–67.

[2] Alfred Schofield, *Nerves in Disorder: A Plea for Rational Treatment*, London, Hodder & Stoughton, 1927, p. xi.

[3] Anne Rogers and David Pilgrim, *Mental Health Policy in Britain*, Basingstoke, Palgrave, 2000, 54.

[4] 82nd AR, 1930–1, RMS, 17.

[5] 91st AR, 1939–40, RMS, 18.

[6] Kathleen Jones, *Mental Health and Social Policy 1845–1959*, London, Routledge & Kegan Paul, 1960, 124. *Report of the Proceedings of the Mental Treatment Conference held at the Central Hall, Westminster*, London, HMSO, 1930, 8–11.

[7] Mathew Thomson, *The Problem of Mental Deficiency*, Oxford, Clarendon Press, 1998.

[8] *73rd Annual Report of the Commissioner of the Board of Control, for the Year 1921*, 12.

[9] Board of Control, *Eleventh Annual Report for the Year 1924*, appendix 1, 436.

[10] 76th AR, 1924–5, RMS, 19.

[11] Ibid., 20.

[12] *The Twenty-First Annual Report of the Board of Control for the Year 1934*, London, HMSO, 1935, 9; *Twenty-Fifth Annual Report of the Board of Control for the Year 1938*, London, HMSO, 1939, 7.

[13] *21st Annual Report of the Board of Control*, 9.

[14] 73rd AR, 1921, RVC, 13.

[15] M. Lomax, *Experiences of an Asylum Doctor*, London, Allen & Unwin, 1921.

[16] Cmd. 1730, Ministry of Health, *Report of the Committee on Administration of Public Mental Hospitals*, London, HMSO, 1922, 80, 77.

[17] Clive Unsworth, *The Politics of Mental Health Legislation*, Oxford, Clarendon Press, 1987, 181.

[18] *The Eighteenth Annual Report of the Board of Control for the Year 1931*, London, HMSO, 1932, 1.

[19] DRO, HD/1/16, minutes of meeting of the house and building committee, 19 January 1931, 5.

[20] Ibid., 6.

[21] 76th AR, 1923–4, RCV, 6.

[22] DRO, HD/1/16, minutes of meeting of the house and building committee, 5 November 1931.

[23] 86th AR, 1934–5, RCV, 7.

[24] Ibid., 11.

[25] *Twenty-Third Annual Report of the Board of Control for the Year 1936*, London, HMSO, 1937, appendix A, 232–3.

26   *25th Annual Report of the Board of Control*, 4.

27   Ibid., 20.

28   86th AR, 1934–5, RCV, 9.

29   George Rosen, 'Patterns of discovery and control in mental illness', in *Madness in Society*, University of Chicago Press, 1968; London, Phoenix edn, 1980, 248–58.

30   Edward M. Brown, 'Why Wagner-Jauregg won the Nobel Prize for discovering malaria therapy for General Paresis of the Insane', *History of Psychiatry*, 11, 2000, 371–82; Magda Whitrow, 'Wagner-Jauregg and fever therapy', *Medical History*, 34, 1990, 294–310.

31   PRO, MH/51/537 – 1928–43, correspondence on malarial treatment including Dr Meagher's report and a history of GPI by Hubert Bond.

32   82nd AR, 1930–1, RMS, 22.

33   78th AR, 1926–7, RMS, 17.

34   79th AR, 1927–28, RMS, 17.

35   81st AR, 1929–30, RMS, 20.

36   Edward Shorter, *A History of Psychiatry*, New York, John Wiley & Sons, 1997, 193–5, where he suggests that Wagner-Jauregg's fever treatment 'broke the therapeutic nihilism that had dominated psychiatry in previous generations'.

37   82nd AR, 1930–1, RMS, 19.

38   89th AR, 1937–8, RMS, 17.

39   90th AR, 1938–9, RMS, 17.

40   Interview with charge nurse Kearns, North Wales Hospital History Group Collection.

41   83rd AR, 1931–2, RMS, 20.

42   90th AR, 1938–9, RMS, 22.

43   G. Windholz and L. H. Witherspoon, 'Sleep as a cure for schizophrenia: a historical episode', *History of Psychiatry*, 4, 1993, 83–93, 84.

44   90th AR, 1938–9, 17.

45   Gerald Grob, *The Mad Among Us: A History of the Care of America's Mentally Ill*, London, Harvard University Press, 1994, 180–1; Renato Sabbatini, *The History of Shock Therapy in Psychiatry*, *http://www.epub.org.br/cm/n04/historia/shock_i.htm*

46   Isabel Wilson, *A Study of Hypoglycaemic Shock Treatment in Schizophrenia*, Board of Control, London, HMSO, 1936.

47   W. Rees Thomas and Isabel Wilson, *Report on Cardiazol Treatment and on the Present Application of Hypoglycaemic Shock Treatment in Schizophrenia*, Board of Control, London, HMSO, 1938.

48   Ibid.

49   In 1938 the Board of Control circulated a questionnaire regarding the use of insulin, cardiazol and triazol. The treatments were employed in 92 institutions: 3 used insulin only, 61 used cardiazol only, 16 used insulin and cardiazol combined, and 12 used insulin and cardiazol not combined. *25th Annual Report of the Board of Control*, 1939, 36.

50   Interview with charge nurse Kearns.

51   87th AR, 1935–6, RVC, 14.

52   *Nineteenth Annual Report of the Board of Control for the Year*, Pt. 1, p. 25.

[53]   89th AR, 1937–8, RMS, 22.
[54]   90th AR, 1938–9.
[55]   73rd Annual Report of the commissioner, 13.
[56]   76th AR, 1924–5, report of the dental surgeon, 23.
[57]   Andrew Scull, 'Focal sepsis and psychosis: the career of Thomas Chivers Graves, BSc, MD, FRCS, MRCVS (1964–1993)', in G. E. Berrios and H. Freeman (eds), *150 Years of British Psychiatry, The Aftermath*, ii, London, Gaskell, 1996, 517–36.
[58]   79th AR, 1927–8, report of the dental surgeon, 18.
[59]   *17th Report of the Board of Control*, appendix C, 165–6.
[60]   88th AR, 1936–7, RMS, 22.
[61]   89th AR, 1937–8, RMS, 21.
[62]   90th AR, 1938–9, RVC, 10.
[63]   91st AR, 1939–40, RVC, 9.
[64]   91st AR, 1939–40, RVC, 11.

10   PATIENTS AND STAFF IN THE INTER-WAR YEARS

[1]   73rd AR, 1921–2, RMS, 27.
[2]   84th AR, 1932–3, RMS, 23.
[3]   78th AR, 1926–7, RMS, 17.
[4]   Personal information from Dr Ceinwen Evans in 1994.
[5]   Glynne R. Jones, 'The King Edward VII Welsh National Memorial Association, 1912–1948', in John Cule (ed.), *Wales and Medicine*, Llandysul, British Society for the History of Medicine, 1975, 30–41.
[6]   Personal interview, May 1994.
[7]   83rd AR, 1931–2, RVC, 14.
[8]   84th AR, 1932–3, RVC.
[9]   Ann Ceinwen Evans, MB, BSc Wales, 'Dysentery due to bacterium dysenteriae (Schmitz): first known outbreaks in Great Britain', *The Lancet*, 23 July 1938, 187.
[10]   83rd AR, 1931–2, RMS, 21–2.
[11]   S. Lyle Cummins and A. Ceinwen Evans, 'The intradermal tuberculin test in non-tuberculous adults', *BMJ*, 13 May 1933, 815–17.
[12]   Isobel Hutton, *Memories of a Doctor in War and Peace*, London, Heinemann, 1960.
[13]   Author's interview with Dr Ceinwen Evans, May 1994.
[14]   DRO, HD/1/17, minutes of house and finance committee, 15 November 1937.
[15]   Julie Grier, 'Eugenics and birth control: contraceptive provision in north Wales, 1918–1939', *Social History of Medicine*, 11, 3, 1998, 443–58, 451.
[16]   Contemporary Medical Archives Centre at the Wellcome Library, SA/FPA/A11/62A, quoted by Grier, 'Eugenics and birth control'.
[17]   John MacNicol, 'Eugenics and the campaign for voluntary sterilization in Britain between the wars', *Social History of Medicine*, 2, 2, August 1989, 147–70.
[18]   DRO, HD/1/16, minutes of the house and finance committee, 28 April 1930.
[19]   DRO, HD/1/16, minutes of the house and finance committee, 21 July 1930.
[20]   DRO, HD/1/16, minutes of finance committee, 18 August 1930, 5.

21   *Committee for Legalising Eugenic Sterilization*, London, Eugenics Society, n.d. (*c.*1930); John MacNicol, 'Eugenics', 157–8.

22   Contemporary Medical Archives Centre at the Wellcome Library, SA/FPA/A11/62A, statement signed by Dr Herbert entitled *Family Limitations*. My thanks to Julie Grier for identifying this leaflet.

23   Grier, 'Eugenics and birth control', 443–58, 453–5.

24   Interview with Tom Hughes conducted by members of the North Wales Hospital staff history team.

25   Ibid. and 76th Annual Report for the year 1924–5.

26   *Handbook for Mental Nurses*, London, Bailliere, Tindall & Cox, 1942. Originally entitled *Handbook for Attendants of the Insane*, this textbook was first issued in 1884, a 2nd edn was produced in 1893, a third in 1896, a fourth in 1898, fifth in 1908, sixth in 1911, seventh in 1923, and this was the version which was still being reprinted in 1942.

27   75th AR, 1923–4, RVC, 13.

28   86th AR, 1934–5, RVC, 11.

29   Interview with Tom Hughes, Bangor.

30   Interview with Kearns.

31   81st AR, 1929–30, RVC, 13.

32   Interviews with Tom Hughes, Bangor, and Kearns and information confirmed by many conversations with past members of staff. It was one of the main points highlighted in many interviews.

33   Interview with Tom Hughes, Bangor.

34   88th AR, 1936–7, RCV, 9.

35   84th AR, 1932–3, clerk and steward's report, 28–9.

36   74th AR, 1922–3, RCV, 10.

37   80th AR, 1927–8, RMS, 26.

38   76th AR 1924–5, RMS, 21.

39   85th AR, 1933–4, RMS, 21–2.

40   86th AR, 1934–5.

41   75th AR, 1923–4, RVC, 10.

42   86th AR, 1934–5, RVC, 10.

43   *Report of the Departmental Committee Appointed to Inquire into Certain Matters Relating to the Diet of Patients in County and Borough Mental Hospitals*, London, HMSO, 1924.

44   Uncatalogued material consulted in the hospital before closure.

45   77th AR, 1925–6, RVC, 13.

46   Ibid., RMS, 21.

47   79th AR, 1927–8, RMS, 19.

48   86th AR, 1934–5, RVC, 11.

49   82nd AR, 1930–1, RMS, 18.

50   81st AR, 1929–0, RCV, 7. On the Act see Kathleen Jones, *Mental Health and Social Policy 1845–1959*, London, Routledge & Kegan Paul, 1960, 39.

51   DRO, HD/1/343, admittance no. 6000, date of admission 30 April 1902.

52   DRO, HD/1/357, admittance no. 11,892, date of admission 17 February 1932.

53   DRO, HD/1/395, admittance no. 896 (private), date of admission 29 November 1920.

[54] DRO, HD/1/386, admittance no. 9841, date of admission 17 December 1919.

[55] DRO, HD/1/385, admittance no. 12731, date of admission 25 March 1936.

[56] Caradog Prichard, *One Moonlit Night/Un Nos Ola Leuad*, London, Penguin Books, 1999.

[57] *New Welsh Review*, 30, 1999, 88–9.

[58] Caernarfon Archives, PE/12/3, Glanogwen Parish, Register of Baptisms, 1849–1909.

[59] Caradog Prichard, *Afal Drwg Adda*, Denbigh, Gwasg Gee, 1973, 15.

[60] Menna Baines, 'Ffaith a dychymyg yng ngwaith Caradog Prichard', M.Phil., Bangor, 1992. Mihangel Morgan, *Caradog Prichard*, Caernarfon, Gwasg Pantycelyn, 2000.

[61] DRO, HD/1/310 and 316, dated 24 October 1924, 28 October 1925, 25 October 1927, 5 November 1935.

[62] DRO, HD/1/330, date of admission 1 July 1903, date of death 22 April 1941.

[63] Caradog Prichard, *Afal Drwg Adda*: 'In a fit of the old anger I had refused to have any flowers on mam's coffin.'

[64] Robert Hughes Parry, *Within Life's Span*, Ilfracombe, Arthur Stockwell, 1973, 93–5.

[65] 87th AR, 1935–6, RVC, 14.

[66] 88th AR, 1936–7, RMS, 33.

[67] For Runwell see *Twenty-Fourth Annual Report of the Board of Control for the Year 1937*, London, HMSO, 1938, 1.

11 The Second World War

[1] *Denbighshire Free Press*, 21 January 1939, 'Mental hospital enlargement scheme', 6.

[2] 91st AR, 1939–40, RCV, 5.

[3] 91st AR, 1939–40, RMS, 17–18.

[4] 92nd AR, 1940–1, RCV, 6.

[5] 92nd AR, 1940–1, RMS, 51.

[6] Ibid., RCV, 6.

[7] The Nuffield Trust, *Hospital Survey: The Hospital Services of the North-Western Area*, London, HMSO, 1942. This showed that the total number of hospital beds in Anglesey was 173, in Caernarfonshire 597, in Merioneth 195, in Flintshire 789 and in Denbighshire 447 (excluding the Llangwyfan Sanatorium, owned by the Welsh National Memorial Fund, and the Abergele Sanatorium, owned by Manchester City Borough, which had 259 and 247 beds respectively). The majority of hospitals (32 out of the 46 excluding the sanatoria) had fewer than fifty beds. The average number of patients resident in the North Wales Counties Mental Hospital during 1942 was 1,355. (94th AR for 1942–3, Report of the medical superintendent, 18.)

[8] 94th AR, 1942–3, RCV, 13.

[9] Ibid., 8–9.

[10] 92nd AR, 1940–1, 25.

[11] Clwyd Wynne, *The North Wales Hospital Denbigh 1842–1995*, Denbigh, Gee & Sons, 1995, 47.

12 93rd AR, 1941–2, RCV, 10, and RMS, 29.
13 Ibid.
14 93rd AR, 1941–2, RCV, 8.
15 Ibid., 9.
16 93rd AR, 1941–2, RMS, 20–1.
17 92nd AR, 1940–1, RMS, 29.
18 Ibid.
19 Ibid., 28–9.
20 G. E. Berrios, 'Early electroconvulsive therapy in Britain, France and Germany: a conceptual history', in Hugh Freeman and German E. Berrios (eds), *150 Years of British Psychiatry, ii: The Aftermath*, London, Athlone, 1996, 3–15. Edward Shorter, *A History of Psychiatry*, New York, John Wiley & Sons, 1997, 218–21.
21 Shorter, *History of Psychiatry*, 388. L. Kalinowsky, 'Electric-convulsion therapy in schizophrenia', *The Lancet*, 2, 9 December 1939.
22 G. W. T. H. Fleming, F. L. Golla and W. G. Walter, 'Electric-convulsion therapy of schizophrenia', *The Lancet*, 2, 30 December 1939, 1353–5.
23 Jonathan Andrews, Asa Briggs, Roy Porter, Penny Tucker and Keir Waddington, *The History of Bethlem*, London, Routledge, 1997, 693.
24 92nd AR, 1940–1.
25 93rd AR, 1941–2, RMS, 25–6.
26 G. E. Berrios, 'Early electroconvulsive therapy', 3–15.
27 Ibid., 5.
28 94th AR, 1942–3, RMS, 24.
29 R. E. Hemphill and W. G. Walter, 'The treatment of mental disorders by electrically induced convulsions', *Journal of Mental Science*, 87, 256–75, 1941, quoted in Berrios, 'Early electroconvulsive therapy', 10.
30 R. Freudenberg, 'On the curability of mental diseases by "shock" treatment', *Journal of Mental Science*, 87, 529–44, quoted by Berrios, 'Early electroconvulsive therapy', 10.
31 95th AR, 1943–4, RMS, 19.
32 DRO, HD/1/284, book of newspaper cuttings, see esp.: *Denbigh Free Press*, 24 January 1942, entitled 'Shock treatment'; *North Wales Times*, 24 April 1948, entitled 'Shock for hospital committee'.
33 99th AR, 1947–8, RMS, 23.
34 91st AR, 1939–40, RMS, 22.
35 92nd AR, 1940–1, RMS, 29.
36 95th AR, 1943–4, RMS, 21.
37 91st AR, 1939–40, RMS, 22.
38 93rd AR, 1941–2, RMS, 26.
39 G. Windholz and L. H. Witherspoon, 'Sleep as a cure for schizophrenia', *History of Psychiatry*, 4, 1993, 83–93, 91.
40 Ibid., and 95th AR, 1943–4, RMS, 20.
41 95th AR, 20.
42 German E. Berrios, 'Psychosurgery in Britain and elsewhere: a conceptual history', in German E. Berrios and Hugh Freeman (eds), *150 Years of British Psychiatry, 1841–1991*, London, Gaskell, 1991, 180–96; Shorter, *History of Psychiatry*, 225–9.

[43] W. Freeman and J. Watts, *Psychosurgery: Intelligence, Emotion and Social Behaviour Following Prefrontal Lobotomy for Mental Disorders*, Springfield, IL: Charles C. Thomas, 1942.

[44] E. L. Hutton, G. W. T. H. Fleming and F. E. Fox, 'Early results of prefrontal leucotomy', *The Lancet*, 241, 1941, 3–7.

[45] 94th AR, 1942–3, RMS, 25.

[46] 99th AR, 1947–8, RMS, 23.

[47] 96th AR, 1944–5, RVC, 13–14.

[48] Ibid., RMS, 19.

[49] D. G. Duff, 'Leucotomy technique', *The Lancet*, 2 November 1946, 639.

[50] Ibid.

[51] Interview with Dr Evans, 1994.

[52] Duff, 'Leucotomy technique'.

[53] Ibid., 640.

[54] E. Schwarz, 'Depression in Parkinsonism treated by prefrontal leucotomy', *Journal of Mental Science*, 91, 1945, 503.

[55] Andrew Scull, 'Somatic treatments and the historiography of psychiatry', *History of Psychiatry*, 5, 1994, 1–12.

[56] Elliot S. Valenstein, *Great and Desperate Cures: The Rise and Decline of Psychosurgery and Other Radical Treatments for Mental Illness*, New York, Basic Books, 1986.

[57] J. D. Pressman, 'Uncertain promise: psychosurgery and the development of scientific psychiatry in America, 1935 to 1955', unpublished Ph.D. dissertation, University of Pennsylvania, 1986; A. Scull, 'Somatic treatments and the historiography of psychiatry', 10–11.

[58] This career move may offer support to Valenstein's arguments regarding professional advancement.

[59] 99th AR, 1947–8, RMS, 25.

[60] Information obtained from J. D. Williams and D. B. Jones, March 2002.

[61] AR, 1945.

[62] David Crossley, 'The introduction of leucotomy: a British case history', *History of Psychiatry*, 4, 1995, 560.

[63] Deirdre Beddoe, *Out of the Shadows: A History of Women in Twentieth-Century Wales*, Cardiff, University of Wales Press, 2000, 133.

12 Welfare State Years – A New Dawn?

[1] Charles Webster, *The National Health Service: A Political History*, Oxford, Oxford University Press, 1998.

[2] Ministry of Health, *National Health Service Act, 1946, Provisions Relating to the Mental Health Services*, London, HMSO, 1948.

[3] Ibid., para. 30.

[4] *North Wales Times*, March 1948, DRO, HD/1/284, newspaper cuttings.

[5] PRO, BD 18/1850, 'Disposal and/or use of Abblett Testimonial Fund', 1948–54.

[6] *North Wales Times*, July 1947, under the title 'On the Map', DRO, HD/1/284, collection of newspaper cuttings.

7   *The Free Press*, Denbigh, 26 January 1945. DRO, HD/1/284, newspaper cuttings.
8   *North Wales Times*, 3 August 1946, under the title 'National awards', and *North Wales Times*, 18 April 1947, under heading 'Urgently required', HD/1/284.
9   *Yr Herald*, 30 July 1947, 'Y Clorianydd, Ysbyty Dinbych'. English version published in *North Wales Times*, July 1947.

> Although it was a truism to state that mental and physical wellbeing go together, the treatment of illness both of mind and body had in the past suffered from an artificial separation brought about in the first instance by erroneous conceptions and perpetuated by administrative convenience. The placing of all hospitals under one authority should facilitate the re-union of two branches of medicine which ought never to have strayed so far apart. An early outcome of the re-union was likely to be the easier entry of the general physician into the Mental Hospital and of the psychiatric physician into the general hospital. This was already being done in America and on the continent. The more the public realised the close connection of the two services the easier would it be to get those suffering from mental trouble to take treatment early.

10 *North Wales Times*, 18 April 1947, under the title 'Urgently required: colony for mental defectives'. DRO/HD/1/284.
11 Ibid.
12 Ibid., quoting Dr Roberts the medical superintendent of the North Wales Counties Mental Hospital.
13 PRO, MH/95/1, report of Board of Control commissioners, 14 April 1950.
14 Ibid., 24 and 25 June 1952.
15 PRO, MH/95/1, medical superintendent's annual report for 1954, in Board of Control Report for 1954.
16 DRO, HD/1/12, medical superintendent's annual report for 1947, 29.
17 99th AR, 1947–8, report of commissioners of the Board of Control, 13.
18 DRO, HD/1/284, newspaper cuttings, *North Wales Times*, July 1947.
19 Minutes of meeting of finance committee held on 27 October 1947. Miscellaneous collection from hospital.
20 Millennium Memory Bank, C900/00065 C1, year of recording 1999. Interview Farrukh Hashmi, 12 September 1927, speaker a male consultant psychiatrist.
21 PRO, MH/96/1868, Board of Control report for 1949.
22 PRO, MH/95/1, report of the Board of Control commissioners, 24 and 25 June 1952.
23 DRO, HD/1/12, medical superintendent's annual report for 1948, 26.
24 Information provided by J. D. Williams.
25 PRO, MH/96/1868, report of the commissioners of the Board of Control, 1 and 2 April 1958.
26 Liam Clarke, 'The opening of doors in British mental hospitals in the 1950s', *History of Psychiatry*, 4, 1993, 527–51.
27 Edward Shorter, *A History of Psychiatry*, New York, John Wiley & Sons, 1997, 231.
28 PRO, MH/95/1, report of Board of Control commissioners, 14 April 1950.
29 DRO, HD/1/12, medical superintendent's annual report for 1947, 15.

[30] PRO, MH/51/1, Board of Control report, 4 April 1951.

[31] PRO, MH/51/1, Board of Control report, 24 and 25 June 1952.

[32] Minutes of meeting of finance committee held on 15 December 1947 – Denbigh hospital.

[33] PRO, MH/96/1868, Board of Control report, 1 and 2 April 1958.

[34] DRO, HD/1/12, medical superintendent's annual report for 1948, 18.

[35] PRO, MH/95/1/, Board of Control report, 4 April 1951.

[36] Kathleen Jones, *Mental Health and Social Policy 1845–1959*, London, Routledge & Kegan Paul, 1960, 159.

[37] Douglas Bennett, 'The drive towards the community', in G. E. Berrios and H. Freeman (eds), *150 Years of Psychiatry*, London, Gaskell, 1991, 321–32, 325.

[38] PRO, MH/95/1, report on inspection of service patients, by M. A. Collins, 22 August 1950.

[39] Ibid., June 1951.

[40] Ibid., 2 July 1958.

[41] DRO, HD/1/12, 99th AR, 1947–8, report of the committee of visitors, 8.

[42] PRO, MH/96/1937, deputation received on 23 June 1955.

[43] PRO, MH/95/1, report of visiting commissioners of the Board of Control for 1951.

[44] DRO, HD/1/523, minutes of the medical officers' meetings, 19 January 1970.

[45] E. H. Griffiths, *Seraff yr Efengyl Seml*, Caernarfon, Llyfrfa'r Methodistiaid Calfinaidd, 1968, 168.

[46] Ibid.

[47] Ibid.

[48] This account of his treatment in the North Wales Hospital, Denbigh is based entirely upon the account given by E. H. Griffiths, *Seraff yr Efengyl Seml*, 169–75.

[49] *The Chronicle (North Wales)*, 30 December 1949.

[50] Ibid.

[51] 'One of the greatest men that the twentieth century has seen', Iorwerth Peate, *Syniadau*, Llandysul, Gwasg Gomer, 1969, Chapter 7: George M. Ll. Davies (1880–1949), 117–18.

[52] 'Ysbyty i'r meddwl – fel y corff – Colli'r hen arswyd yn y cynhesrwydd newydd' (A hospital for the mind – like the body – the old terror disappears in the new warmth of caring), *Y Cymro*, 25 Chwefror 1960, 12–14.

[53] 'Here is Your Opportunity, Daughters and Sons of Wales to serve Wales in a modern and adventurous career – a career with a brilliant future to it, and widespread advantages.' Ibid., 13.

13 New Directions

[1] Kathleen Jones, *Mental Health and Social Policy 1845–1959*, London, Routledge & Kegan Paul, 1960, 178–85; Clive Unsworth, *The Politics of Mental Health Legislation*, Oxford, Clarendon Press, 1987.

[2] Cmd. 7320, *Review of the Mental Health Act 1959*, Department of Health and Social Security, London, HMSO, 1978.

3   Kathleen Jones, *Mental Health and Social Policy*, 204–5.
4   See for instance the Granada Television programme *Insanity or Illness?* broadcast on Wednesday 28 January 1959, at 8.30 p.m., which was prepared with help from the National Association of Mental Health, transcript published by Granada Television, London, 1959.
5   Ibid., 27.
6   *Liverpool Post*, 27 October 1960.
7   Shulamit Ramon and Maria Grazia Geannichedda (eds), *Psychiatry in Transition: The British and Italian Experiences*, London, Pluto Press, 1991.
8   M. Rolf Olsen, 'The personal and social consequences of the discharge of the long-stay psychiatric patient from the North Wales Hospital, Denbigh, 1956–66', Ph.D. thesis, University of Wales, 1976, 41.
9   Annual report of the medical superintendent for the year 1962.
10 DRO HD/6/50, report of the Inquiry team appointed to investigate the admission and discharge policy at North Wales Hospital, Denbigh; submission by Dr T. Gwynne Williams, Physician Superintendent, App. 3, p. 4, 30 September 1970.
11 M. Rolf Olsen, 'An analysis of the accumulation, discharge and characteristics of a long-stay psychiatric patient population (the North Wales Hospital, Denbigh 1842–1966)', M.Sc. dissertation, University of Wales, 1972, 107.
12 Ibid.
13 Ibid., 76.
14 D. Alun Jones and H. Lewis Miles, 'The Anglesey mental health survey', in Gordon McLachlan (ed.), *Problems and Progress in Medical Care*, Nuffield Provincial Hospitals Trust, Oxford, Oxford University Press, 1964, 205–63.
15 Quoted by Olsen, 'Analysis', 106–7.
16 Jones and Miles, 'Anglesey mental health survey', p. 262.
17 DRO, HD/1, report of the Welsh Hospitals Board team of investigation, 1970, 5.
18 *Abergele Visitor*, 19 March 1966, see Olsen, 'Personal and social consequences of discharge', *Western Mail*, 16 March 1966.
19 *Western Mail*, 17 March 1966.
20 *Rhyl Journal*, 13 November 1969.
21 N. Davies, 'Well, then I met these lunatics . . .', chapter 5 in D. Brandon and B. Jordan (eds), *Creative Social Work*, Oxford, Blackwell, 1979.
22 *Guardian*, 2 May 1970; *Liverpool Daily Post*, 2 May 1970; *Western Mail*, 2 May 1970.
23 Ibid., 16 March 1970.
24 *News of the World*, 'Nursing home drama', 20 December 1970; *The Sunday Times*, 'Inquiry into lodgings for ex-mental patients', 20 October 1970.
25 *Hansard*, House of Commons Official Report, Fifth Series, 17 December 1970, Vol. 808, 434; *Liverpool Daily Post*, 'Boarding-house a scandal says M.P.', 17 December 1970.
26 Jones and Miles, 'Anglesey mental health survey', 8–9.
27 DRO, HD/1/523, minutes of medical committee, 18 January 1971, minute 7.
28 Ibid., 2 March 1970.
29 HD/1/523, minutes of medical officers' meeting, 13 May 1968.

30   Ibid.
31   Ibid., 7 October 1968.
32   Ibid., 13 October 1969.
33   Ibid., 20 October 1969.
34   Ibid., 13 May 1968.
35   Ibid., 18 March 1968.
36   Ibid., 20 May 1968, item 3.
37   Ibid., 22 December 1969.
38   Ibid., 20 May 1968.
39   Ibid., 20 September 1968.
40   Ibid., 22 July 1968.
41   *Daily Post*, Wednesday, 30 May 2001, 9.
42   DRO HD/1/523, minutes of medical officers' meetings, 19 January 1970.
43   Ibid., 24 June 1968.
44   Ibid., 20 January 1969.
45   Ibid., 1 July 1968.
46   Ibid., 30 September 1968.
47   Oral information obtained from senior charge nurse, Clwyd Wynne.
48   Ibid., 19 January 1970.
49   Ibid., 25 November 1968.
50   Ibid., 23 December 1968.
51   Ibid., 7 July 1969.
52   Ibid., 11 August 1969.
53   Ibid., 25 August 1969.
54   Information obtained from Dai Bryn Jones, Clwyd Wynne and John Davey.
55   DRO HD/1/523, medical officers' meeting, 29 July 1968.
56   Ibid., 18 November 1968.
57   Ibid., 24 May 1971.
58   Ibid., 29 July 1968.
59   Ibid., 7 October 1968.
60   Ibid., 18 January 1972, item 6.

14 THE FINAL YEARS

1   *Care in Wales for People with a Mental Illness and People with a Mental Handicap, Report Prepared Pursuant to Section 11 of the Disabled Persons (Services, Consultation and Representation) Act 1986*, House of Commons, London, HMSO, 1995, 2.
2   Stephen Croad, 'Recent emergency recording', *Ancient Monuments Society Transactions*, 41, 1997, 93–4.
3   *Daily Post*, 3 July 1996, 'Stalemate on plans for former hospital'.
4   *Daily Post*, 3 April 1997, 'Threat to pull out as hospital plan is scrapped'.
5   *Daily Post*, 24 July 1997, 1–2, '350 jobs for hospital site'.
6   *Daily Post*, 21 May 1998, 'New bid to solve hospital site row'.
7   *Daily Post*, 5 May 1999, 8, 'Former hospital site goes for a song and a promise'.
8   *Daily Post*, 17 May 1999, 'Site in running for sports centre'; 19 May 1999,

'Hospital war goes on'; 27 May 1999, 'School in protest over sale of former hospital'.

⁹ *Daily Post*, 18 June 1999, 'Inquiry call over site sale'.

¹⁰ *Daily Post*, 14 July 1999, 'Auditors probe £100,000 profit on hospital deal'.

¹¹ Ibid.

¹² *Daily Post*, 10 September 1999, 'Pottery craft centre plan for hospital site'; 17 September 1999, ' "Horror" at plans for 160 houses'.

¹³ *Daily Post*, 17 September 1999.

¹⁴ *Daily Post*, 31 March 2001, 'How on earth did thieves manage to steal our clock?'.

CONCLUSION

¹ Norbert Elias, *The Civilizing Process: State Formation and Civlization*, London, Blackwell, 1982.

² Jonas Larsson, 'Behandlingstanken inom svensk simnessjudvard under borjan av 1800-talet' (The idea of treatment in Swedish mental health care at the beginning of the 19th century), Ph.D. thesis, Historical Institute, University of Uppsala, Sweden, 1973.

³ Lindsay Prior, *The Social Organization of Mental Illness*, London, Sage, 1993.

⁴ The National Assembly for Wales, *Health Statistics*, appendix 1, Cardiff, 2001, 240–2. This included 70 beds at the Hergest Unit, Ysbyty Gwynedd, Bangor, 16 beds at the Minffordd Hospital, Bangor, 92 beds at the Llwyn y Groes Unit at Wrexham Maelor, 74 beds at the Ablett Unit, Ysbyty Glan Clwyd, Bodelwyddan, 15 beds at the Gwynfryn Unit, Denbigh, 16 elderly mentally ill beds at the Bodnant Unit, Llandudno, and 146 beds, some for learning disability and some for more severe psychiatric cases, at Bryn-y-Neuadd, Llanfairfechan.

⁵ There is no psychiatric unit on Anglesey, only a small support bed unit.

⁶ David Healy et al., 'Psychiatric bed utilization: 1896 and 1996 compared', *Psychological Medicine*, 31, 2001, 779–90; and other forthcoming publications.

⁷ Charles Crosby et al., *Changing Care, Changing Lives: Resettlement from North Wales Psychiatric Hospital*, Bangor, University of Wales Bangor, n.d. (*c.*1993).

⁸ Charles Crosby in *Ar ôl Dinbych*, documentary film produced by Medwen Roberts, Ffilmiau Hiraethog, 1995.

⁹ Helen Madog, MIND, in *Ar ôl Dinbych*. 'Just find the right place and the right people and everything can work out o.k.'

¹⁰ Emlyn, in *Ar ôl Dinbych*. 'I never want to go back to Denbigh.'

¹¹ Kelly Flynn, in a documentary shown on HTV Wales, *A Question of Balance*, Hiraethog, produced and directed by Medwen Roberts, 1995.

¹² Diana Gittens, *Madness in its Place*, London, Routledge, 1998, 220.

¹³ Charles Webster, 'Psychiatry and the early National Health Service: the role of the Mental Health Standing and Advisory Committee', in G. E. Berrios and H. Freeman (eds), *150 Years of Psychiatry*, London, Gaskell, 1998, 115.

Index